Neuroendovascular Surgery

Progress in Neurological Surgery

Vol. 17

Series Editor

L. Dade Lunsford *Pittsburgh, Pa.*

KARGER

Neuroendovascular Surgery

Volume Editors

Michael B. Horowitz *Pittsburgh, Pa.*
Elad I. Levy *Buffalo, N.Y.*

55 figures and 8 tables, 2005

KARGER

Basel · Freiburg · Paris · London · New York ·
Bangalore · Bangkok · Singapore · Tokyo · Sydney

Michael B. Horowitz, MD
Department of Neurosurgery
Director, Neuroendovascular Surgery
UPMC Presbyterian
Suile B–400, 200 Lothrop Street
Pittsburgh, PA 15213–2582 (USA)

Elad I. Levy, MD
Millard Filmore Hospital
Dept. of Neurosurgery
3 Gates Circle
Buffalo, NY 14209–1194

Library of Congress Cataloging-in-Publication Data

Neuroendovascular surgery / volume editors, Michael Horowitz, Elad Levy.
p. ; cm. – (Progress in neurological surgery, ISSN 0079-6492 ; v. 17)
Includes bibliographical references and index.
ISBN 3-8055-7781-8 (hard cover : alk. paper)
1. Nervous system–Blood-vessels–Endoscopic surgery.
[DNLM: 1. Nervous System Diseases–surgery. 2. Vascular Diseases–surgery. 3. Neurosurgical Procedures. 4. Vascular Surgical Procedures. WL 368 N4942 2004] I. Horowitz, Michael S. II. Levy, Elad. III. Series.
RD594.2.N455 2004
617.4′8–dc22

2004013518

Bibliographic Indices. This publication is listed in bibliographic services, including Current Contents® and Index Medicus.

Drug Dosage. The authors and the publisher have exerted every effort to ensure that drug selection and dosage set forth in this text are in accord with current recommendations and practice at the time of publication. However, in view of ongoing research, changes in government regulations, and the constant flow of information relating to drug therapy and drug reactions, the reader is urged to check the package insert for each drug for any change in indications and dosage and for added warnings and precautions. This is particularly important when the recommended agent is a new and/or infrequently employed drug.

www.karger.com
Printed in Switzerland on acid-free paper by Reinhardt Druck, Basel
ISSN 0079–6492
ISBN 3–8055–7781–8

Contents

Series Editor's Note

Perhaps the most profound change in the delivery of neurosurgical health care in the last ten years represents the rapid incorporation of endovascular techniques into the armamentarium of options for neurosurgical patients with cerebrovascular and spinal disease. Based on the histological principles of intravascular localization begun by the neurologist, Egas Moniz, in Portugal in the late 1920's, and pursued by both neurosurgeons, radiologists and neurologists over the ensuing 80+ years, the ability to perform miracles from within the blood vessels has now become a reality. The myriad of applications ranges from treatment of acute strokes ('brain attack', a condition with much greater morbidity than heart attack), aneurysm management, carotid occlusive disease, adjuvant tumor embolization prior to planned surgical excision, management for arteriovenous malformations, and now the insertion of stents, coils, and adhesive agents. By partnering with industry, we see the examples of this remarkable trend in minimally invasive (or as the series editors prefer '*minimally intrusive*') options. We see a concomitant reduction in hospital stays, lessening of hospital costs, reduced morbidity, and increasingly better outcomes. Stroke is no longer an event with severe long term repercussions, it represents instead an opportunity to emergently intervene to keep the blood vessel open, restore cerebral blood flow function, and maintain quality of life. These technologies continue to mature and to progress. The enclosed volume represents a state of the art summary of current techniques, and also provides glimpses of the future. Pioneers in the usage of these technologies have preceded this work. I hope that the knowledge contained in this book will spur the next generation onto even greater achievements. All of us, the present and the future generation, needs to become educated in these techniques, as the world of brain and spinal surgery matures, grows, and transforms.

L. Dade Lunsford, MD

Foreword

Many surgical subspecialties over the past decades have moved towards what has been termed *minimally invasive* approaches to traditionally *open* procedures. Endoscopy comes to mind whenever one considers this trend as it has either revolutionized or has begun to revolutionize General Surgery, Otolaryngology, Urology, Neurosurgery, and Cardiothoracic Surgery. Endovascular surgical procedures first drastically altered the surgical landscape as they pertained to coronary bypass and are now providing alternatives for repair of other cardiac and vascular anomalies such as septal defects, peripheral arterial occlusions and stenoses, peripheral aneurysms, and carotid disease. With the advent of improved technology and smaller maneuverable devices more delicate procedures have been developed such as those to occlude cerebral aneurysms, occlude arteriovenous malformations, eliminate blood supply to tumors, and treat extracranial and intracranial arterial stenoses. However, because all of these procedures carry risk and are ultimately as invasive as open surgical procedures we prefer to use the term *minimally intrusive surgery* for those endovascular procedures that are discussed in the coming chapters. These procedures gain access to the target lesion without disrupting or destroying surrounding tissues such as skin, muscle, bone, and brain. As a result pain is minimized and recovery is ideally facilitated and shortened.

The purpose of this text is to discuss the most common neuroendovascular procedures currently practiced. Less commonly performed procedures such as intra-arterial chemotherapy and sclerotherapy have been omitted not because we consider them unimportant but because space was limited. We hope that the readers find this book to be a useful resource when investigating the most frequently conducted endovascular procedures.

We would like to thank the many chapter authors for their contributions and encourage all entering this field to expand the horizons as this field is limited only by our imaginations and the abilities of talented engineers.

Michael B. Horowitz, MD
Elad I. Levy, MD

Horowitz MB, Levy EI (eds): Neuroendovascular Surgery.
Prog Neurol Surg. Basel, Karger, 2005, vol 17, pp 1–17

Current and Future Management Strategies for Intracranial Aneurysms and Carotid Artery Stenosis

Eric M. Deshaies, Alan S. Boulos

Department of Surgery, Division of Neurosurgery, Albany Medical Center, Albany, N.Y., USA

Introduction

Surgical clip ligation for intracranial saccular aneurysms and carotid artery endarterectomies for carotid stenosis valiantly triumphed as cures for cerebrovascular disease in the days of microneurosurgery. These open microsurgical techniques still have their place in modern neurosurgery but are expected to wane as further advancements are made in the field of neuroendovascular surgery. The future of neuroendovascular surgery is promising with the advent of novel modifications in bioengineering, biomaterials, and surface-coating techniques. Coil embolization and stent placement for intracranial cerebrovascular pathology offers alternative therapeutic options to patients who are not open surgical candidates where none had previously existed. However, the current limitations of neuroendovascular therapy are apparent with thromboembolic complications, aneurysm perforations, aneurysm recurrences or incomplete embolization, and in-stent stenosis being the major causes of concern for the neuroendovascular surgeon.

Currently, neuroendovascular techniques provide a complimentary therapy for patients with comorbidities that place them at high risk for open microneurosurgical techniques. With the advent of three-dimensional angiography to view cerebrovascular pathology, improvements in angiographic magnification to detect subtle changes in flow and microcatheter positioning, and development of softer microcatheters and coils, the complications of neuroendovascular surgery will be lowered and the benefits may surpass that of open surgical techniques. Recent studies, such as the International Subarachnoid Aneurysm

Trial (ISAT) study [Molyneux et al., 2002], have provided prospective randomized evidence that coil embolization of small ruptured predominantly anterior circulation intracranial saccular aneurysms significantly reduces morbidity and mortality in certain groups of patients compared to surgical clip ligation at 1 year's follow-up.

In this chapter, we will discuss the current and future management strategies, complications, and effectiveness of neuroendovascular surgery as it pertains to the management of cerebral aneurysms and carotid artery stenosis.

Saccular Cerebral Aneurysms

Current Management Strategy

Choosing the optimal treatment for a patient with an intracranial aneurysm can be complicated because it is based on perpetually evolving endovascular technology. Unruptured saccular intracranial aneurysms carry an accumulative 0.05–1%/year risk of rupture over an individual's lifetime [Juvela et al., 1993; Tsutsumi et al., 2000; Juvela, 2002]. This small, but real risk of aneurysm rupture makes the management decision of unruptured saccular aneurysms more challenging than for ruptured cerebral aneurysms because observational management must be balanced against surgical and endovascular intervention. On the contrary, a ruptured intracranial saccular aneurysm has a rehemorrhage rate of 5.7% within 3 days and 20% within 30 days of the initial hemorrhage [Kassell et al., 1990a,b]. Here the decision to exclude the aneurysm from the circulation is clear as the risks of intervention are less than that of observation in a majority of cases (though there remain a certain number of aneurysms where treatment may still carry higher risks than observation).

Surgical clip ligation of a ruptured intracranial aneurysm is highly effective in preventing rerupture of the aneurysm and is still considered the gold standard for the treatment of both unruptured and ruptured intracranial aneurysms. However, this is controversial with the advent of the FDA-approved Guglielmi detachable coils (GDC; Boston Scientific Target, Fremont, Calif., USA) for endosaccular coil embolization. There are numerous retrospective and prospective studies supporting a role for neuroendovascular treatment of intracranial aneurysms showing that endosaccular coil embolization of unruptured and ruptured intracranial saccular aneurysms is effective and safe [Byrne, 1999; Byrne et al., 1999; Lot et al., 1999; Richling et al., 1995; Raymond and Roy, 1997; Raymond et al., 1997; Vinuela et al., 1997; Roy et al., 2001]. The ISAT study is the most recent prospective randomized study to show that endovascular aneurysm coil embolization is effective and associated with a lower morbidity rate than surgical clip ligation in patients with a ruptured intracranial aneurysm [Molyneux et al., 2002]. This study consisted of 2,143 patients with ruptured aneurysms deemed amenable to either surgical clip ligation or endosaccular coil embolization. In this study, 50% of these aneurysms were located at the anterior communicating artery site, 20% at the posterior communicating artery site, and only a small group at the middle cerebral artery and basilar bifurcation sites. The ISAT study concluded that the relative risk for dependency or death was reduced by 22.6% in those patients who underwent coil embolization rather than clip ligation. This significantly decreased relative risk is further evidence demonstrating the improved safety of coil embolization over clip ligation in this specific subpopulation of patients whose aneurysm is amenable to either coil embolization or clip ligation.

Many factors enter the decision when selecting whether or not aneurysm clip ligation or endosaccular embolization is the optimal treatment for aneurysm obliteration. The natural history must be balanced against the risks and effectiveness of each form of intervention. There is increasing evidence that endosaccular coil embolization provides some advantages to clip ligation in particular subsets of patients. Aneurysm location, size, and the fundus-to-neck ratio are also important factors when deciding whether coil embolization or surgical clip ligation is the optimal treatment modality for an aneurysm [Richling et al., 1995; Fertl et al., 1999; Lot et al., 1999; Regli et al., 1999; Vanninen et al., 1999; Raftopoulos et al., 2000; Richling et al., 2000]. The International Cooperative Study on the Timing of Aneurysm Surgery showed that poorer surgical outcomes in patients with ruptured saccular aneurysms were associated with older age, severe medical comorbidities, poor Hunt-Hess grade, peak onset of vasospasm (5–10 days postrupture), and posterior circulation aneurysms [Kassell and Torner et al., 1990a,b]. It logically follows that patients with these risk factors would benefit from a less strenuous, minimally invasive, endovascular approach to saccular aneurysm therapy.

Our intracranial aneurysm treatment algorithm is based on a combination of patient characteristics, aneurysm morphology, and aneurysm location (table 1) [Boulos et al., 2002]. In analyzing our results, approximately 50% of ruptured aneurysms are treated via an endovascular technique. We aggressively use the endovascular technique in patients who are in poor neurological or medical condition as long as their aneurysm is amenable to it. To some degree patient preference is also changing the selection process. Many of the benefits of either microsurgical versus endovascular techniques can be discussed with the patient and family and the decision can be made by them. In the future, endovascular techniques will likely play a larger role in aneurysm management. Though it is still a long way from entirely replacing microsurgical aneurysm treatment, improvements in medications, embolization agents, and imaging technology will reduce many of the current endovascular limitations.

Table 1. Indications for selecting different therapeutic options

	Endovascular			Surgery		
Characteristic	absolute	relative	possible	possible	relative	absolute
Technique						Unable to obtain adequate working projection
Clinical presentation	Coagulopathy	Age >65 years Medical comorbidities Peak period of vasospasm In vasospasm	Unruptured aneurysm Hunt-Hess grade III, IV			Intracerebral hematoma with mass effect
Aneurysm morphology		Fusiform Dissecting Calcification/ atherosclerotic neck		Giant	Wide-necked fundus: neck ratio < 1 Mass effect	
Aneurysm site		Basilar apex Basilar trunk Cavernous	Paraclinoidal Anterior communicator	Superior cerebellar	MCA ICA	

MCA = Middle cerebral artery; ICA = internal carotid artery (posterior communicator, anterior choridal).

Thromboembolic Events

Thromboembolic events are the most common (5–12% risk) causes of periprocedural neurological morbidity during neuroendovascular procedures and may be related to the amount of thrombus within the aneurysm and the degree of coil impingement within the parent vessel [Raymond and Roy, 1997; Raymond et al., 1997; Vinuela et al., 1997; Brilstra et al., 1999]. Periprocedural anticoagulation with heparin and antiplatelet agents reduced the risk of thromboembolic events to 5.9% with heparin and 6.4% with aspirin [Qureshi et al., 2000]. However, antithromboembolic treatment modalities may increase the risk or severity of aneurysm rupture and the risk of hematoma formation at the arterial access site. Improvements in periprocedural medication management may reduce the risks of thromboembolic complications and access site complications. Bivalirudin, a direct noncompetitive thrombin inhibitor, has recently been demonstrated to reduce the risk of access site complications owing to its short half-life (20 min) and the risk of thromboembolic complications in comparison to unfractionated heparin in percutaneous coronary interventions [Lincoff et al., 2003]. Utilization of this medication in neuroendovascular techniques is currently under investigation. By achieving higher levels of anticoagulation with bivalirudin than that possible with unfractionated heparin (as measured by activated clotting times), periprocedural thromboembolic events may be reduced. Unfractionated heparin is also a platelet activator while bivalirudin is a weak platelet inhibitor thereby making it potentially effective at reducing ischemic events. Owing to its short half-life, access site complications (groin hematomas or pseudoaneurysms) are also less likely. In addition, the use of glycoprotein receptor IIb/IIIA inhibitors has been used in several case reports to resolve thrombus identified on angiography with good success and reduced hemorrhagic complications in comparison to recombinant tissue plasminogen activators (alteplase). These agents have thus reduced the use of ëbailout' thrombolysis that was associated with a higher morbidity. Lastly, the addition of clopidogrel (an oral platelet inhibitor) to anticoagulation regimens prior to aneurysm coil embolization may also reduce the risks of thromboembolic complications by increasing the platelet inhibition in the periprocedural time period. None of the above medications have been proven in randomized or prospective trials.

Aneurysm Perforation or Intraoperative Rupture

Studies have demonstrated that intraprocedural aneurysm perforation occurs at a rate of 1.74–8% (average rate of 2.8%) [Tummala et al., 2001; Cloft and Kallmes, 2002]. In one retrospective study, 80% of the aneurysms with intraprocedural rupture were smaller than 2 mm (smaller than the smallest available coil) [Raymond and Roy, 1997; Vinuela et al., 1997]. Several technological advances may reduce these risks. Softer and more flexible coils, microcatheters, and microwires may further decrease the risk of aneurysm rupture. The use of balloon assistance to tamponade potential rupture has been advocated by Ross [2004] to limit the injury related to aneurismal perforations. Lastly, the ability to more accurately identify catheter location with high definition, highly magnified fluoroscopy may reduce the incidence of perforations.

Wide Neck Aneurysm

Wide neck aneurysms with a fundus-to-neck ratio of less than 1.5 pose a special problem to the neuroendovascular surgeon because coil herniation into the parent vessel is more likely to occur. Stent-assisted coiling of wide-necked aneurysms provides a buttress for the coils to rest upon and prevents coil herniation into the parent vessel. Stents divert flow from inflow zone of the aneurysm neck and allow for tighter coiling [Aenis et al., 1997; Lieber et al., 1997]. Following stent-assisted coiling of wide-necked aneurysms, optimal

(>90%) angiographic results can be seen [Higashida et al., 1997; Lylyk et al., 1998; Mericle et al., 1998; Sekhon et al., 1998; Lanzino et al., 1999].

Aneurysm Recurrence

Current limitations of endovascular therapy include the inability to prevent recurrence in giant and wide-necked aneurysms (delayed complications). Studies on giant (>25 mm), large (10–25 mm), and wide-necked aneurysms found a high recurrence rate with incompletely occluded giant and large aneurysms and aneurysms with wide necks [Hayakawa et al., 2000]. Maintenance of aneurysm occlusion required multiple treatments in most cases [Gruber et al., 1999]. Although the aforementioned reports indicate that current neuroendovascular therapy is limited in its ability to successfully occlude giant and large wide-necked aneurysms, clipping of giant aneurysms poses a significant risk with complication rates for surgical clipping of giant, unruptured aneurysms being 26.7% in the anterior circulation and 37.9% in the posterior circulation [Raaymakers et al., 1998]. Aneurysms with a neck size greater than 4 mm were at a significantly higher risk of recurrence because a distance of 4 mm or less is necessary for proper bridging of the coil mass across the aneurysm neck, allowing for endothelialization to occur [Hilal and Solomon, 1992]. Several technological advances have been made to reduce giant, large, and wide-necked aneurysm recurrence rates including coils coated with biodegradable proteins or hydrogels, stents, and liquid embolic agents [Higashida et al., 1997; Levy and Ku, 1997; Mericle et al., 1998; Sekhon et al., 1998; Lanzino et al., 1999; Lefkowitz et al., 1999; Murayama et al., 1999; Aletich et al., 2000; Cloft et al., 2000; Moret et al., 2000; Piotin et al., 2000; Cottier et al., 2001; Murayama et al., 2001; Mawad et al., 2002].

Several of these devices are currently being investigated. In particular the hydrocoil, Matrix coils, radiation-emitting coils and Onyx (ethanol covinyl copolymer) are being used to reduce the risk of aneurysm recurrence. Two basic strategies in reducing aneurysm recurrence rates include increasing the percent of the aneurysm filled during embolization with embolic material or altering the biochemical or hematological milieu around the aneurysm resulting in more persistent occlusion.

The use of liquid embolic agents to embolize aneurysms has been examined for several years. The feasibility of Onyx embolization for the treatment of giant aneurysms was recently examined. In this clinical trial, patients were randomly selected to receive either Onyx (20% ethylene-vinyl alcohol polymer; Micro Therapeutics, Irvine, Calif., USA), a precipitating agent, or GDCs for aneurysm embolization [Al-Mubarak et al., 2001]. In the patients receiving Onyx, a stent was placed to reconstruct the parent vessel and Onyx was administered after a balloon was inflated within the stent to prevent Onyx from protruding or migrating into the parent vessel [Murayama et al., 2000; Hayakawa et al., 2000]. Of the 11 patients, 1 died, 1 suffered a watershed infarct (presumably from balloon inflations during Onyx administration), and 1 demonstrated recanalization at 6-month follow-up angiography; the other 8 patients demonstrated good results at 6-month follow-up angiography without evidence of recanalization. This method of treatment, although clearly preliminary, suggests a possible alternative to coil embolization or surgery. In experiments with wide-necked bifurcation aneurysms in canines, we found that high (30%) concentrations of EVAL (Ethylene-Vinyl Alcohol Copolymer), which possess increased viscosity, may allow for safe aneurysm embolization without the need for balloon protection. The use of a stent, coil framework, or a GDC Tri-Span coil (Boston Scientific Target, Fremont, Calif., USA) prevented untoward migration or protrusion of the polymer into the parent vessel. Onyx could be administered slowly, and complete embolization of the aneurysm was possible. The intrinsic advantage of liquid embolization is the elimination of the coil interstices that allow for recanalization and regrowth.

To reduce the degree of recanalization and aneurysm regrowth and therefore achieve more durable results, platinum coils have been reengineered to include an outer biodegradable coating on platinum coils, growth factor-impregnated biodegradable coils, and coils that emit irradiation with implantation. In a series of studies by Murayama et al. [2001], biodegradable-coated platinum coils induced a more pronounced endothelialization than bare platinum coils in sidewall aneurysms in swine. Moreover, the compaction of the aneurysms treated by embolization with coated coils resembled the contraction that occurs with scarring, possibly decreasing mass effect of the aneurysm [Lefkowitz et al., 1999; Murayama et al., 2001]. A cellular reaction to the coating may promote closure and scarring of the aneurysm. This robust cellular response, in conjunction with balloon or stent-assist techniques, appears to facilitate the occlusion of wide-necked aneurysms. Although the interpretation of these results is limited because the swine sidewall aneurysm model does not accurately reflect the histology or rheology of human intracranial saccular aneurysms, modified platinum coils have the potential to be more effective at occluding aneurysms than bare coils.

Abrahams et al. [2001] presented several experiments in ligated vessels of the rat demonstrating the feasibility of the use of endovascular coils to deliver recombinant human vascular endothelial growth factors (rhVEGF). Significant reductions in lumen diameters were observed in ligated arteries that were treated with rhVEGF-impregnated collagen coils compared with those treated with either bare platinum or collagen coils alone. Furthermore, vessel walls were thickest in the ligated arteries treated with rhVEGF-impregnated coils. By using endovascular techniques to alter the biochemical milieu around aneurysms, permanent aneurysm closure may be achieved. One additional important result of such an alteration will be an improved understanding of the pathophysiology of aneurysm formation and expansion. By understanding these biochemical changes, aneurysm prevention may be possible.

Another modification of coils that is undergoing laboratory investigation includes the use of radiation-emitting platinum coils. The radiation dose is low and is thought to inhibit endothelialization. The process of early endothelialization may be the precursor to recanalization of embolized aneurysms. By inhibiting this process, thrombosis and subsequent organization of thrombus might promote continued closure of the aneurysm and improve the long-term results of the endovascular procedure.

The hydrocoil uses the concept of increasing the volume of occupancy of the aneurysm and potentially affecting the biochemical milieu within the aneurysm. Piotin et al. [2000] demonstrated that in aneuryms embolized without any further visualization of contrast during angiography correlated with 34% volume filled with platinum coils within the aneurysm. The hydrocoil may potentially increase the volume filled as the platinum core of the coil is coated with a hydrogel that expands when in contact with blood. Several preclinical animal studies demonstrated persistent occlusion of aneurysms. This coil is currently being investigated for its efficacy and safety, and holds promise in its ease of delivery.

New Advances in Stent Technology

Stent placement can be used in giant and wide-necked intracranial aneurysms to prevent coil herniation into the parent vessel that would result in an ischemic event. Intracranial stenting is a novel technique and still in its early developmental stages. Novel modifications of stent surfaces using biomaterial science and surface-coating techniques have opened a new area in stent research. Investigators have demonstrated some promising results in both human and animal studies with the use of heparin-coated stents. Although rates of subacute thrombosis with heparin-coated stents are lower in some series, consistently significant reductions in restenosis rates have not been demonstrated. Stents that have shown promise in the cardiac literature are those coated with antiproliferative agents such as paclitaxel (Taxol) and rapamycin (Sirolimus). The Asian Paclitaxel-Eluting Stent Clinical Trial (ASPECT) compared the safety and efficacy of high-dose and low-dose paclitaxel-coated stents versus uncoated stents in patients with single lesions in coronary arteries and showed that restenosis rates had dropped from 27% in the control group to 4% in the high-dose paclitaxel group after 6 months [Park, 2001; Hong et al., 2003]; these findings were attributed to reductions in neointimal hyperplasia since paclitaxel alters microtubule stability and inhibits mitosis.

The Randomized Study with the Sirolimus-Eluting Bx Velocity Balloon-Expandable Stent study demonstrated that in patients with single lesions in the coronary vasculature who were treated with sirolimus-coated balloon expandable stents, no restenosis occurred at 6 months out and neointimal volume was 2 versus 37% in those treated with noncoated stents [Sousa et al., 2001a,b; Degertekin, 2002; Puel, 2002; Toutouzas et al., 2002].

Although intracranial stents are being used with increasing frequency, it is important to remember that there are no long-term data regarding rates of patency, restenosis, or vessel injury. Additionally, the effects of stent-induced intimal hyperplasia are not known in the cerebral vasculature, and the treatment for in-stent stenosis may be problematic. Another important limitation to stent placement remains the increased tortuosity of the cerebral vessels compared to vasculature throughout the body. The skull base confines these vessels in certain turns and curves that can make navigating a stent intracranially difficult. Recently, several stents are being investigated that are self-expanding and advanced intracranially through the microcatheter [Byrne et al., 2000; Nakayama et al., 2003]. By making the stents more flexible and with finer designs, the difficultly in placing these stents intracranially will be resolved. The advantages stents provide are altering the anatomical constraints of coil embolization techniques alone and changing the hemodynamics around the aneurysm to possibly make it more favorable to occlude the aneurismal dilatation. More recently, a self-expanding nitinol stent is being used for intracranial treatment of aneurysm with coil embolization. Promising initial experiences suggest this technology may play a large role in future aneurysm and intracranial atherosclerosis management. Drug-coated self-expanding stents that inhibit restenosis are going to alter the safety and effectiveness of endovascular therapy. In addition, knowledge regarding the pathophysiology and formation of aneurysm and atherosclerosis may be learned by using these stents which alter the biochemical milieu of the vessel.

Conclusions

Endovascular treatment of saccular aneurysms has become an alternative effective treatment to surgical clip ligation. Current literature and experience suggest that endovascular techniques should be used particularly in the patient at higher risk of surgical complications related to microsurgical clip ligation. By continuing to utilize clip ligation for aneurysms unfavorable to endovascular treatment and to patients who require a long-term effective treatment albeit at a potentially higher immediate morbidity, a complementary solution is provided that results in an overall decrease in morbidity for patients. Of the current technological advances, intracranial stent placement and biologically altered coils provide an attractive solution to several of the current limitations of endovascular techniques (namely aneurysm morphology and limiting aneurysm recurrence and rehemorrhaging). There is a paucity of literature demonstrating improved effectiveness with these techniques. Only speculation regarding their effectiveness in improving endovascular outcomes can be made at this time.

Carotid Artery Stent Placement

The North American Symptomatic Carotid Endarterecomy Trial (NASCET) showed that patients with a neurological deficit and at least 70% carotid artery stenosis on the ipsilateral side to the deficit are candidates for a carotid endarterectomy [NASCET, 1991]. Subsequent reports by NASCET investigators have demonstrated efficacy of carotid endarterectomy with stenosis greater than 50% by angiographic criteria ipsilateral to the neurological deficit [Barnett et al., 1998]. The Asymptomatic Carotid Atherosclerosis Study (ACAS) demonstrated that carotid endarterectomies are indicated for asymptomatic patients with carotid artery stenosis of greater than or equal to 60% [ACAS, 1995]. Carotid endarterectomy remains the gold standard for treatment of carotid artery stenosis despite the development of percutaneous methods of carotid artery stenting [Mullenix et al., 2002]. The reported perioperative stroke rate ranges from 2.2 to 5.8% for carotid endarterectomy overall [Mullenix et al., 2002]. These relatively low stroke death rates have made it difficult for some to accept the new percutaneous techniques of carotid artery stenting. Most vascular specialists feel it should only be used in the highest-risk patients and those patients enrolled in clinical trials. However, with the development of distal protection devices and advances in stent coating to prevent restenosis, carotid stenting may soon become the optimal treatment for carotid artery stenosis.

Studies have shown that carotid artery stenting is safer than carotid endarterectomy in patients with high risk factors for surgery such as advanced age (>80 years), cardiopulmonary disease, carotid restenosis after an endarterectomy, vasculopathy, complex carotid lesions, and radiation-induced stenosis [Al-Mubarak et al., 2000; Colombo, 2001; Mukherjee et al., 2001; Roubin, 2001; Sievert, 2001; Ailawadi et al., 2002; Chaturvedi, 2002; Drescher et al., 2002; Mukherjee and Yadav, 2002]. Shawl et al. [2000] and Shawl [2002] reports a prospective study evaluating the safety and efficacy of carotid artery stenting in patients who are at high surgical risk. They looked at 299 consecutive patients who underwent carotid artery stenting with high risk factors including age >80 years old, unstable angina, previous ipsilateral carotid endarterectomy, contralateral carotid artery occlusion, and other severe comorbidities [Shawl et al., 2000]. Mean carotid stenosis in these patients was

75 ± 12% before and 7 ± 8% after carotid stenting. Thirty-day postprocedural outcome analysis showed that there were two (0.6%) major and seven (2.3%) minor strokes, no myocardial infarctions, or deaths; none of the NASCET-eligible patients had a stroke. At 26-month follow-up visit (26 ± 13 months), 8 patients (2.7%) had asymptomatic restenosis [Shawl, 2002]. A recent industry-sponsored trial investigated in a randomized prospective fashion the effectiveness and morbidity of carotid endarterectomy versus carotid angioplasty and stent placement in high risk patients [Yadav, 2002]. This single study demonstrated reduced morbidity associated with stent placement in comparison to endarterectomy. In the 307 patients randomized, the stent group suffered a 5.8% risk of myocardial infarction, stroke, or death within 30 days of the procedure, while the surgical group suffered a 12.6% risk. The majority of this difference in morbidity could be attributed to periprocedural myocardial infarction (stent group 2.5%, endarterectomy group 7.3% with comparable nonsignificant rates of death and stroke). The higher incidence of myocardial infarction could largely be explained by differences in anesthetic technique or the treatment of myocardial ischemia during endovascular techniques using higher doses of intravenous heparin, aspirin, clopidogrel, and the occasional use of IIb/IIIA inhibitors. This trial is the first to randomize patients with the use of a distal protection device when placing the stent. Two prior randomized trials were stopped early because the neurological morbidity associated with stent placement was higher than with endarterectomy. Both trials were completed in the last several years and done without distal protection devices [Naylor et al., 1998].

Proponents of carotid stenting are interested in the safety and efficacy in patients without premorbid conditions so that this minimally invasive procedure can be offered to all patients with carotid artery stenosis who meet the NASCET and ACAS criteria. Kastrup et al. [2003] performed a study to look at the safety and outcome of carotid artery stenting versus carotid endarterectomy. In this study, they prospectively compared early outcome from carotid stenting to a retrospective review of 142 patients who underwent carotid endarterectomies over the same period of time. The occurrence of major and minor stroke, myocardial infarction, and death was analyzed over the initial 30 days after surgical or procedural intervention. 63 of the patients (63%) in the carotid artery stented patients and 92 (65%) of the carotid endarterectomy patients had symptomatic carotid artery stenosis. In the carotid stented group for symptomatic patients, the overall complication rate (any stroke or death) was 8% (2 minor strokes, 2 major strokes, and 1 death) while that of the surgical group was 6.5% (3 minor and 3 major strokes). For asymptomatic patients there were no strokes or deaths in the stented group and one minor stroke (2%) in the endarterectomized group. Three groin hematomas developed in the stented patients and were surgically treated, while 3 endarterectomized patients had to return to the operating suite for evacuation of a neck hematoma at the surgical site. Overall, the 30-day outcome in both the symptomatic and asymptomatic carotid stenosis groups was similar in those patients treated with carotid stents or endarterectomies.

Carotid endarterectomies remain the gold standard for treatment of carotid artery stenosis at this time. It should continue to be utilized in the patients at low perioperative risk of complications given its longevity. As with aneurysm treatment, patients who are high risk for surgical treatment may benefit from this alternative method of percutaneous revascularization. By combining the strategies to optimize outcomes, both treatments will flourish and morbidity will be reduced.

There are several promising technologies to making carotid artery stent placement safer and potentially with less risk of restenosis. Multiple techniques of distal protection to reduce the neurological morbidity of stent placement already exist. We are only beginning to see trials investigating these devices conclude. Their long-term ability to be utilized safely and reduce morbidity still needs to be proven. Several prospective series have been published suggesting the neurological morbidity with utilization of distal protection devices is reduced to 0–3% [Parodi et al., 2000; Ohki et al., 2001; Ohki and Veith, 2001; Reimers et al., 2001; Guimaraens et al., 2002; Sievert and Rabe, 2002; Yadav, 2002; Grube et al., 2003]. Even though the risk of in-stent restenosis remains low (2–10% in most series) [Roubin et al., 2001] the drug-eluting stents utilized currently in the peripheral and coronary circulations will certainly be investigated in the carotid artery. There indeed may be a time when carotid artery stent placement may become the optimal treatment of both high and low risk patients. In order to determine this however, large, multicenter, prospectively randomized trials must be performed comparing the efficacy, safety, and cost-effectiveness of carotid artery stenting versus carotid endarterecomies [Hobson et al., 1997; Hobson, 2002].

Conclusion

Despite new surgical approaches to cerebrovascular surgery and the durability of open surgical techniques, neuroendovascular surgery is here to stay. The optimal management strategy for cerebral aneurysms and carotid artery stenosis persistently changes on account of the technological inertia that drives research and development in the fields of endosaccular coil embolization, stenting technology, and periprocedural antithrombolytics. Overall, the literature suggests that endovascular techniques are safer than surgical techniques, shorten the patient's length of hospital stay, and decrease medical costs, morbidity, and mortality.

However, there are limitations to neuroendovascular surgery which include the inability to effectively embolize certain aneurysms and the durability of coil embolization and stent patency. The technological advancements are aimed at curing these complications by altering the biochemical milieu of the embolized aneurysm to give a more durable result, creating drug-eluting stents to reduce the incidence of in-stent stenosis, and developing better antithrombolytic agents to reduce thromboembolic and access site complications.

Clearly, long-term, prospective data are needed to better understand and define the safety, efficacy, and durability of neuroendovascular surgery. As we are at a crossroads regarding the best management of these patients, we need three types of prospective studies. First, we need to look at the long-term effectiveness and durability of neuroendovascular techniques in the areas of coil embolization of aneurysms and carotid artery stent placement. Second, we need prospective well-designed studies evaluating the complimentary techniques of endovascular and open surgical treatment in comparison to historical series of patients treated with open surgical therapy alone [Sturaitis et al., 2000]. This method may allow us to understand if these complimentary techniques truly improve patient outcomes and if so how we need to modify current treatment paradigms to reproduce these results. Lastly, we need to answer the question as to whether or not carotid stent placement would be beneficial in patients who do not meet the ACAS or NASCET criteria for carotid endarterectomy, but do have carotid stenosis; for example, would stent placement in a symptomatic patient with 40% stenosis reduce stroke risk?

Ultimately, the tumultuous pendulum will find its equilibrium at a point where the strategies of neuroendovascular surgery and open surgical techniques will compliment each other and optimize patient outcome.

References

Beneficial effect of carotid endarterectomy in symptomatic patients with high-grade carotid stenosis. North American Symptomatic Carotid Endarterectomy Trial Collaborators. N Engl J Med 1991; 325:445–453.

Endarterectomy for asymptomatic carotid artery stenosis. Executive Committee for the Asymptomatic Carotid Atherosclerosis Study. JAMA 1995;273:1421–1428.

Abrahams JM, Forman MS, Grady MS, Diamond SL: Delivery of human vascular endothelial growth factor with platinum coils emances wall thickening and coil impregnation in a vat aneurysm model. J Biomech Eng 2001;119:206–212.

Aenis M, Stancampiano AP, et al: Modeling of flow in a straight stented and nonstented side wall aneurysm model. J Biomech Eng 1997;119/2:206–212.

Ailawadi G, Stanley JC, et al: Carotid stenosis: Medical and surgical aspects. Cardiol Clin 2002;20: 599–609.

Aletich VA, Debrun GM, et al: The remodeling technique of balloon-assisted Guglielmi detachable coil placement in wide-necked aneurysms: Experience at the University of Illinois at Chicago. J Neurosurg 2000;93:388–396.

Al-Mubarak N, Roubin GS, et al: Carotid stenting for severe radiation-induced extracranial carotid artery occlusive disease. J Endovasc Ther 2000;7/1:36–40.
Al-Mubarak N, Roubin GS, et al: Effect of the distal-balloon protection system on microembolization during carotid stenting. Circulation 2001;104:1999–2002.
Barnett HJ, Taylor DW, et al: Benefit of carotid endarterectomy in patients with symptomatic moderate or severe stenosis. North American Symptomatic Carotid Endarterectomy Trial Collaborators. N Engl J Med 1998;339:1415–1425.
Boulos AS, Bendok BR, et al: Endovascular aneurysm treatment: A proven therapy. Neurol Res 2002;24(suppl 1):S71–S79.
Brilstra EH, Rinkel GJ, et al: Treatment of intracranial aneurysms by embolization with coils: A systematic review. Stroke 1999;30:470–476.
Byrne JV: Long-term outcomes of Guglielmi detachable coil packing for acutely ruptured cerebral aneurysms. AJNR Am J Neuroradiol 1999;20:1184.
Byrne JV, Bashiri M, et al: A novel flexible endovascular stent for use in small and tortuous vessels. Neuroradiology 2000;42/1:56–61.
Byrne JV, Sohn MJ, et al: Five-year experience in using coil embolization for ruptured intracranial aneurysms: Outcomes and incidence of late rebleeding. J Neurosurg 1999;90:656–663.
Chaturvedi S: Carotid artery stenting for high-risk patients. Neurol Res 2002;24(suppl 1):S63–S65.
Cloft HJ, Joseph GJ, et al: Use of three-dimensional Guglielmi detachable coils in the treatment of wide-necked cerebral aneurysms. AJNR Am J Neuroradiol 2000;21:1312–1314.
Cloft HJ, Kallmes DF: Cerebral aneurysm perforations complicating therapy with Guglielmi detachable coils: A meta-analysis. AJNR Am J Neuroradiol 2002;23:1706–1709.
Colombo A: Extra cranial carotid arteries: A unique field for self-expanding stents. J Invasive Cardiol 2001;13:736–737.
Cottier JP, Pasco A, et al: Utility of balloon-assisted Guglielmi detachable coiling in the treatment of 49 cerebral aneurysms: A retrospective, multicenter study. AJNR Am J Neuroradiol 2001;22:345–351.
Degertekin M, Regar E, et al: Sirolimus eluting stent in the treatment of atherosclerosis coronary artery disease. Minerva Cardioangiol 2002;50:405–418.
Drescher R, Mathias KD, et al: Clinical results of carotid artery stenting with a nitinol self-expanding stent (SMART stent). Eur Radiol 2002;12:2451–2456.
Fertl E, Killer M, et al: Long-term functional effects of aneurysmal subarachnoid haemorrhage with special emphasis on the patient's view. Acta Neurochir 1999;141:571–577.
Grube E, Colombo A, et al: Initial multicenter experience with a novel distal protection filter during carotid artery stent implantation. Catheter Cardiovasc Interv 2003;58/2:139–146.
Gruber A, Killer M, et al: Clinical and angiographic results of endosaccular coiling treatment of giant and very large intracranial aneurysms: A 7-year, single-center experience. Neurosurgery 1999;45: 793–804.
Guimaraens L, Sola MT, et al: Carotid angioplasty with cerebral protection and stenting: Report of 164 patients (194 carotid percutaneous transluminal angioplasties). Cerebrovasc Dis 2002;13/2: 114–119.
Hayakawa M, Murayama Y, et al: Natural history of the neck remnant of a cerebral aneurysm treated with the Guglielmi detachable coil system. J Neurosurg 2000;93:561–568.
Higashida RT, Smith W, et al: Intravascular stent and endovascular coil placement for a ruptured fusiform aneurysm of the basilar artery. Case report and review of the literature. J Neurosurg 1997;87:944–949.
Hilal SK, Solomon RA: Endovascular treatment of aneurysms with coils. J Neurosurg 1992;76:337–339.
Hobson RW II: Update on the Carotid Revascularization Endarterectomy versus Stent Trial (CREST) protocol. J Am Coll Surg 2002;194(suppl 1):S9–S14.
Hobson RW II, Brott T, et al: CREST: Carotid revascularization endarterectomy versus stent trial. Cardiovasc Surg 1997;5:457–458.
Hong MK, Mintz GS, et al: Paclitaxel coating reduces in-stent intimal hyperplasia in human coronary arteries: A serial volumetric intravascular ultrasound analysis from the Asian Paclitaxel-Eluting Stent Clinical Trial (ASPECT). Circulation 2003;107:517–520.
Juvela S: Natural history of unruptured intracranial aneurysms: Risks for aneurysm formation, growth, and rupture. Acta Neurochir Suppl 2002;82:27–30.

Juvela S, Porras M, et al: Natural history of unruptured intracranial aneurysms: A long-term follow-up study. J Neurosurg 1993;79/2:174–182.
Kassell NF, Torner JC, et al: The International Cooperative Study on the Timing of Aneurysm Surgery. 1. Overall management results. J Neurosurg 1990a;73/1:18–36.
Kassell NF, Torner JC, et al: The International Cooperative Study on the Timing of Aneurysm Surgery. 2. Surgical results. J Neurosurg 1990b;73/1:37–47.
Kastrup ASM, Krapf H, Nagele T, Dichgans J, Schulz JB: Early Outcome of Carotid Angioplasty and Stenting versus Carotid Endarterectomy in a Single Academic Center. Cerebrovasc Dis 2003; 15/1–2:84–89.
Lanzino G, Wakhloo AK, et al: Efficacy and current limitations of intravascular stents for intracranial internal carotid, vertebral, and basilar artery aneurysms. J Neurosurg 1999;91:538–546.
Lefkowitz MA, Gobin YP, et al: Balloon-assisted Guglielmi detachable coiling of wide-necked aneurysma. II. Clinical results. Neurosurgery 1999;45:531–538.
Levy DI, Ku A: Balloon-assisted coil placement in wide-necked aneurysms. Technical note. J Neurosurg 1997;86:724–727.
Lieber BB, Stancampiano AP, et al: Alteration of hemodynamics in aneurysm models by stenting: Influence of stent porosity. Ann Biomed Eng 1997;25:460–469.
Lincoff AM, Bittl JA, et al: Bivalirudin and provisional glycoprotein IIb/IIIa blockade compared with heparin and planned glycoprotein IIb/IIIa blockade during percutaneous coronary intervention: REPLACE-2 randomized trial. JAMA 2003;289:853–863.
Lot G, Houdart E, et al: Combined management of intracranial aneurysms by surgical and endovascular treatment. Modalities and results from a series of 395 cases. Acta Neurochir 1999;141:557–562.
Lylyk P, Ceratto R, et al: Treatment of a vertebral dissecting aneurysm with stents and coils: Technical case report. Neurosurgery 1998;43:385–388.
Mawad ME, Cekirge S, et al: Endovascular treatment of giant and large intracranial aneurysms by using a combination of stent placement and liquid polymer injection. J Neurosurg 2002;96:474–482.
Mericle RA, Lanzino G, et al: Stenting and secondary coiling of intracranial internal carotid artery aneurysm: Technical case report. Neurosurgery 1998;43:1229–1234.
Molyneux A, Kerr R, et al: International Subarachnoid Aneurysm Trial (ISAT) of neurosurgical clipping versus endovascular coiling in 2143 patients with ruptured intracranial aneurysms: A randomised trial. Lancet 2002;360:1267–1274.
Moret J, Ross IB, et al: The retrograde approach: A consideration for the endovascular treatment of aneurysms. AJNR Am J Neuroradiol 2000;21/2:262–268.
Mukherjee D, Kalahasti V, et al: Self-expanding stents for carotid interventions: Comparison of nitinol versus stainless-steel stents. J Invasive Cardiol 2001;13:732–735.
Mukherjee D, Yadav JS: Percutaneous treatment for carotid stenosis. Cardiol Clin 2002;20:589–597.
Mullenix PS, Andersen CA, et al: Carotid endarterectomy remains the gold standard. Am J Surg 2002; 183:580–583.
Murayama Y, Suzuki Y, et al: Development of a biologically active Guglielmi detachable coil for the treatment of cerebral aneurysms. I. In vitro study. AJNR Am J Neuroradiol 1999;20:1986–1991.
Murayama Y, Vinuela F, et al: Endovascular treatment of experimental aneurysms by use of a combination of liquid embolic agents and protective devices. AJNR Am J Neuroradiol 2000;21:1726–1735.
Murayama Y, Vinuela F, et al: Bioabsorbable polymeric material coils for embolization of intracranial aneurysms: A preliminary experimental study. J Neurosurg 2001;94:454–463.
Nakayama Y, Nishi S, et al: Fabrication of micropored elastomeric film-covered stents and acute-phase performances. J Biomed Mater Res 2003;64A/1:52–61.
Naylor AR, Bolia A, et al: Randomized study of carotid angioplasty and stenting versus carotid endarterectomy: A stopped trial. J Vasc Surg 1998;28:326–334.
Ohki T, Parodi J, et al: Efficacy of a proximal occlusion catheter with reversal of flow in the prevention of embolic events during carotid artery stenting: An experimental analysis. J Vasc Surg 2001; 33:504–509.
Ohki T, Veith FJ: Carotid artery stenting: Utility of cerebral protection devices. J Invasive Cardiol 2001;13/1:47–55.
Park S-J: The clinical effectiveness of paclitaxel-coated coronary stents for the reduction of stenosis in the ASPECT Trial. American Heart Association Scientific Session, Anaheim, 2001.

Parodi JC, La Mura R, et al: Initial evaluation of carotid angioplasty and stenting with three different cerebral protection devices. J Vasc Surg 2000;32:1127–1136.

Piotin M, Mandai S, et al: Dense packing of cerebral aneurysms: An in vitro study with detachable platinum coils. AJNR Am J Neuroradiol 2000;21:757–760.

Puel J: The best of 2001. Coronary angioplasty or post-interventional cardiology (in French). Arch Mal Coeur Vaiss 2002;95(Spec No 1):45–48.

Qureshi AI, Luft AR, et al: Prevention and treatment of thromboembolic and ischemic complications associated with endovascular procedures. II. Clinical aspects and recommendations. Neurosurgery 2000;46:1360–1376.

Raaymakers TW, Rinkel GJ, et al: Mortality and morbidity of surgery for unruptured intracranial aneurysms: A meta-analysis. Stroke 1998;29:1531–1538.

Raftopoulos C, Mathurin P, et al: Prospective analysis of aneurysm treatment in a series of 103 consecutive patients when endovascular embolization is considered the first option. J Neurosurg 2000; 93/2:175–182.

Raymond J, Roy D: Safety and efficacy of endovascular treatment of acutely ruptured aneurysms. Neurosurgery 1997;41:1235–1246.

Raymond J, Roy D, et al: Endovascular treatment of acutely ruptured and unruptured aneurysms of the basilar bifurcation. J Neurosurg 1997;86/2:211–219.

Regli L, Uske A, et al: Endovascular coil placement compared with surgical clipping for the treatment of unruptured middle cerebral artery aneurysms: A consecutive series. J Neurosurg 1999;90:1025–1030.

Reimers B, Corvaja N, et al: Cerebral protection with filter devices during carotid artery stenting. Circulation 2001;104:12–15.

Richling B, Gruber A, et al: GDC-system embolization for brain aneurysms – Location and follow-up. Acta Neurochir 1995;134/3–4:177–183.

Richling B, Gruber A, et al: Treatment of ruptured saccular intracranial aneurysms by microsurgery and electrolytically detachable coils: Evaluation of outcome and long-term follow-up. Operative Tech Neurosurg 2000;3/4:282–299.

Ross IB: Endovascular Treatment of Cerebral Aneurysms with Routine Balloon Assistance. American Association of Neurological Surgeons, Orlando, Fl., 2004.

Roubin GS, New G, et al: Immediate and late clinical outcomes of carotid artery stenting in patients with symptomatic and asymptomatic carotid artery stenosis: A 5-year prospective analysis. Circulation 2001;103:532–537.

Roy D, Milot G, et al: Endovascular treatment of unruptured aneurysms. Stroke 2001;32:1998–2004.

Sekhon LH, Morgan MK, et al: Combined endovascular stent implantation and endosaccular coil placement for the treatment of a wide-necked vertebral artery aneurysm: Technical case report. Neurosurgery 1998;43/2:380–384.

Shawl F: Carotid artery stenting: Acute and long-term results. Cardiol Clin 2002;17:672–676.

Shawl F, Kadro W, et al: Safety and efficacy of elective carotid artery stenting in high-risk patients. J Am Coll Cardiol 2000;35:1721–1728.

Sievert H: Carotid artery stenosis: Who should undergo surgery and who should undergo stenting? J Interv Cardiol 2001;14:625–628.

Sievert H, Rabe K: Role of distal protection during carotid stenting. J Interv Cardiol 2002;15:499–504.

Sousa JE, Costa MA, et al: Lack of neointimal proliferation after implantation of sirolimus-coated stents in human coronary arteries: A Quantitative Coronary Angiography and Three-Dimensional Intravascular Ultrasound Study. Circulation 2001a;103/2:192–195.

Sousa JE, Costa MA, et al: Sustained suppression of neointimal proliferation by sirolimus-eluting stents: One-year angiographic and intravascular ultrasound follow-up. Circulation 2001b;104:2007–2011.

Sturaitis MK, Rinne J, et al: Impact of Guglielmi detachable coils on outcomes of patients with intracranial aneurysms treated by a multidisciplinary team at a single institution. J Neurosurg 2000;93:569–580.

Toutouzas K, Di Mario C, et al: Sirolimus-eluting stents: A review of experimental and clinical findings. Z Kardiol 2002;91(suppl 3):49–57.

Tsutsumi K, Ueki K, et al: Risk of rupture from incidental cerebral aneurysms. J Neurosurg 2000;93: 550–553.

Tummala RP, Chu RM, et al: Outcomes after aneurysm rupture during endovascular coil embolization. Neurosurgery 2001;49:1059–1067.

Vanninen R, Koivisto T, et al: Ruptured intracranial aneurysms: Acute endovascular treatment with electrolytically detachable coils – A prospective randomized study. Radiology 1999;211:325–336.
Vinuela F, Duckwiler G, et al: Guglielmi detachable coil embolization of acute intracranial aneurysm: Perioperative anatomical and clinical outcome in 403 patients. J Neurosurg 1997;86:475–482.
Yadav J: Stenting and Angioplasty with Protection in Patients at High Risk for Endarterectomy (The SAPPHIRE Study). American Heart Association Scientific Session, Chicago, Ill., 2002.

Eric M. Deshaies
Department of Surgery, Division of Neurosurgery, Albany Medical Center
Albany, NY 12208 (USA)
Tel. +1518 262 5884, Fax +1518 262 5400, E-Mail deshaie@mail.amc.edu

Horowitz MB, Levy EI (eds): Neuroendovascular Surgery.
Prog Neurol Surg. Basel, Karger, 2005, vol 17, pp 18–31

The Use of Stents in the Management of Neurovascular Disease: A Historical and Present Status Review

Michael B. Horowitz, Phillip D. Purdy

Center for Cranial Nerve Disorders, UPMC Presbyterian, Pittsburgh, Pa., USA

Definition and Original Role

The origin of the term 'stent' is controversial. According to Kutryk and Serruys [33] and Dyet [17], 'stent' may refer to a device used to hold a skin graft in position that was composed of a substance invented by British dentist Charles Thomas Stent (1807–1885) called Stent's mass that was originally employed to make impressions of the teeth and oral cavity. Alternatively, the term 'stent' could have developed from the term 'stint' which means to restrain within certain limits [33].

According to Palmaz [54], a stent is a coil or mesh tube that is introduced into the body via a catheter in a small or constrained form. Once the device reaches its destination it is deployed by a variety of mechanisms. The device's role was originally felt to be (1) to prevent elastic recoil of a vessel following balloon angioplasty by holding a vessel open to a predetermined diameter, (2) to prevent dissection following balloon angioplasty by pushing the dissected layers against one another and against the arterial wall, and (3) to provide a cylindrical vessel lumen by forcing asymmetrical plaques eccentrically [54]. Palmaz felt that in order to meet these goals a stent had to have five mechanical characteristics. First, it had to have a high ratio between its expanded and collapsed diameter to allow for delivery via a small diameter catheter system. Second, it had to have a low postdeployment wall thickness or profile. Third, it had to have a low postdeployment surface area so as to reduce thrombus formation. Fourth, it had to have high postdeployment circumferential strength to prevent collapse. Finally, the stent had to be radiopaque to allow for precise positioning under fluoroscopy [54].

Early Experimental Work

In 1969 Dotter [14] began work on stents by placing a spiral coil into a dog's popliteal artery and demonstrating long-term vessel patency. In 1983 Dotter et al. [15] and Cragg et al. [10] published separate reports relating to the endovascular placement of nitinol stents into canine arteries. These pioneering efforts were followed by additional experimental efforts in the mid to late 1980s by Wright et al. [80], Palmaz et al. [55], Rousseau et al. [62], Roubin et al. [61], and Schatz et al. [64], each of whose groups placed either self-expanding or balloon-expandable stents into canine peripheral or coronary arteries demonstrating good patency rates thus ushering in new, nonsurgical treatments for peripheral and coronary artery stenoses.

The first placement of a stent into a human coronary artery was accomplished by Puel and published in 1987 [33]. That same year, Puel's group [68] published their experience with 24 self-expanding stents placed into the coronary arteries of 19 patients thus introducing in a new therapy for ischemic cardiac disease that in many cases obviated the need for coronary artery bypass grafting.

Neurovascular Applications for Arterial Stenting

Review of Published Surgical Series

The NASCET trial has investigated surgical results for the treatment of symptomatic 70–99% internal carotid artery stenosis and 30–69% stenosis [5, 52]. In patients with 70–99% stenosis the risk of ipsilateral stroke after surgery was 9 versus 26% in those patients treated with maximum medical therapy. Patients with 50–69% symptomatic stenoses had a 5-year ipsilateral stroke rate of 15.7% after surgery versus 22.2% after maximal medical therapy. In the 70–99% group 5.5% of patients suffered cerebrovascular events and 0.6% died. Cranial nerve injury was noted in 7.6%, wound hematoma in 5.5%, wound infection in 3.4%, and myocardial infarction in 0.9%.

The ACAS study and Veteran's Affairs Cooperative Study looked at the effects of carotid endarterectomy (CEA) in asymptomatic patients with ≥60% internal carotid artery stenosis [1, 24]. Thirty-day postoperative complications in the Veteran's Study were as follows: mortality 1.9%, stroke 2.4%, transient ischemic event (TIA) 0.9%, and cranial nerve injury 3.8%. Including the risk of angiography the 30-day stroke and death rate was 4.7%. In the Veteran's Study the surgical results at a mean follow-up of 47.9 months was 4.3% TIA, and 8.1% stroke while results with medical therapy were 7.3% TIA and 12% stroke.

These three North American studies have clearly demonstrated the superiority of surgery in comparison to best medical therapy in the management of certain types of symptomatic and asymptomatic carotid disease. Patient selection for these studies, however, was governed by a number of medical and demographic issues. Exclusion criteria in ACAS included age over 79, prior ipsilateral carotid or any vertebrobasilar symptoms, contralateral carotid symptoms within the previous 45 days, contraindication to aspirin therapy, a serious medical condition that would make surgery dangerous or limit survival to less than 5 years. NASCET exclusion criteria included age over 79, intracranial arterial stenosis more severe than the extracranial lesion, systemic disease limiting life span to less than 5 years, prior cerebral infarct that resulted in hemiplegia, and prior ipsilateral CEA. Patients were temporarily ineligible for a variety of conditions which had to be stable for at least 6 months prior to surgery, if they had undergone a contralateral CEA within the prior 4 months or a major surgical procedure within the previous 30 days.

Cervical and Extradural Internal Carotid Artery Angioplasty and Stenting

The application of stenting to internal carotid artery disease grew out of the success that such procedures had in both the peripheral and coronary arenas. While CEA has been shown the be an excellent means of reducing the risk of subsequent stroke in carefully selected individuals, many patients fall out of the NASCET selection criteria based upon concomitant vascular disease, age, or health-related issues as described above. Those patients have often been referred for carotid stenting and it is these cohorts that make up a large percentage of the patients studied retrospectively by investigators that will be listed below. While it is clear that no randomized, prospective trials relating to carotid angioplasty and stenting have to date been reported a number of retrospective series are available for review. Because these are retrospective studies in a selected population it is impossible to make any comparisons between the results seen with stenting and those with CEA. Nevertheless, the data on stenting does provide the reader with a glimpse at what the future might hold if an organized randomized prospective study demonstrates comparable short- and long-term results.

In 1996, Roubin et al. [60] published a series of 210 stents placed in 152 vessels. Sixty-three percent of treated individuals were symptomatic, 8% had contralateral occlusions, 11% had restenosis following a prior endarterectomy, and 69% had severe symptomatic coronary artery disease. More than 40% of patients were referred because they were considered poor CEA candidates and 80% of the study group would have been excluded from the NASCET and ACAS trials because of medical or anatomical considerations. Despite the relative poor quality of the patient pool the reported results were promising. Technical success was achieved in 99% of cases. Stent thrombosis was

0.4% per stent and 0.6% per treated vessel. The 30-day postprocedure incidence of death was 0.6%, major stroke 1.2%, minor stroke 4.8%, and minor stroke with residual weakness 1.2%. Seventy-four patients were eligible or available for 6-month follow-up. Restenosis was 5% with a considerable portion of these secondary to Palmaz stent (Johnson & Johnson Interventional Systems, Warren, N.J., USA) deformation. No strokes occurred in the follow-up group while the incidence of TIA was 1.3%.

A multicenter study on angioplasty and stenting published in 1996 by Iyer et al. [27] reviewed results in 543 cases. Technical success was achieved in 97% of cases with a 3.3% incidence of major stroke, a 2.2% incidence of minor stroke, and a 0.6% incidence of death.

In 1996, Diethrich et al. [12] reported their series of 110 patients with 117 involved vessels. Seventy-two percent of the group was asymptomatic. All symptomatic patients had either a 70% or greater stenosis or a severely ulcerative lesion. Asymptomatic patients had a 75% or greater stenosis. Technical success was achieved in 99% of the procedures. Neurologic complications included major stroke (1.7%), TIA (4.3%), conversion to CEA (2.6%), and stroke-related death (0.9%). Two stents occluded without associated symptoms during the 30-day postprocedural period (1.7% of treated vessels). At a mean follow-up of 7.6 months in 98 eligible patients no new neurologic events occurred, one additional stent occluded at 2 months, and one case of significant intimal hyperplasia was seen at 7 months. Patency after 27–30 months was 89%.

Theron et al. [76] in 1996 described results in 259 endovascular procedures performed to treat carotid stenoses. Sixty-nine of these cases were performed using stents. The authors chose to conduct 136 of their procedures using distal balloon occlusion ('protection') to reduce the chance of distal emboli during balloon inflation and plaque manipulation. A 13% incidence of neurologic complications occurred after angioplasty without 'protection' while a 0% complication rate followed angioplasty with 'protection'. Unprotected stent placement was accompanied by a 1% complication rate and a 0% complication rate when using proximal balloon occlusion. Restenosis rate was 16% without and 4% with stent placement.

In 1997 Vozzi et al. [78] published their results with 24 angioplasties in 22 patients using 19 stents. Ninety-six percent of cases were technically successful with stenoses being reduced from 85.6 ± 8.5 to 5.7 ± 3.2%. Only one major stroke and one minor stroke (normal within 72 h) were noted for the entire series for a permanent neurologic complication rate of 4.2%.

Smedema and Saaiman [70] also reported favorable results in a series of 48 stents deployed in 43 carotid arteries (5 common and 38 internal carotid arteries). Technical success was achieved in 100% of cases. All stenoses were reduced from greater than 60% to less than 10%. Clinical success was noted in

97.7% with one procedure-related stroke, no TIAs or deaths and no late restenoses at a mean follow-up of 9 months.

In 1997, Yadav et al. [82] published a series of 107 patients who underwent stenting of 126 vessels. A 6-month clinical follow-up was obtained in all patients 76% of whom had follow-up imaging. Technical success was achieved in 100% of the procedures with mean stenosis reduced from 78 ± 14 to 2 ± 5%. Thirty-day morbidity/mortality was 7.9% (7 minor strokes, 2 major strokes and 1 death). Ipsilateral major stroke was 1.6%. No strokes occurred after 30 days. Mean stenosis at 6 months in 81 patients was 18 ± 16%. Asymptomatic restenosis was recorded in 5 vessels (3.9%), 4 of which were retreated interventionally and 1 of which was treated with CEA.

In 1997 Mathur et al. [43] looked at a part of their patient group to see whether or not restenosis could be in some way device related. In the group's 1996 review they had noted that a significant number of their restenoses were in patients with Palmaz stents [60]. Review of 222 patients showed that balloon-expandable Palmaz stents because of their stainless steel composition and compressibility were more prone to the effects of external forces and subsequent deformation. As a result of their findings, the authors recommended that whenever possible self-expanding stents be used in the relatively unprotected cervical region.

In 1998 Naylor et al. [50] published their results with a randomized prospective study comparing carotid angioplasty and stenting with CEA. The authors aborted the study prior to its planned course because of significant differences between outcomes following each procedure. Of 10 patients who underwent CEA no morbidity or mortality was experienced during the 30-day postoperative period. Of 7 patients who underwent angioplasty and stenting 5 suffered ipsilateral strokes, 4 of which occurred during angioplasty and 1 of which occurred 8 days after the procedure.

Shawl's 1998 series [66] of 124 stented patients is of interest. Ninety-four percent of the author's patients did not meet ACAS/NASCET medical criteria for a surgical procedure. Procedural success was recorded in 99% of cases with carotid stenosis reduced from 86 ± 7 to 2 ± 2%. The major postprocedure stroke rate was 0.8% and the minor stroke rate (resolved within 7 days) was 2%. Of 92 patients eligible for the 6-month follow-up, only 2% had asymptomatic restenosis as determined by angiography or duplex studies.

In 1999 Mericle et al. [47] addressed the management of critical carotid stenosis in 23 patients with contralateral carotid occlusion. Twenty-one stents were placed. The average pretreatment stenosis was 78% while the post-procedure stenosis was 5%. The 30-day poststenting stroke and death rate was 0%. No neurologic deaths occurred over the follow-up period while 2 patients died of systemic illnesses. These results compared favorably to a 14.3% stroke rate for similar anatomic findings in surgically treated patients under the NASCET trial.

In addition to the larger series discussed above, a number of other case reports have been published regarding the use of stents in the treatment of carotid stenosis, recurrent carotid stenosis as well as vertebral artery stenosis [2, 5, 18, 19, 22, 28, 29, 35, 44, 67, 71, 72]. Most of these reports are favorable although risks of intimal hyperplasia and Palmaz stent deformation are brought to light. The reports of Yadav et al. [81] and Lanzino et al. [35] relating to stent treatment of recurrent carotid artery stenosis following CEA are particularly interesting. Recurrent carotid stenosis following CEA is reportedly 10% in the first year, 3% in the second year, and 2% in the third year followed by 1% per year from year 4 on [20]. The combined rates of major morbidity and mortality in the series of Meyer et al. [48] of 82 recurrent stenoses that underwent repeat CEA was 10.8% with an additional reversible ischemic event incidence of 3.3%. These findings pointed to a 5- to 6-fold increase in overall risk compared to a routine CEA at the authors' institution. The series of Yadav et al., of 25 carotid arteries treated with angioplasty and stenting following postendarterectomy restenosis demonstrated a 4% periprocedural complication rate per treated artery. The series of Lanzino et al., of stents for the treatment of recurrences in 18 patients demonstrated no major periprocedural complications. Sixteen patients underwent at least 6 months of follow-up and no new neurologic events referable to the treated artery had occurred over a mean period of 27 months. One stented patient had restenosis to 55%. From these limited reports, stenting appears to be a safer option in the management of recurrent carotid stenosis following CEA.

In comparison to outcomes from the NASCET and ACAS trials most published results of stenting series show competitive results in terms of overall short- and long-term morbidity and mortality. While a formal prospective randomized study has yet to prove the efficacy of stenting, it is possible that such a trial might provide us with an alternative to the traditional, effective CEA.

Stents for Intradural, Subarachnoid Arterial Stenosis

There are few published cases of intracranial subarachnoid stents for the treatment of arterial stenosis. The concept of using stents along with percutaneous transluminal angioplasty (PTA) for intracranial arterial stenoses comes from the cardiac intervention experience. Coronary balloon angioplasty is accompanied by abrupt closure secondary to elastic recoil and vessel dissection in approximately 5% of patients. In the presence of thrombus the risk of abrupt closure increases to 7.2 to 27.8% [3]. While such closure may be tolerable in the cardiac system it is rarely tolerable intracranially.

The use of stents for the management of intracranial arterial disease has been limited by the interventionalist's inability to negotiate the relatively stiff balloon/stent assembly through the tortuous carotid and vertebral artery systems without damaging the vessel in the process. Recent advances in coronary stents, however, have made a delivery of more flexible systems possible. Hopkins' group in Buffalo, N.Y., USA, has utilized a stent to manage one basilar stenosis [Lanzino, pers. commun.]. At UT Southwestern Medical Center in Dallas we have successfully treated three basilar artery stenoses using coronary stents. In 1999 Phatouros et al. [57] published the first case of intracranial subarachnoid arterial stenting for a basilar stenosis accompanied by acute basilar artery thrombosis. Although the patient died of cardiac disease the procedure itself was successful at restoring a normal basilar artery lumen.

Stents for the Management of Arterial Dissections and Pseudoaneurysms

In the mid 1990s interest grew in the use of stents for the management of arterial dissections and pseudoaneurysms. Experimental work by Geremia et al. [21], Wakhloo et al. [79], Massoud et al. [42], Link et al. [37], Szikora et al. [73, 74], and Turjman et al. [77] all pointed to the effectiveness of stents in bridging side wall aneurysm ostia . Once the neck was covered the aneurysm could be more safely embolized with coils or polymers with reduced risk of errant embolization of the parent vessel and its branches. Experimental studies also showed that when simply left alone with a covered or uncovered stent across its orifice many experimental aneurysms would thrombose secondary to alteration of hemodynamics within the fundus. On the basis of experimental findings endovascular surgeons began using stents in the treatment of extracranial arterial dissections and pseudoaneurysms. Use of covered and uncovered devices with or without the addition of trans-stent aneurysm coil embolization proved a promising means of treating spontaneous and traumatic vessel injuries and their sequelae [7, 11, 13, 16, 25, 26, 32, 39–41, 45, 49, 51, 56, 59, 69, 83]. The majority of aneurysms treated with stents alone ceased to opacify almost immediately after being covered by the device while those that continued to fill did so slowly and thrombosed over a period of days to weeks. When coils were used in conjunction with stents immediate aneurysm thrombosis was achieved without compromise of the parent vessel lumen. When dissections alone were treated with the device the lumen diameter and contour were usually returned to normal with minimal evidence on follow-up angiography of significant delayed intimal hyperplasia. Unfortunately, no large studies have been published pertaining to the topic of stenting for pseudoaneurysms and arterial dissections. Whether or not stenting improves upon the natural history of these disease processes remains to be determined by a large multicenter prospective study that looks to the natural history of untreated lesions as well as the outcomes with medical (antiplatelet and/or anticoagulant therapy) and interventional therapies.

Stents for the Management of Dural Sinus Stenosis and Thrombosis

Stents may be used not only for arterial stenosis but for the remediation of venous sinus stenosis. Two reports, one by Malek et al. [38] and the other by Marks et al. [39] point to the utility of angioplasty and stenting of venous sinuses to help reestablish venous sinus patency and function. Stents in this situation can be useful when thrombolysis and angioplasty alone are unsuccessful in maintaining sinus function.

Stents for the Management of Intracranial Aneurysms

One of the limitations of coil embolization of aneurysms is the effective and permanent obliteration of wide necked or fusiform lesions. Stents may provide a means of covering an aneurysm neck to allow for coil deposition within the fundus without the fear of parent vessel occlusion or stenosis. In 1997 Higashida et al. [23] successfully placed a Palmaz-Schatz PS 1540 articulated stent (Johnson & Johnson Interventional Systems) across the neck of a ruptured fusiform basilar aneurysm and used the stent to hold coils in the aneurysm fundus and out of the basilar artery lumen. In 1998, Lanzino et al. [34] described the use of an AVE coronary stent (Arterial Vascular Engineering, Santa Rosa, Calif., USA) in the management of a paraclinoidal aneurysm. Since that first procedure, this group from Buffalo, N.Y., USA has utilized stents to manage seven intracranial aneurysms [Lanzino, pers. commun.]. Sekhon et al. [65] have also used a stent to assist with successful coil embolization of a wide-necked vertebral artery aneurysm. In this case the authors introduced the stent not from a femoral route but rather through the vertebral artery following direct surgical exposure.

Pharmaceutical Manipulations to Improve Stenting Outcomes

Patient preparation prior to and after stent placement is integral to achieving a good outcome with stenting procedures. The rationale for a number of interventions will be discussed below.

The major etiology of acute and subacute stent thrombosis is platelet deposition on stent struts and damaged intima/media following PTA and stent placement. Exuberant platelet deposition takes place within 1 h of deployment. By 1 week stents are covered by a thin layer of thrombus, fibrin, and neointimal cells and by 4–8 weeks stents are fully covered by proliferating smooth muscle cells and fibroblasts, making subsequent thrombosis unlikely [4, 63]. Acute stent thrombosis within the first 24 h is rare. Subacute thrombosis occurs at a median of 5–6 days but is rarely observed after 21 days [4]. Multiple series have found coronary stent thrombosis rates of 0.3–18% [4].

In order to reduce the incidence of stent thrombosis a variety of pharmaceutical manipulations have been tried. The use of clopidogrel and aspirin is one strategy. The use of clopidogrel is based upon the CAPRIE study which demonstrated a 8–10% relative risk reduction of ischemic stroke, myocardial infarction, or vascular death in patients taking 75 mg/day clopidogrel compared to those ingesting 325 mg/day of aspirin [8]. The Stent Anticoagulation Regimen Study (STARS) also supported the use of thienopyridine derivative antiplatelet substances like ticlopidine and clopidogrel which inhibit platelet-fibrinogen binding. The STARS study demonstrated a reduction in stent thombosis in patients treated with 350 mg aspirin/day and 250 mg ticlopidine following stent placement as compared to those managed with coumdin alone or coumadin and aspirin [33]. We use clopidogrel as opposed to ticlopidine because of its greater antithrombotic properties as well as its better patient tolerance [8].

Abciximab (ReoPro, Eli Lilly, Indianapolis, Ind., USA) is another antiplatelet agent that is useful when placing stents intra- or extracranially. Abciximab binds to the human platelet glycoprotein IIb/IIIa receptor and inhibits platelet aggregation. It also binds to the vitronectin receptor found on platelets and vessel wall endothelial and smooth muscle cells thus inhibiting wall deposition [36]. The EPIC study demonstrated a significantly lower rate of 30-day coronary stent thrombosis, death, nonfatal myocardial infarction, unplanned surgical revascularization, unplanned repeat PTA, and unplanned stent implantation in patients treated with abciximab bolus (0.25 mg/kg over 10–60 min) followed by a 12-hour infusion (0.125 mg/kg/min; maximum 10 mg/min) versus those treated with placebo (12.8 vs. 8.3%) [75].

In addition to antiplatelet medications, fibrinolytics still retain favor with some investigators while others consider them dangerous in the setting of angioplasty and stenting. Urokinase (UK) is a protein that promotes the dissolution of thrombi by stimulating the activation of endogenous plasminogen to plasmin, which in turn hydrolyzes fibrin [53]. Prior to cervical internal carotid angioplasty Lanzino et al. [34] suggest a 150,000-unit UK infusion at 50,000 units/min. The aim of this infusion is to both dissolve any debris from the plaque face which might have a propensity to break free when the wire and the balloon/stent system are advanced across the stenosis and to possibly increase the available working vessel lumen. A UK infusion, however, runs the risk of creating emboli from a plaque. It also may increases the risk of a hemorrhagic event, especially when a thrombolytic agent is combined with a glycoprotein IIb/IIIa receptor blocker [Lange, pers. commun.]. Finally, and most importantly, because of its effects on plasminogen UK also has procoagulant properties which may be mediated through release of clot-bound thrombin and/or through platelet activation. The latter may occur through UK's conversion of plasminogen to plasmin, which in turn activates factor V to Va, which in turn helps to accelerate the generation of thrombin which activates platelets, converts fibrinogen to fibrin, and converts factor XIII to XIIIa which cross-links fibrin monomers [9]. The Thrombolysis and Angioplasty in Unstable Angina

(TAUSA) trial found that abrupt closure of lesions prior to angioplasty was higher in the group receiving prophylactic UK than in the group given placebo (15 vs. 5.9%) [46]. In view of the findings from the TAUSA trial UK administration is controversial.

Heparin infusion is maintained throughout all stenting procedures with activated coagulation time (ACT) kept between 200 and 250 s. ACTs greater than 300 s are associated with increased risk of nonintracranial hemorrhage when patients are also being infused with abciximab [75]. Following completion of the procedure the heparin infusion is generally stopped and the drug's effects allowed to wear off gradually. Most acute and subacute stent failures are secondary to platelet aggregation and as such, postprocedure heparinization is not necessary.

Patient Follow-Up

Assuming the stent remains patent for the initial 30 days following implantation, one must consider the risks of delayed stenosis. There is inadequate literature concerning intracranial stent patency simply because of the paucity of cases. In the cardiology intimal hyperplasia has been shown to be the major component of late lumen loss after stent implantation. Risk factors for restenosis include stent implantation at a site that stenosed following a previous angioplasty, use of multiple stents regardless of whether or not they overlap, extent of residual stenosis following initial stenting, stent placement in a totally occluded vessel, diabetes mellitus, and stent placement in a vessel with a normal diameter less than 3.0 mm [33].

Intimal hyperplasia follows a fairly predictable time course. Serial angiographic studies in humans demonstrate that the greatest smooth muscle proliferation occurs between 1 and 3 months with only a small number of stents exhibiting further narrowing between 6 and 12 months [4, 30, 31]. These findings are supported by experimental work that has shown late replacement of proliferating smooth muscle cells by relatively inactive ground matrix and fibrosis [4, 63].

Experimental Concepts

Investigators have begun to study ways to reduce the incidence of intimal hyperplasia. One such method is through the use of low-dose ionizing radiation. To test this hypothesis two trials have been launched. The Beta-Cath trial aims to assess whether beta radiation can prevent restenosis after coronary angioplasty or stenting. The Beta-Washington Radiation for In-Stent Restenosis Trial also seeks to evaluate the efficacy and safety of beta radiation for the prevention of instent restenosis. Both trials are currently active with results pending. If irradiation proves to reduce the incidence of intimal hyperplasia it is possible stents will be ultimately manufactured which will emit low dose radiation that is delivered directly to the involved arterial segment.

Conclusion

Stenting is an exciting neurointerventional procedure that assists the practitioner with the management of a variety of neurovascular disease processes. As new devices are developed and controlled trials run to assess their effectiveness older surgical procedures may be replaced in favor of less costly and less debilitating endovascular ones. Neurosurgery must stay abreast of this development so as not to lose input over the control of illnesses it uniquely understands and has traditionally managed.

References

1 Asymptomatic Carotid Atherosclerosis Study Committee: Endarterectomy for asymptomatic carotid artery stenosis. JAMA 1995;273:1421–1428.

2 Atar E, Garniek A, Rabi I, Morag B, Rubinstein Z: Angioplasty and stenting of the carotid artery. Harefuah 1997;132:388–391.

3 Baim DS: Coronary angioplasty; in Baim DS, Grossman W (eds): Cardiac Catheterization, Angiography, and Intervention, ed 5. Baltimore, Williams & Wilkins, 1995, chap 27, pp 537–579.

4 Baim DS, Carrozza JP: Coronary stenting; in Baim DS, Grossman W (eds): Cardiac Catheterization, Angiography, and Intervention, ed 5. Baltimore, Williams & Wilkins, 1995, pp 617–639.

5 Barnett HJM, Taylor DW, Eliasziw M, Fox AJ, et al: Benefit of carotid endarterectomy in patients with symptomatic moderate or severe stenosis. N Engl J Med 1998;339:1415–1425.

6 Bergeron P, Chambran P, Benichou H, Alessandri C: Recurrent carotid disease: Will stents be an alternative to surgery? J Endovasc Surg 1996;3:76–79.

7 Bejjani GK, Monsein LH, Laird JR, Satler LF, Starnes BW, Aulisi EF: Treatment of symptomatic cervical carotid dissections with endovascular stents. Neurosurgery 1999;44:755–761.

8 CAPRIE Steering Committee: A randomized, blinded trial of clopidogrel versus aspirin in patients at risk of ischemic events (CAPRIE). Lancet 1996;248:1329–1339.

9 Chesebro JH, Zoldhelyi P, Fuster V: Pathogenesis of thrombosis in unstable angina. Am J Cardiol 1991;68:2B–10B.

10 Cragg A, Lund G, Rysavy J: Nonsurgical placement of arterial endoprostheses: A new technique using nitinol wire. Radiology 1983;147:261–263.

11 DeOcampo J, Brillman J, Levy DI: Stenting: A new approach to carotid dissection. J Neuroimaging 1997;7:187–190.

12 Diethrich EB, Ndiaye M, Reid DB: Stenting in the carotid artery: Initial experience in 110 patients. J Endovasc Surg 1996;3:42–62.

13 Dorros G, Cohn JM, Palmer LE: Stent deployment resolves a petrous carotid artery angioplasty dissection. AJNR Am J Neuroradiol 1998;19:392–394.

14 Dotter CT: Transluminally placed coilspring endarterial tube grafts. Long-term patency in canine popliteal artery. Invest Radiol 1969;4:327–332.

15 Dotter CT, Buschman PAC, McKinney MK, Rosch J: Transluminal expandable nitinol coil stent grafting: Preliminary report. Radiology 1983;147:259–260.

16 Duke BJ, Ryu RK, Coldwell DM, Brega KE: Treatment of blunt injury to the carotid artery by using endovascular stents: An early experience. J Neurosurg 1997;87:825–829.

17 Dyet JF: Review: Endovascular stents in the arterial system – Current status. Clin Radiol 1997;52: 83–108.

18 Emery DJ, Ferguson RD, Williams JS: Pulsatile tinnitus cured by angioplasty and stenting of petrous carotid artery stenosis. Arch Otolaryngol Head Neck Surg 1998;124:460–461.

19 Feldman RL, Trigg L, Gaudier J, Galat J: Use of coronary Palmaz-Schatz stent in the percutaneous treatment of an intracranial carotid artery stenosis. Catheter Cardiovasc Diagn 1996;38:316–319.

20 Frericks H, Kievit J, van Baalen JM, van Bockel JH: Carotid recurrent stenosis and risk of ipsilateral stroke. A systematic review of the literature. Stroke 1998;29:244–250.
21 Geremia G, Haklin M, Brennecke L: Embolization of experimentally created aneurysms with intravascular stent devices. AJNR Am J Neuroradiol 1994;15:1223–1231.
22 Guterman LR, Budny JL, Gibbons KJ, Hopkins LN: Throbolysis of the cervical internal carotid artery before balloon angioplasty and stent. Neurosurgery 1996;38:620–624.
23 Higashida RT, Smith W, Gress D, Urwin R, Dowd C, Balousek PA, Halbach VV: Intravascular stent and endovascular coil placement for a ruptured fusiform aneurysm of the basilar artery. J Neurosurg 1997;87:944–949.
24 Hobson RW, Weiss DG, Fields WS, Goldstone J, et al: Efficacy of carotid endarterectomy for asymptomatic carotid stenosis. N Engl J Med 1993;328:221–227.
25 Horowitz MB, Miller G, Meyer Y, Carstens G, Purdy PD: Use of intravascular stents in the treatment of internal carotid and extracranial vertebral artery pseudoaneurysms. AJNR Am J Neuroradiol 1996;17:693–696.
26 Huang A, Al-Kutoubi A, Mansfield AO: Endovascular stenting of internal carotid artery false aneurysm. Eur J Vasc Endovasc Surg 1996;12:375–377.
27 Iyer SS, Roubin GS, Yadav JS, Dietrich EB, Whorley MH, Shawl FA: Angioplasty and stenting for extracranial carotid stenosis: Multicenter experience. Circulation 1996;94(8 suppl I):1–58.
28 Johnson SP, Fujitani RM, Leyendecker JR, Joseph FB: Stent deformation and intimal hyperplasia complicating treatment of a post-carotid endarterectomy intimal flap with a Palmaz stent. J Vasc Surg 1997;25:764–768.
29 Joseph G, Baruah DK, Zacharias TU, Krishnaswami S: Combined percutaneous coronary and carotid artery stenting. Indian Heart J 1997;49:425–426.
30 Kastrati A, Schomig A, Dietz R, Neumann FJ, Richardt G: Time course of restenosis during the first year after emergency carotid stenting. Circulation 1993;87:1498.
31 Kimura T, Nosaka H, Yokoi H, Iwabuchi M, Nobuyoshi M: Serial angiography follow-up after Palmaz-Schatz stent implantation: Comparison with conventional balloon angioplasty. J Am Coll Cardiol 1993;21:1557.
32 Klein GE, Szolar DH, Raith J, Fruhwirth H, Pascher O, Haussegger KA: Posttraumatic extracranial aneurysm of the internal carotid artery: Combined endovascular treatment with coils and stents. AJNR Am J Neuroradiol 1997;18:1261–1264.
33 Kutryk MJB, Serruys PW: Stenting; in Topol EJ (ed): Comprehensive Cardiovascular Medicine. Philadelphia, Lippincott-Raven, 1998, pp 2307–2338.
34 Lanzino G, Fessler RD, Mericle R, Wakhaloo AK, Guterman LR, Hopkins LN: Angioplasty and stenting for carotid artery stenosis: Indications, techniques, results, and complications. Neurosurg Focus 1998;5:1–23.
35 Lanzino G, Mericle RA, Lopes DK, Wakhloo AK, Guterman LR, Hopkins LN: Percutaneous transluminal angioplasty and stent placement for recurrent carotid artery stenosis. J Neurosurg 1999;90:688–694.
36 Lefkovits J, Plow EF, Topol EJ: Platelet glycoprotein IIb/IIIa receptors in cardiovascular medicine. N Engl J Med 1995;332:1553–1559.
37 Link J, Fayerabend B, Grabener M, Linstedt U, Brossman J, Thomsen H, Heller M: Dacron-covered stent grafts for the percutaneous treatment of carotid artery aneurysms: Effectiveness and biocompatibility – Experimental study in swine. Radiology 1996;200:397–401.
38 Malek AM, Higashida RT, Balousek PA, Phatouros CC, Smith WS, Dowd CF, Halbach VV: Endovascular recanalization with balloon angioplasty and stenting of an occluded occipital sinus for treatment of intracranial venous hypertension: Technical case report. Neurosurgery 1999;44:896–901.
39 Marks MP, Dake M, Steinberg GK, Norbash AM, Lane B: Stent placement for arterial and venous cerebrovascular disease: Preliminary experience. Radiology 1994;191:441–446.
40 Marotta TR, Buller C, Taylor D, Morris C, Zwimpfer T: Autologous vein-covered stent repair of a cervical internal carotid artery pseudoaneurysm: Technical case report. Neurosurgery 1998;42:408–413.
41 Mase M, Banno T, Yamada K, Katano H: Endovascular stent placement for multiple aneurysms of the extracranial internal carotid artery: Technical case report. Neurosurgery 1995;37:832–835.

42 Massoud TF, Turjman F, Ji C, Vinuela F, Guglielmi G, Gobin P, Duckwiler GR: Endovascular treatment of fusiform aneurysms with stents and coils: Technical feasibility in a swine model. AJNR Am J Neuroradiol 1995;16:1953–1963.
43 Mathur A, Dorros G, Iyer SS, Vitek JJ, Yadav SS, Roubin GS: Palmaz stent compression in patients following carotid stenting. Catheter Cardiovasc Diagn 1997;41:137–140.
44 Mathur A, Roubin GS, Yadav JS, Iyer SS, Vitek J: Combined coronary and bilateral carotid stenting. Catheter Cardiovasc Diagn 1997;40:202–206.
45 Matsuura JH, Rosenthal D, Jerius H, Clark MD, Owens DS: Traumatic carotid artery dissection and pseudoaneurysm treated with endovascular coils and stent. J Endovasc Surg 1997;4:339–343.
46 Mehran R, Ambrose JA, Bongu RM, Almeida O, Israel DH, Torre S, Sharma SK, Ratner DE: Angioplasty of complex lesions in ischemic rest angina: Results of the Thrombolysis and Angioplasty in Unstable Angina (TAUSA) trial. J Am Coll Cardiol 1995;26:961–966.
47 Mericle RA, Kim SH, Lanzino G, Lopes DK, Wakhloo AK, Guterman LR, Hopkins LN: Carotid artery angioplasty and use of stents in high risk patients with contralateral occlusions. J Neurosurg 1999;90:1031–1036.
48 Meyer FB, Piepgras DG, Fode NC: Surgical treatment of recurrent carotid artery stenosis. J Neurosurg 1994;80:781–787.
49 Miyachi S, Ishiguchi T, Taniguchi K, Miyazaki M, Mueda K: Endovascular stenting of a traumatic dissecting aneurysm of the extracranial internal carotid artery. Case report. Neurol Med Chir (Tokyo) 1997;37:270–274.
50 Naylor AR, Bolia A, Abbott RJ, Pye IF, et al: Randomized study of carotid angioplasty and stenting versus carotid endarterectomy: A stopped trial. J Vasc Surg 1998;28:326–334.
51 Nicholson A, Cook AM, Dyet JF, Galloway JM: Case report: Treatment of a carotid artery pseudoaneurysm with a polyester covered nitinol stent. Clin Radiol 1995;50:872–873.
52 North American Symptomatic Endarterectomy Trial Collaborators: Beneficial effect of carotid endarterectomy in symptomatic patients with high grade stenosis. N Engl J Med 1991;325:445–453.
53 O'Reilly RA: Anticoagulant, antithrombotic, and thrombolytic drugs; in Gilman AG, Goodman LS, Rall TW, Murad F (eds): The Pharmaceutical Basis of Therapeutics. New York, Macmillan, 1985, pp 1338–1359.
54 Palmaz JC: Intravascular stenting: From basic research to clinical application. Cardiovasc Intervent Radiol 1992;15:279–284.
55 Palmaz JC, Sibbit RR, Reuter SR: Expandable intraluminal graft: A preliminary study. Radiology 1985;156:73–77.
56 Perez-Cruet MJ, Patwardhan RV, Mawad ME, Rose JE: Treatment of dissecting pseudoaneurysms of the cervical internal carotid artery using a Wall stent and detachable coils: Case report. Neurosurgery 1997;40:622–626.
57 Phatouros CC, Higashida RT, Malek AM, Smith WS, Mully TW, DeArmond SJ, Dowd CF, Halbach VV: Endovascular stenting of an acutely thrombosed basilar artery: Technical case report and review of the literature. Neurosurgery 1999;44:667–673.
58 Price RF, Sellar R, Leung C, O'Sullivan MJ: Traumatic vertebral arterial dissection and vertebrobasilar thrombosis successfully treated with endovascular thrombolysis and stenting. AJNR Am J Neuroradiol 1998;19:1677–1680.
59 Reubben A, Merlo M, Verri A, Rossato D, Savio D, Tettoni S, Muratore PL, Rabbia C: Exclusion of an internal carotid aneurysm by a covered stent. J Cardiovasc Surg 1997;38:301–303.
60 Roubin GS, Yadav S, Iyer SS, Vitek J: Carotid stent-supported angioplasty: A neurovascular intervention to prevent stroke. Am J Cardiol 1996;78/3A:8–12.
61 Roubin GS, Robinson KA, King SB III: Early and late results of intracoronary arterial stenting after coronary angioplasty in dogs. Circulation 1987;76:841–897.
62 Rousseau H, Puel J, Joffre F: Self-expanding endovascular prosthesis: An experimental study. Radiology 1987;164:709–714.
63 Schatz RA: A view of vascular stents. Circulation 1989;79:445.
64 Schatz RA, Palmaz JC, Tio FOR: Balloon-expandable intracoronary stents in the adult dog. Circulation 1987;76:450–457.

65 Sekhon LHS, Morgan MK, Sorby W, Grinnell V: Combined endovascular stent implantation and endosaccular coil placement for the treatment of a wide-necked vertebral artery aneurysm: Technical case report. Neurosurgery 1998;43:380–384.
66 Shawl FA: Carotid artery stenting: Technical considerations and results. Indian Heart J 1998; 50(supp I):138–144.
67 Shawl FA, Efstratiou A, Hoff S, Dougherty K: Combined percutaneous carotid stenting and coronary angioplasty during acute ischemic neurologic and coronary syndromes. Am J Cardiol 1996; 77:1109–1112.
68 Sigwart U, Puel J, Mirkovitch V: Intravascular stents to prevent occlusion and restenosis after transluminal angioplasty. N Engl J Med 1987;316:701–706.
69 Singer RJ, Dake MD, Norbash A, Abe T, Marcellus ML, Marks MP: Covered stent placement for neurovascular disease. AJNR Am J Neuroradiol 1997;18:507–509.
70 Smedema JP, Saaiman A: Carotid stent-assisted angioplasty. S Afr Med J 1997;87(suppl 1):C0–14.
71 Storey GS, Marks MP, Dake M, Norbash AM, Steinberg GK: Vertebral artery stenting following percutaneous transluminal angioplasty. J Neurosurg 1996;84:883–887.
72 Sullivan TM, Grey BH, Bacharach JM, Perl J, Childs MB, Modzelewski L, Beven EG: Angioplasty and primary stenting of the subclavian, innominate, and common carotid arteries in 83 patients. J Vasc Surg 1998;28:1059–1065.
73 Szikora I, Guterman LR, Standard SC, Wakhloo AK, Hopkins LN: Endovascular treatment of experimental aneurysms with liquid polymers: The protective potential of stents. Neurosurgery 1996;38:339–347.
74 Szikora I, Guterman LR, Wells KM, Hopkins LN: Combined use of stents and coils to treat experimental wide necked carotid aneurysms: Preliminary result. AJNR Am J Neuroradiol 1994;15: 1091–1102.
75 Use of a monoclonal antibody directed against the platelet glycoprotein IIb/IIIa receptor in high risk coronary angioplasty. The EPIC Investigation. N Engl J Med 1994;330:956–961.
76 Theron JG, Payelle GG, Coskun O, Huet HF, Guimaraens L: Carotid artery stenosis: Treatment with protected balloon angioplasty and stent placement. Radiology 1996;201:627–636.
77 Turjman F, Massoud TF, Ji C, Guglielmi G, Vinuela F, Robert J: Combined stent implantation and endovascular coil placement for treatment of experimental wide necked aneurysms. A feasibility study in swine. AJNR Am J Neuroradiol 1994;15:1087–1090.
78 Vozzi CR, Rodriguez AO, Paolantonio D, Smith JA, Wholey MH: Extracranial carotid angioplasty and stenting. Initial results and short-term follow-up. Tex Heart Inst J 1997;24:167–172.
79 Wakhloo AK, Schellhammer F, de Vries J, Habersroh J, Schumaker M: Self-expanding and balloon expandable stents in the treatment of carotid aneurysms: An experimental study in a canine model. AJNR Am J Neuroradiol 1994;15:493–502.
80 Wright KC, Wallace S, Charnsangavej C: Percutaneous endovascular stents: An experimental evaluation. Radiology 1985;156:69–72.
81 Yadav JS, Roubin GS, King P, Iyer S, Vitek J: Angioplasty and stenting for restenosis after carotid endarterectomy. Initial experience. Stroke 1996;27:2075–2079.
82 Yadav JS, Roubin GS, Iyer S, Vitek J, King P, Jordan WD, Fisher WS: Elective stenting of the extracranial carotid arteries. Circulation 1997;95:376–381.
83 Yamashita K, Okamoto S, Kim C, Nakatsu S, Miyasaki A, Hojo M: Emergent treatment of iatrogenic dissection of the internal carotid artery with the Palmaz-Schatz stent. Case report. Neurol Med Chir (Tokyo) 1997;37:336–339.

Dr. Michael B. Horowitz
Department of Neurosurgery
Director, Neuroendovascular Surgery
UPMC Presbyterian
Suite B-400, 200 Lothrop Street, Pittsburgh, 15213-2582, USA
Tel. +1 412 647 3685, Fax +1 412 647 7000, E-Mail horowitzmb@upmc.edu

Horowitz MB, Levy EI (eds): Neuroendovascular Surgery.
Prog Neurol Surg. Basel, Karger, 2005, vol 17, pp 32–53

Carotid Angioplasty with Stenting and Carotid Endarterectomy: Both Are Here to Stay

Ricardo A. Hanel, Elad I. Levy, Lee R. Guterman, L. Nelson Hopkins

Department of Neurosurgery and Toshiba Stroke Research Center, School of Medicine and Biomedical Sciences, University at Buffalo, State University of New York, Buffalo, N.Y., USA

Introduction

Stroke is the third leading cause of death, ranking behind heart diseases and cancer [1, 2]. It is also an important cause of severe and permanent disability [3]. Approximately 750,000 people experience a stroke annually, costing an estimated USD 40 billion in direct and indirect costs. By the year 2050, an estimated 1 million persons will suffer from stroke every year because of changes in age and ethnic distribution [4].

Approximately 25% of the 750,000 strokes occurring annually are attributable to ischemic events related to occlusive disease of the cervical internal carotid artery (ICA) [5]. Carotid stenosis caused by atherosclerotic disease increases the risk of ischemic stroke by acting either as an embolic source and/or causing hypoperfusion of the ipsilateral cerebral hemisphere. Introduced in the early 1950s [6], carotid endarterectomy (CEA) involves the performance of an arteriotomy of the cervical carotid artery with subsequent removal of the atherosclerotic plaque. This operation was performed with increasing frequency after its introduction [7]; however, in 1985, when the Extracranial/Intracranial (EC/IC) Bypass Study [8] failed to show the benefits of surgical revascularization of the intracranial circulation, concerns were raised about the value of CEA [2]. These concerns ultimately led to the performance of numerous large, randomized trials to test the efficacy of CEA, including the North American Symptomatic Carotid Endarterectomy Trial (NASCET) [9], and the

Asymptomatic Carotid Atherosclerosis Study (ACAS) [10]. With some limitations, these studies have shown that CEA substantially reduces the stroke risk and increases the survival rate for patients with symptomatic carotid stenosis greater than 50% and asymptomatic stenosis greater than 60% [9–11]. During the past few years, carotid angioplasty with stenting (CAS) has evolved as an alternative to CEA, particularly for those patients in whom CEA is associated with a higher risk of complications [12–14]. The aim of this paper is to provide a brief review of the relative indications and limitations for both CEA and CAS, illustrating how the two approaches are actually complementary, rather than mutually exclusive. A general description of the endovascular technique used for carotid revascularization at our center is also provided.

Carotid Endarterectomy

Several randomized, multicenter, prospective trials have demonstrated evidence of the safety and efficacy of CEA in patients with both symptomatic and asymptomatic carotid stenosis. Since the publication of the NASCET results in 1991 [9], CEA has been considered the 'gold standard' for revascularization of extracranial carotid stenosis. However, it is being increasingly recognized that certain patients who undergo CEA have a higher risk of perioperative complications with increased mortality and morbidity [12].

Symptomatic Patients

In the NASCET trial, 2,885 patients with recently symptomatic (ischemic stroke or transient ischemic attack, TIA) carotid stenosis were stratified into two groups: 2,226 patients with moderate-grade (30–69%) stenosis [15] and 659 patients with high-grade (70–99%) stenosis [9]. The results of this study demonstrated a highly significant benefit for CEA over medical treatment in symptomatic patients with high-grade carotid stenosis at a mean follow-up of 2 years (fig. 1) [9]. Moreover, a significant benefit was shown for CEA over medical treatment in patients with 50–69% stenosis at a mean follow-up of 5 years (fig. 2) [15]. However, the NASCET selection criteria were restrictively defined. Exclusion criteria included a previous ipsilateral endarterectomy, an intracranial lesion that was more severe than the surgically accessible lesion, no angiographic depiction of the carotid arteries and their intracranial branches, and organ failure of the lung, liver or kidney. Temporary exclusion criteria included uncontrolled hypertension, diabetes mellitus, or unstable angina pectoris, myocardial infarction (MI) within the previous 6 months, contralateral CEA within the previous 4 months, signs of progressive neurological dysfunction, and a major surgical procedure within the previous 30 days. These patients

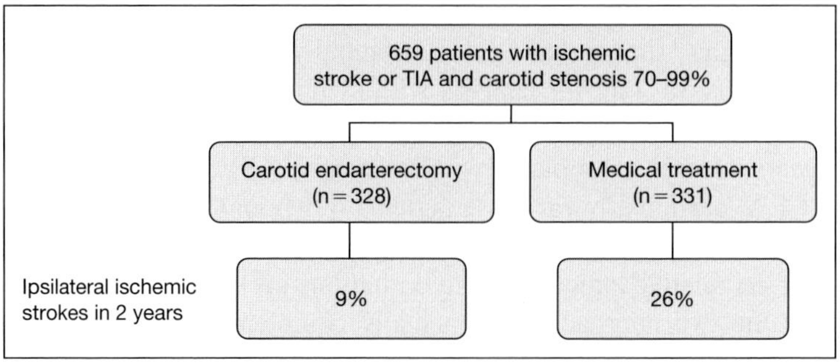

Fig. 1. Diagram showing reduction of ipsilateral ischemic stroke in NASCET patients with symptomatic high-grade carotid stenosis at the completion of 2 years of follow-up [9].

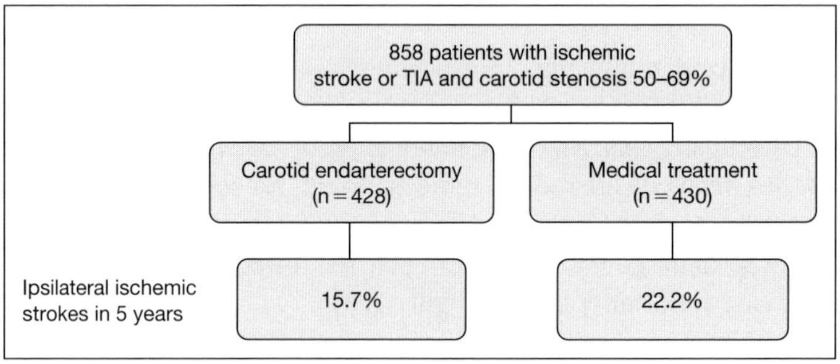

Fig. 2. Diagram showing reduction of ipsilateral ischemic stroke in NASCET patients with symptomatic moderate-grade carotid stenosis at the completion of 5 years of follow-up [15].

could be included in the trial if the disorder responsible for their ineligibility resolved within 120 days of their qualifying cerebrovascular event. In effect, these criteria excluded the highest-risk group of patients from the trial.

In the ECST, 3,024 patients were enrolled at 97 centers in Europe and Australia, with a mean follow-up of 6.1 years [11]. In this trial, which was begun in 1981, patients with TIA, retinal embolic phenomenon, or nondisabling stroke occurring within 180 days were randomized to receive medical therapy (usually aspirin alone) or medical therapy plus CEA. The final results of this trial showed a reduction in the 3-year risk of major stroke or death in patients with symptomatic carotid stenosis equal to or greater than 80% (60% according to the NASCET method for calculating angiographic stenosis [9]) from 26.5% in the medically managed group to 14.9% in the surgical treatment group, an absolute rate reduction of 11.6% in 3 years.

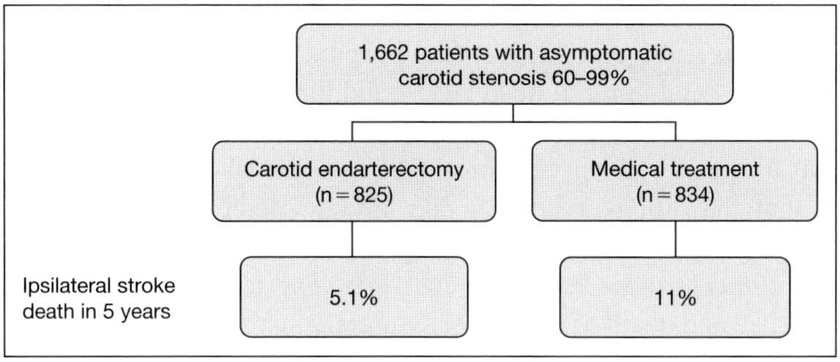

Fig. 3. Diagram showing reduction of ipsilateral ischemic stroke and death in ACAS patients with asymptomatic carotid stenosis (60–99%) at the completion of 5 years of follow-up [10].

Asymptomatic Patients

In the ACAS, 1,662 asymptomatic patients with more than 60% carotid stenosis (measured by the NASCET method [9]) were randomized to receive CEA or medical treatment [10]. As in the NASCET, the inclusion criteria were very strict. Follow-up data for 1,659 patients was available (median duration, 2.7 years). The composite rates of ipsilateral stroke and death at 5 years were 5.1% in the CEA group (825 patients) and 11% in the medical group (834 patients) (fig. 3). These results were obtained in conjunction with very low rates of death (0.1%) and stroke (2.3%) at 30 days in the CEA group.

Justification for Another Carotid Revascularization Procedure

Risk-to-Benefit Ratio

The benefits of carotid revascularization surgery demonstrated by NASCET [9, 15], ACAS [10], and ECST [16] are lost if the 30-day rate of perioperative stroke or death exceeds 6% for patients with symptomatic carotid stenosis or 3% for those with asymptomatic carotid stenosis. Moreover, the stringent criteria used to select patient in these trials excluded those with the highest risk of complications, i.e. the group in whom the benefits of CEA might not have been evident.

Trials versus the 'Real World'

There is now substantial evidence in the literature showing that the 'trials world' is different from the real world. Complication rates in clinical practice often exceed those obtained in clinical trials. Wennberg et al. [17], when comparing the perioperative mortality among 113,300 Medicare patients submitted to CEA during 1992 and 1993 at trial hospitals (those participating in NASCET and ACAS) and nontrial hospitals, found that the mortality rate was 2 times greater at nontrial hospitals. The mortality rate was 2.5% in nontrial hospitals versus a rate of 1.4% in trial hospitals. In a similar study, Hsia et al. [18] reported that the 30-day mortality rate among Medicare beneficiaries undergoing CEA was 2.5%, a figure much higher than the 1.0% mortality rate described in the clinical trials. Chaturvedi et al. [19] reported 30-day combined rates of major stroke and death of 11.1% for symptomatic patients and 5.6% for asymptomatic patients in a prospective, small series of patients receiving operations and routine neurological examinations at an academic center, suggesting an underestimation of complication rates in clinical trials.

Operator experience is probably an important factor contributing to this significant difference in complication rates. However, careful patient selection has been found to be the key determinant in maintaining a low perioperative complication rate. Certain patient groups have been found to have a higher risk for perioperative complications with CEA [12, 20–22]. CAS is an alternative method for carotid revascularization that could benefit these high-risk patients.

High-Risk Surgical Candidates

The risk of CEA associated with medical comorbidities has been well documented in the literature. This is true for both neurological complications like stroke and nonneurological complications such as MI [23]. In an analysis of the NASCET results, CEA was approximately 1.5 times more likely to be associated with medical complications in patients with a previous history of MI, angina, or hypertension [22]. Because patients with other significant coexistent diseases were excluded from the major CEA trials, the indications for and the results of surgery in this subgroup of patients have not been established. The factors that increase the risk of perioperative morbidity and mortality associated with CEA are reviewed here.

Age

Older patients appear to have a higher rate of perioperative complications with CEA. When assessing perioperative mortality of 113,300 Medicare patients, Wennberg et al. [17] found that patients 85 years or older were 3 times more likely to die than those younger than 70 years. In a multicenter review of 1,160 CEA procedures, Goldstein et al. [20, 21] reported a postoperative stroke or death rate of 7.5% in asymptomatic patients 75 years or older versus a rate of 1.8% in patients younger than 75 years. Similarly, the risk of postoperative MI associated with CEA was 6.6% in symptomatic patients 75 years or older versus 2.3% in patients younger than 75 years [20, 21]. However, a NASCET subgroup analysis performed by Alamowitch et al. [24] found that patients aged 75 years or older actually derived a greater benefit from CEA than those in younger age groups. The absolute risk reduction was 28.9% for patients aged 75 years or older (n = 71), 15.1% for those between 65 and 74 years (n = 285), and 9.7% for patients younger than 65 years (n = 303). Hence, although CEA definitely appears to benefit older individuals, it is reasonable to ask the question whether CAS could achieve similar benefits with a lower perioperative complication rate in older patients [20].

Congestive Heart Failure

Patients with congestive heart failure have a higher rate of perioperative stroke or death with CEA. A multicenter review of patients undergoing CEA found a perioperative stroke or death rate of 8.6% in patients with congestive heart failure as opposed to 2.3% in patients without this condition [20, 21]. CAS might be considered an alternative to CEA in this patient population.

Severe Coronary Artery Disease

Coronary artery disease is one of the most important factors to consider when evaluating the perioperative risk of CEA. The coexistence of severe carotid artery stenosis and symptomatic coronary artery disease presents the physician with a management dilemma [22, 25]. The surgical repair of one condition cannot be accomplished without a substantial risk of complications from the other. In an analysis of the NASCET results, a history of treatment of coronary artery disease was associated with a lower CEA complication rate, when compared with previously undiagnosed coronary artery disease [26]. This incongruity may be the result of improved cardiac and general medical care in patients undergoing treatment for coronary artery disease, many of whom may have had no regular, long-term medical care previously.

Adjunct to Coronary Bypass Surgery

Significant carotid artery disease places patients who are undergoing coronary artery bypass grafting (CABG) at an increased risk for stroke or embolization (air or atheromatous) or both. Faggioli et al. [27] reported on a series of 539 patients who underwent noninvasive evaluation (with carotid Doppler ultrasonography and ocular pneumoplethysmography) for the detection of carotid artery occlusive disease before undergoing CABG. They found that greater than 75% carotid artery stenosis was an independent predictor of stroke risk (odds ratio, 9.9) during CABG.

For patients with significant coexistent disease of the carotid and coronary arteries, there is little debate that revascularization is appropriate for both conditions; however, controversy exists regarding the timing of the procedures.

Surgical options include the performance of a simultaneous procedure or a staged approach in which one procedure is performed several days after the other. Published reports on combined CEA and CABG suggest that the risk of stroke or death ranges from 7.4 to 9.4%, which is roughly 1.5 to 2.0 times the independent risk of each operation [22]. In a multicenter review, the composite risk of stroke and death was higher in patients who had CEA performed in conjunction with CABG (18.7%), compared with those who had CEA alone (2.1%) [21].

Conversely, patients who undergo CEA before CABG also have a higher risk of perioperative complications [25, 28]. In this high-risk subgroup, avoiding a major operation or general anesthesia by performing angioplasty with stenting may represent a valid alternative to CEA [29]. The CEA guidelines published by the American Heart Association report a composite incidence of stroke, MI, and death of 16.4% for combined carotid and coronary operations, 26.2% for CEA proceeded by CABG, and 16.4% for CABG proceeded by CEA [30]. These high rates of complications would clearly offset the long-term benefit from secondary stroke prevention. Revascularization with CAS was performed in 49 patients with concomitant coronary artery and carotid artery diseases (carotid artery stenosis 70% or greater) at our center [29]. These patients underwent CAS before planned CABG. The 30-day mortality rate for the combined procedure was 8%, and the stroke rate for the same period was 2%. These complication rates appear to be substantially lower than those associated with either combined CABG and CEA or with CABG followed by CEA. In addition, no clinically significant recurrent stenosis was noted during a mean follow-up period of 27 months. Although the numbers in this report are small, the data supports the consideration of CAS as a valid alternative to CEA in patients with coexistent symptomatic coronary artery disease that requires CABG.

Anatomic Features and Tandem Lesions

Anatomic variations may increase the technical difficulty of CEA and adversely impact the results. A high carotid bifurcation near the skull base, especially in a patient with a short or thick neck, or a long carotid artery stenosis that extends to the skull base can be difficult to expose surgically. Surgical dissection of the carotid artery in these cases can be very difficult and at times extremely traumatic. These patients could be candidates for CAS.

The presence of tandem lesions, where the distal lesion is more severe than the proximal lesion, was an exclusion criterion for the NASCET [9]. Among symptomatic patients with ipsilateral carotid siphon stenosis, the risk of postoperative stroke or death associated with CEA in a multicenter review of 1,160 procedures was 13.9% versus 7.9% in patients without distal stenosis [20]. Angioplasty was performed with and without stent placement at our center in 11 patients with tandem lesions [31]. The proximal lesion was considered to be the flow-limiting lesion and was the only lesion treated in 10 of these patients. In the remaining patient, both lesions were treated. No perioperative stroke or cardiac event or deaths occurred in this series. Hence, angioplasty with or without stenting could be considered as a safe and viable alternative to CEA for patients with surgically inaccessible tandem carotid artery lesions.

Ipsilateral Intraluminal Thrombus

In a multicenter review of 1,160 procedures, Goldstein et al. [20] found that the risk of postoperative stroke or death with CEA was 17.9% in symptomatic patients with ipsilateral intraluminal thrombus versus 8.1% in those without thrombus. In a subgroup analysis of 53 patients enrolled in the NASCET who had intraluminal clot superimposed on atherosclerotic plaque identified by angiographic procedures, the 30-day risk of stroke was 10.7% in those randomly assigned to receive medical treatment and 12% in those who underwent CEA [32]. The high morbidity rate in this subgroup is related to the presence of fresh clot and the substantial risk of emboli dislodgment during surgical dissection of the carotid artery. CAS is an attractive theoretical alternative for these patients. An endovascular approach affords the opportunity to combine intra-arterial thrombolysis with CAS. In addition, antiplatelet agents [such as glycoprotein (GP) IIb–IIIa inhibitors] can be administered to patients who experience embolization of carotid artery thrombus into the intracranial circulation during the endovascular procedure; this may not be an option during CEA because of potential bleeding complications.

Contralateral Carotid Occlusion

Patients with recent symptoms referable to severe carotid artery stenosis and coexistent contralateral carotid artery occlusion have a high risk of ipsilateral ischemic stroke [33]. In the NASCET, the risk of ipsilateral stroke in medically treated patients with severe stenosis of the symptomatic carotid artery and occlusion of the contralateral carotid artery was 69.4% at 2 years [33]. Although CEA significantly reduced the stroke risk in this group, the perioperative risk of stroke or death in the presence of contralateral carotid artery occlusion was a high 14.3%. This increased risk may be related to the use of carotid artery shunting during CEA for patients with contralateral occlusions in up to 83% of cases [33]. In this subgroup, CAS represents a valid alternative to CEA, obviating the need for temporary occlusion in the presence of an already reduced cerebrovascular reserve.

Restenosis after CEA

Postendarterectomy recurrent carotid artery stenosis is being increasingly recognized [34]. Technically, a repeat operation is far more challenging than the initial procedure because of scarring around the arteries, friability of the recurrent plaque, and the necessity for more complex anastomosis techniques. The Mayo Clinic experience in 82 patients receiving operations for recurrent carotid stenosis showed a combined rate of major morbidity and mortality of 10.8%, which was 5 times the risk posed by primary CEA at the same institution [34]. AbuRahma et al. [35] found an increased risk of cerebral ischemic events associated with CEA for recurrent stenosis. The 30-day rates of perioperative stroke and TIAs were 4.8 and 4%, respectively, in the reoperation group, as compared with 0.8 and 1%, respectively, in the primary endarterectomy group. They also found a very high rate (17%) of cranial nerve palsy with reoperation. However, in a review of the results of CAS performed at our center in a similar group of 18 patients with postendarterectomy recurrent carotid stenosis, only a single case of TIA and no perioperative stroke was identified [36].

Recently presented, the results of the Acculink® for Revascularization of Carotids in High Risk Patients (ARCHeR) Trial suggest that CAS is a technically feasible alternative to surgical reexploration for patients with recurrent carotid artery stenosis [37]. The 30-day composite rate of stroke, MI, and death for the 141 patients receiving treatment with CAS in this study was 0.7% [37]. Further analysis of the data is pending the publication of the study results.

Radiation-Induced Carotid Stenosis

Patients who develop radiation-induced, accelerated carotid stenosis represent a similar high-risk group, primarily because of the technical pitfalls associated with a surgical approach. The presence of a long lesion, lack of well-defined dissection planes, and scarring around the vessels make the surgery more difficult [38, 39], exposing these patients to a higher risk of wound infections and cranial nerve palsies. Carotid angioplasty and stent placement can provide a more effective method for treatment of carotid stenosis associated with radiation.

Carotid Angioplasty and Stenting

Background and Preliminary Results

Two major issues compelled the development of CAS: (1) the need for a better therapeutic option for high-risk patients (as described above) and (2) the wave of minimally invasive surgery. After its introduction about 20 years ago by such pioneers as Kerber et al. [40], Mathias [41], and Mullan et al. [42], the field of endovascular treatment of carotid occlusive disease did not evolve, whereas the field of coronary and peripheral percutaneous transluminal angioplasty was developing rapidly. Kachel [43], in a review of the literature published up to 1996, found only 523 carotid angioplasty procedures performed from 1980 to 1995.

Publication of the results with stent-assisted balloon angioplasty in the coronary literature undoubtedly provided a new impetus for endovascular treatment of carotid artery occlusive disease [44] and prompted the conduct of studies in which carotid angioplasty with or without stenting and CEA were compared. The proposed advantages of stent placement over simple angioplasty include avoidance of plaque dislodgment, intimal dissection, and late recurrent stenosis, as well as diminution of vessel recoil.

The Carotid and Vertebral Artery Transluminal Angioplasty Study (CAVATAS), the results of which were published in 2001, was the first randomized comparison of endovascular versus surgical treatment in patients with carotid artery stenosis [45]. Between March 1992 and July 1997, 505 patients in 22 centers in Europe, Australia, and Canada were randomized. One patient was excluded from participation in the study owing to complete carotid artery occlusion before treatment. Of 504 patients, 251 were assigned for endovascular treatment and 253 to CEA. Stents suitable for use in carotid arteries were developed during the course of the study. Despite the fact that the use of a stent in this trial was approved from 1994 onward, only 55 (26%) of the patients in the endovascular treatment group received a stent. Similar rates of stroke and death were reported for endovascular and surgical treatment. The number of recurrent strokes, with a mean follow-up period of approximately 2 years, was also similar in both groups. The 8-year follow-up report, which was recently presented, showed equivalent efficacy in stroke prevention for both therapeutic options [46].

Several other groups have reported on the effectiveness, safety, and durability of CAS. Roubin et al. [13], in a review of their 5-year experience with a series of 528 consecutive patients undergoing CAS, described a 30-day major stroke or death of 2.6%. In 1996, Gil-Peralta et al. [47] reported a series of 85 patients who underwent percutaneous angioplasty for symptomatic carotid artery stenosis over the course of a 4-year period. No deaths occurred within 30 days postprocedure, and the major morbidity rate at 30 days was 4.9%. Our group [48] has reported a 30-day major stroke or death rate of 5% in 80 high-risk patients who were considered NASCET-ineligible according to the exclusion criteria of that study.

Distal protection, initially introduced by Theron et al. [49], is considered to be an important advance in the endovascular treatment of carotid occlusive disease. The rationale for using this technique is based on the concept that an embolic shower released from carotid plaque during CAS causes neurological deficits in the periprocedural period [49]. Preliminary studies have demonstrated the potential benefit of distal embolic protection. Jaeger et al. [50]

reported the occurrence of cerebral lesions (detected by diffusion-weighted magnetic resonance images) in 20 (29%) of 70 patients submitted to CAS without cerebral embolic protection. This percentage dropped to 7.1% with the use of embolic protection devices [51]. Whitlow et al. [52] reported a multicenter experience in which a balloon device (PercuSurge GuardWire; PercuSurge, Sunnyvale, Calif., USA) was used during CAS. Among the 75 patients treated with this device, no single case of periprocedural death or major stroke was noted.

The Stent and Angioplasty with Protection for Patients at High Risk for Endarterectomy (SAPPHIRE) trial also demonstrated the benefit of distal embolic protection [53, 54]. Patients from 29 centers in the United States were enrolled in this trial. Eligible study patients were those who were either asymptomatic with greater than 80% stenosis (by Doppler) or symptomatic with greater than 50% stenosis plus at least one feature that would make them high-risk for CEA: older than 80 years, congestive heart failure, severe chronic obstructive pulmonary disease, postendarterectomy recurrent carotid stenosis, previous radiation therapy, or previous radical neck surgery. Eligible patients were then screened by a team that included a vascular surgeon, an interventionist, and a neurologist. Consensus that patients were good candidates for either procedure was required before randomization; those rejected as candidates for surgery underwent stenting and were included in a stent registry, whereas those rejected for stenting had surgery and were included in a surgical registry. At the end of the enrollment period in June 2002, 409 patients had been included in the stenting registry (surgical risk considered excessively high) and 7 patients in the surgical registry (considered too risky for CAS). A total of 307 patients were randomized: 156 to CAS and 151 to CEA. The devices used for CAS in this trial were the Precise® nitinol stent (Johnson & Johnson, Warren, N.J., USA) and the AngioGuard® (Johnson & Johnson) distal protection device. The preliminary results have been presented but not published. The 30-day stroke and death rate was similar for both groups (4.5% CAS group vs. 6.6% CEA group). When the rate of MI was taken into consideration, the CAS group did better, with a major adverse cardiovascular event rate of 5.8% compared with a 12.6% event rate in the CEA group. Further analysis of the data is pending the publication of the results of this study and completion of study follow-up.

The preliminary results of the ARCHeR Trial were recently presented [37]. In this trial, 437 patients were enrolled at 41 sites in the US, Europe, and South America. Eligibility criteria included carotid artery stenosis that was either asymptomatic and greater than 80% (by angiography) or symptomatic and greater than 50%. The high-risk factors established for inclusion in this trial were two or more of the following criteria: (1) two or more coronary vessels with 70% or greater stenosis, (2) MI within 30 days, (3) CABG or valve surgery within 30 days, (4) unstable angina, and (5) contralateral carotid occlusion, and/or one or more of the following criteria: (1) ejection fraction less than 30% or New York Heart Association Functional Class III or greater, (2) FEV_1 less than 30% (predicted), (3) dialysis-dependent renal failure, (4) uncontrolled diabetes, (5) postendarterectomy recurrent stenosis, (6) history of radical neck surgery and/or radiation therapy, (7) surgically inaccessible lesion, (8) spinal immobility, (9) tracheostomy stoma, and (10) contralateral laryngeal nerve paralysis. Eligible patients were assessed by an independent neurologist before enrollment and throughout the duration of follow-up. After enrollment in the trial, the patients were submitted to CAS using the Acculink™ stent (Guidant/Advanced Cardiovascular Systems, Temecula, Calif., USA) and the Accunet™ filter (Guidant) for distal embolic protection. The 30-day combined rate of stroke and death rate was 6.6% and the major adverse cardiovascular event rate was 7.8%. The ipsilateral stroke rate was 5.1% (0.2% contralateral) and the death rate 2.3% [one (0.7%) was stroke-related]. Further data analysis will be possible after the results of the study have been published.

Several other carotid stent registries are being maintained in the United States, and one randomized, controlled trial currently under way is the Carotid Revascularization Endarterectomy versus Stent Trial (CREST), which is jointly sponsored by the National Institutes of Health and Guidant Corporation (Indianapolis, Ind., USA) (table 1). The results of these studies are expected to provide the level I evidence necessary for Food and Drug Administration approval for CAS as an optimal technique for carotid revascularization.

Endovascular Management Protocol and Procedural Technique

The technique of CAS varies slightly from case to case, depending on the clinical situation. The following description is of the management protocol and procedural technique used for most patients at our center.

Medical Management

Endovascular procedures carry an inherent risk of intimal injury and subsequent thrombosis and vessel occlusion. Furthermore, all stents are thrombogenic [55]. Thus, patient preparation for stenting centers on adequate antiplatelet and anticoagulation therapy. Consideration must be given not only to the selection and dosing of the antithrombotic medications but also to minimizing the potential for associated hemorrhagic complications. Most information about treatment with these medications must be gleaned from the cardiac literature because clinical data in the neurosurgical literature is limited. Aspirin is a cyclooxygenase-1 inhibitor that irreversibly inhibits platelet aggregation but does not impede platelet adhesion or platelet-activated mitogenic activity.

Table 1. CAS trials

Study (sponsor)	Design	Clinical characteristics and percentage of stenosis	Stent	Distal protection device
ARCHeR RX (Guidant)	Prospective single-arm registry	High risk Asymptomatic >80% Symptomatic >50%	Acculink RX	Accunet RX
BEACH (Boston Scientific)	Prospective single-arm registry	High risk Asymptomatic >80% Symptomatic >50%	Monorail Wallstent	EPI FilterWire EZ
CABERNET (Boston Scientific and EndoTex)	Prospective single-arm registry	High risk Asymptomatic >60% Symptomatic >50%	NexStent	EPI FilterWire
CARESS (NIH) (excludes CREST patients)	Prospective double-arm registry; physician chooses treatment – 2:1 CEA:CAS	Asymptomatic >75% Symptomatic >50%	Physician's choice	Physician's choice
CREST (NIH, Guidant)	Randomized trial	Symptomatic >50%	Acculink	Accunet
MAVEriC 2 (Medtronic AVE)	Prospective single-arm registry	High risk Asymptomatic >80% Symptomatic >50%	Maverick	PercuSurge
SECURITY (ABBOTT/ MEDNOVA)	Prospective single-arm registry	High risk Asymptomatic >80% Symptomatic >50%	X.act	NeuroShield

ARCHeR = Acculink for Revascularization of Carotids in High Risk Patients; BEACH = Boston Scientific EPI: A Carotid Stent for High Risk Surgical Patients; CABERNET = Carotid Artery Revascularization using Boston Scientific EPI FilterWire and EndoTex Stent; CARESS = Carotid Revascularization with Endarterectomy or Stenting Systems; CREST = Carotid Revascularization Endarterectomy vs. Stent Trial; MAVEriC = Evaluation of the Medtronic AVE Self-Expanding Carotid Stent System with Distal Protection in the Treatment of Carotid Stenosis [this table was modified with permission from 60].

Clopidogrel is a thienopyridine derivative with potent antiplatelet action that inhibits adenosine phosphate-induced platelet aggregation. This drug works synergistically with aspirin, and evidence from the cardiac literature supports the use of combination antiplatelet regimens [56]. Clopidogrel, in combination with aspirin, has become the standard treatment for patients undergoing coronary angioplasty and stenting. When possible, patients should receive aspirin (325 mg daily) and clopidogrel (75 mg daily) for at least 3 days before CAS or be given a loading dose of clopidogrel (300–600 mg) early on the day of the procedure.

For most stenting procedures, an intravenous bolus dose of heparin (50 U/kg) is administered after catheterization of the common carotid artery (CCA). In addition, all saline solutions to be used for irrigation of catheters should be prepared with heparin (1 unit/ml). The activated coagulation time should be kept in the range of 250–300 s for the duration of the procedure.

The use of platelet GP IIb–IIIa inhibitors, such as abciximab or eptifibatide, in conjunction with CAS is controversial. These agents block the final common pathway of platelet aggregation by preventing the binding of fibrinogen to platelets and are the most potent of the antiplatelet drugs [57]. Our preliminary experience suggests that the administration of GP IIb–IIIa inhibitors places patients with chronic cerebral ischemia at an elevated risk of intracranial hemorrhage; therefore, these drugs should be reserved for patients who experience thromboembolic complications during or soon after the procedure [57]. Abciximab can be given as an initial loading dose of 0.25 mg/kg followed by a 12-hour intravenous infusion at a rate of 10 μg/min. Eptifibatide may be administered as a loading dose of 180 μg/kg, followed by a 20- to 24-hour infusion of 0.5 μg/kg. When GP IIb–IIIa inhibition is used, we recommend obtaining a computed tomographic scan immediately after the procedure to check for intracerebral hemorrhage before proceeding with the postprocedure infusion.

Bradycardia occurs occasionally during angioplasty, particularly when the plaque involves the carotid sinus. Atropine and a prepared dopamine solution are kept available should significant bradycardia and hypotension appear. Medical management of bradycardia during angioplasty is usually sufficient; we do not place transvenous pacemakers before performing CAS.

Following stent placement, heparin therapy is usually discontinued but not reversed with protamine. In some situations, such as when an angiographically visible dissection or thrombosis is present, continued infusion of heparin to maintain the activated prothrombin time at 1.5–2.3 times the baseline value is appropriate. Aspirin (325 mg daily) and clopidogrel (75 mg daily) should be administered for at least 4 weeks to allow for complete endothelialization of the stent [58]. Aspirin is continued indefinitely.

Preparation for the Procedure

The procedure is performed in an angiography suite with biplane digital subtraction and fluoroscopic imaging capabilities. The patient is kept awake, with local anesthesia and sedatives administered to permit continuous neurological assessment. Dorsalis pedis and posterior tibialis pulses are assessed and marked for later reference, a practice that is particularly important in patients with coexistent peripheral vascular disease. A Foley catheter and two peripheral intravenous lines are placed. Oxygen saturation, cardiac rhythm, and blood pressure are monitored throughout the procedure.

Diagnostic Angiogram

A 5-french sheath is placed in the right femoral artery, and a three-vessel diagnostic angiogram is obtained (if not previously performed) using a 5-french Simmons-2 or angled glide catheter. An intracranial angiogram with the injection of contrast material into the ipsilateral CCA is necessary for later comparison should intracranial thromboembolism be suspected after angioplasty. After a working projection image of the target vessel has been obtained, the vessel diameter proximal and distal to the lesion, lesion length, and severity of stenosis (using the NASCET method [9]) are measured.

Vascular Access

As previously mentioned, the loading dose of heparin is administered before the guide catheter is placed within the CCA. When the activated coagulation time reaches at least 250 s, the diagnostic catheter is positioned in the CCA and is used to advance a 0.035-inch, 300-cm-long stiff glide wire into the distal external carotid artery (ECA). In the setting of stenosis or occlusion of the ECA, an Amplatz exchange 'J' wire (Cook, Bloomington, Ind., USA) is placed in the distal CCA and used to provide support for the guide sheath. With the stiff wire in position, the diagnostic catheter is removed, as well as the femoral artery sheath. A 6-french, 90-cm guide sheath (Cook, Bloomington, Ind., USA) is then advanced over the wire and placed just proximal to the carotid bifurcation. All catheter systems are flushed continuously with heparinized saline. The position of and integrity of the target vessel are assessed by angiography.

Distal Protection Device Placement

Once the guide catheter is in place, we proceed with a four-stage CAS procedure. First, the distal protection device is positioned. Second, if necessary, prestent deployment angioplasty is performed to enlarge the stenotic region sufficiently to permit passage of the stent. Third, the stent is deployed, and fourth, poststent deployment angioplasty is done to remodel and fully expand the stent.

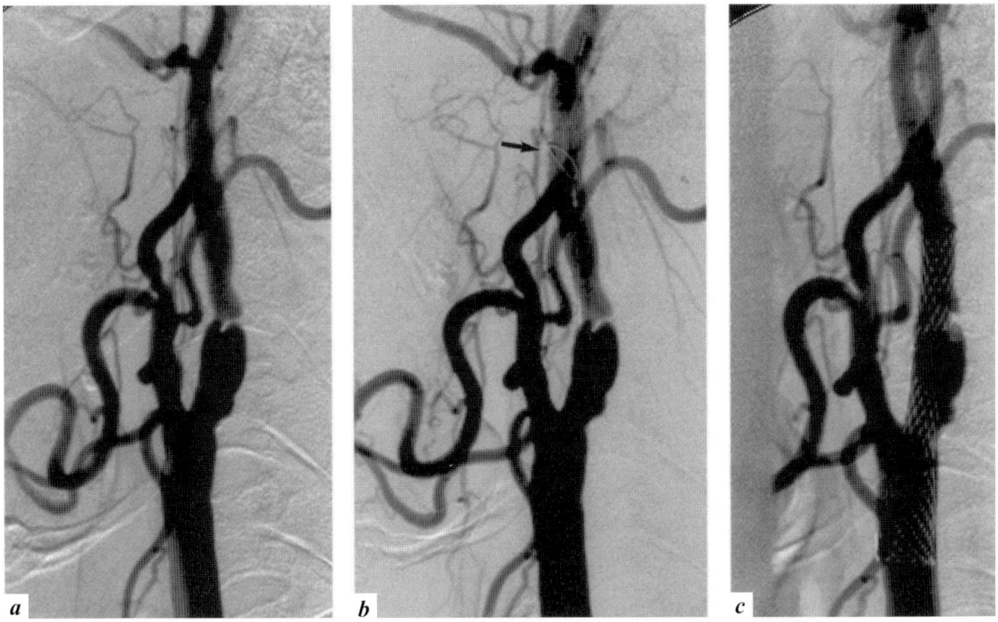

Fig. 4. Lateral angiogram of the left cervical carotid artery in a symptomatic man. ***a*** Pretreatment image demonstrates severe stenosis (large arrow) at left carotid bifurcation. ***b*** After a distal embolic protection device (EPI Filter – arrow) has been deployed distal to the lesion. ***c*** Poststenting image showing an optimal result after endoluminal carotid revascularization.

After each step, high-resolution biplanar angiograms are obtained and neurological examinations are performed to allow for prompt recognition of any changes from the patient's baseline status (fig. 4).

There are three classes of distal protection devices: filtration, balloon occlusion, and flow reversal (fig. 5). Retrievable filters designed to collect debris during CAS are placed distal to the stenotic region without interrupting flow within the ICA. Examples include the EPI FilterWire (Boston Scientific Embolic Protection, San Carlos, Calif., USA) (fig. 6), Accunet (Guidant, Menlo Park, Calif., USA), Angioguard (Cordis, Miami Lakes, Fla., USA), and Mednova (Abbott Laboratories, Abbott Park, Ill., USA). Balloon occlusion techniques involve inflation of a balloon and interruption of flow in the ICA distal to the stenosis for the duration of the stenting procedure. An example is the PercuSurge balloon. The flow-reversal technique involves the placement of balloons in the ECA and CCA to interrupt flow in these vessels and cause retrograde flow in the ICA to prevent embolization into the intracranial circulation [59].

After the guide catheter is positioned, a distal protection device (the authors' preference is to use a retrievable filter) mounted on a 0.014-inch

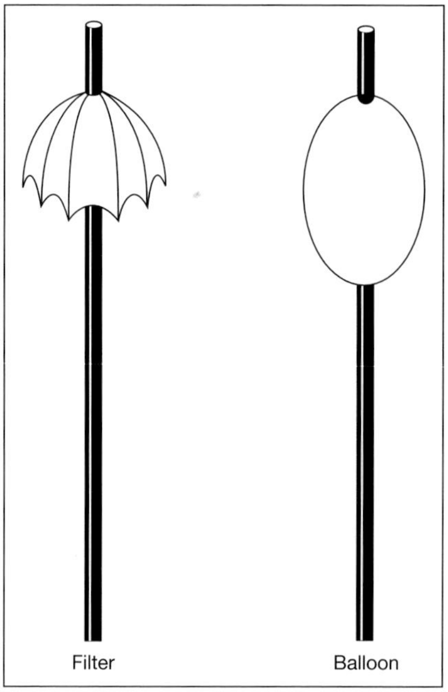

Fig. 5. Schematic illustrating the two devices used most commonly for distal embolic protection – filter and balloon – placed across the lesion in the distal portion of the ICA.

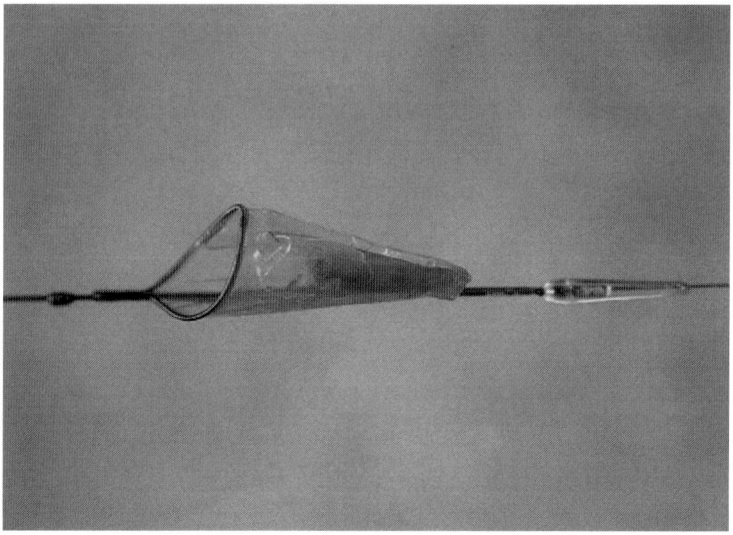

Fig. 6. Illustration of the EPI FilterWire (Boston Scientific Embolic Protection, San Carlos, Calif., USA) after retrieval showing plaque debris captured.

microguidewire is carefully guided across the stenotic region, using a biplanar roadmapping technique, and then deployed.

Predilation Angioplasty

The selection of a predilation angioplasty balloon is based on the dimensions of the lesion. The balloon must be long enough to cover the entire length of the lesion, and the inflation diameter should be undersized to avoid overinflation and to open the artery just enough to allow passage of the stent. With lower grade lesions, predilation angioplasty may not be necessary. After an angiogram of the cervical carotid is obtained with the distal protection device in place, the angioplasty balloon is advanced and centered on the lesion. The balloon is inflated to the manufacturer's recommended nominal pressure for several seconds and then deflated. The blood pressure cuff is set at a continuous mode during angioplasty to allow rapid sequential measurement of blood pressure should bradycardia and hypotension occur.

Stent Placement

Most stents currently in use for CAS are self-expanding stents such as the Wallstent (Boston Scientific Scimed, Maple Grove, Minn., USA), Acculink, and Precise (Cordis) stents. The Wallstent is composed of stainless steel, and the Acculink and Precise stents are made of nitinol, a nickel and titanium alloy. Selection of the stent is determined by the length of the lesion and the normal diameter of the artery. The stent should be oversized by 1–2 mm more than the normal arterial caliber and should cover the lesion completely. At diameters less than full expansion, nitinol stents exert a chronic outward radial force that serves to maintain apposition of the stent to the vessel wall after deployment. Often the stent extends from the CCA into the ICA, crossing the bifurcation and origin of the ECA; in these cases, the stent should be sized according to the larger caliber of the CCA.

When using a retrievable filter for distal protection, the position of the stent should be angiographically verified before the stent is deployed. The use of distal balloon occlusion precludes vessel assessment; in these cases, anatomical landmarks should be carefully analyzed before the stent is deployed to assure precise positioning of the stent.

Postdilation Angioplasty

After the stent is in place, poststent deployment angioplasty is performed. Balloon selection is based on the diameter of the ICA. The balloon should be kept within the segment of stented artery during the angioplasty to avoid the risk of vessel dissection. Slow balloon inflation can be used on those patients with known overresponsive carotid baroreceptors.

Distal Protection Device Retrieval

The distal protection device is withdrawn, and a final series of cervical carotid and intracranial circulation angiograms are obtained. When distal balloon occlusion is used for distal protection, 60 ml of blood is aspirated before the balloon is deflated. The aspiration is accomplished by use of an export catheter placed just proximal to the balloon.

Closure of the Access Site

The catheter systems and femoral sheath are removed, and a percutaneous closure device such as the Perclose device (Redwood City, Calif., USA) or AngioSeal (St. Jude Medical, Minnetonka, Minn., USA) is used to close the femoral artery puncture site.

Periprocedural Management and Discharge Plan

Following the procedure, the patient is admitted to the intensive care unit for monitoring overnight. Hourly neurological assessments and close surveillance of hemodynamic parameters are important. A systolic blood pressure of 110–160 mm Hg is maintained. A baseline carotid Doppler ultrasound study is obtained within 24 h of the procedure to assess vessel patency and to provide a reference for further Doppler evaluations. Most patients are discharged to home on the day after the procedure. As previously mentioned, aspirin and clopidogrel are prescribed.

Limitations of Carotid Angioplasty and Stenting

Several anatomic features can make CAS difficult to undertake. Endovascular access to the carotid system can be problematic in patients with severe peripheral vascular disease that affects the iliac or femoral arteries and in those with a bovine configuration to the aortic arch, a tortuous aortic arch, or an ecstatic CCA. Near-complete occlusion of the carotid artery (string sign), perilesional tortuosity, or kinks can impair safe passage of a distal protection device, and a tortuous distal cervical ICA can make deployment of the distal protection device difficult. Also, because antiplatelet therapy is strongly recommended, an inability to tolerate these agents might be considered a relative contraindication to carotid stent placement.

Conclusions

Carotid angioplasty with stent placement appears to be at least as safe as CEA in the high-risk population. Studies are underway to assess the efficacy and long-term durability of this procedure (with distal protection) in both NASCET- and ACAS-eligible populations.

Acknowledgment

We thank Paul H. Dressel for preparation of the illustrations.

References

1 American Heart Association: Stroke Statistics. http://www.americanheart.org/presenter.jhtml?identifier = 4725 (accessed June 10, 2003).
2 Matchar DB: Cost of stroke. Stroke Clin Update 2002;5:9–12.
3 Bonita R: Epidemiology of stroke. Lancet 1992;339:342–344.
4 Taylor TN, Davis PH, Torner JC: Projected number of strokes by subtype in the year 2050 in the United States (abstract). Stroke 1998;29:322.
5 Dyken ML: Stroke risk factors; in Norris JW, Hachinski VC (eds): Prevention of Stroke. New York, Springer, 1991, pp 83–102.
6 DeBakey ME: Carotid endarterectomy revisited. J Endovasc Surg 1996;3:4.
7 Pokras R, Dyken ML: Dramatic changes in the performance of endarterectomy for diseases of the extracranial arteries of the head. Stroke 1988;19:1289–1290.
8 Failure of extracranial-intracranial arterial bypass to reduce the risk of ischemic stroke. Results of an international randomized trial. The EC/IC Bypass Study Group. N Engl J Med 1985;313:1191–1200.
9 Beneficial effect of carotid endarterectomy in symptomatic patients with high-grade carotid stenosis. North American Symptomatic Carotid Endarterectomy Trial Collaborators. N Engl J Med 1991;325:445–453.
10 Endarterectomy for asymptomatic carotid artery stenosis. Executive Committee for the Asymptomatic Carotid Atherosclerosis Study. JAMA 1995;273:1421–1428.
11 MRC European Carotid Surgery Trial: Interim results for symptomatic patients with severe (70–99%) or with mild (0–29%) carotid stenosis. European Carotid Surgery Trialists' Collaborative Group. Lancet 1991;337:1235–1243.
12 Ouriel K, Hertzer NR, Beven EG, et al: Preprocedural risk stratification: Identifying an appropriate population for carotid stenting. J Vasc Surg 2001;33:728–732.
13 Roubin GS, New G, Iyer SS, et al: Immediate and late clinical outcomes of carotid artery stenting in patients with symptomatic and asymptomatic carotid artery stenosis: A 5-year prospective analysis. Circulation 2001;103:532–537.
14 Yadav JS, Roubin GS, Iyer S, et al: Elective stenting of the extracranial carotid arteries. Circulation 1997;95:376–381.
15 Barnett HJ, Taylor DW, Eliasziw M, et al: Benefit of carotid endarterectomy in patients with symptomatic moderate or severe stenosis. North American Symptomatic Carotid Endarterectomy Trial Collaborators. N Engl J Med 1998;339:1415–1425.
16 Randomised trial of endarterectomy for recently symptomatic carotid stenosis: Final results of the MRC European Carotid Surgery Trial (ECST). Lancet 1998;351:1379–1387.
17 Wennberg DE, Lucas FL, Birkmeyer JD, Bredenberg CE, Fisher ES: Variation in carotid endarterectomy mortality in the Medicare population: Trial hospitals, volume, and patient characteristics. JAMA 1998;279:1278–1281.
18 Hsia DC, Krushat WM, Moscoe LM: Epidemiology of carotid endarterectomies among Medicare beneficiaries. J Vasc Surg 1992;16:201–208.
19 Chaturvedi S, Aggarwal R, Murugappan A: Results of carotid endarterectomy with prospective neurologist follow-up. Neurology 2000;55:769–772.
20 Goldstein LB, McCrory DC, Landsman PB, et al: Multicenter review of preoperative risk factors for carotid endarterectomy in patients with ipsilateral symptoms. Stroke 1994;25:1116–1121.
21 Goldstein LB, Samsa GP, Matchar DB, Oddone EZ: Multicenter review of preoperative risk factors for endarterectomy for asymptomatic carotid artery stenosis. Stroke 1998;29:750–753.

22 Paciaroni M, Eliasziw M, Kappelle LJ, Finan JW, Ferguson GG, Barnett HJ: Medical complications associated with carotid endarterectomy. North American Symptomatic Carotid Endarterectomy Trial (NASCET). Stroke 1999;30:1759–1763.

23 Sundt TM, Sandok BA, Whisnant JP: Carotid endarterectomy. Complications and preoperative assessment of risk. Mayo Clin Proc 1975;50:301–306.

24 Alamowitch S, Eliasziw M, Algra A, Meldrum H, Barnett HJ: Risk, causes, and prevention of ischaemic stroke in elderly patients with symptomatic internal-carotid-artery stenosis. North American Symptomatic Carotid Endarterectomy Trial Group. Lancet 2001;357:1154–1160.

25 Harbaugh RE, Stieg PE, Moayeri N, Hsu L: Carotid-coronary artery bypass graft conundrum. Neurosurgery 1998;43:926–931.

26 Ferguson GG, Eliasziw M, Barr HW, et al: The North American Symptomatic Carotid Endarterectomy Trial: Surgical results in 1415 patients. Stroke 1999;30:1751–1758.

27 Faggioli GL, Curl GR, Ricotta JJ: The role of carotid screening before coronary artery bypass. J Vasc Surg 1990;12:724–731.

28 Del Sette M, Eliasziw M, Streifler JY, Hachinski VC, Fox AJ, Barnett HJ: Internal borderzone infarction: A marker for severe stenosis in patients with symptomatic internal carotid artery disease. For the North American Symptomatic Carotid Endarterectomy (NASCET) Group. Stroke 2000;31:631–636.

29 Lopes DK, Mericle RA, Lanzino G, Wakhloo AK, Guterman LR, Hopkins LN: Stent placement for the treatment of occlusive atherosclerotic carotid artery disease in patients with concomitant coronary artery disease. J Neurosurg 2002;96:490–496.

30 Moore WS, Barnett HJ, Beebe HG, et al: Guidelines for carotid endarterectomy. A multidisciplinary consensus statement from the ad hoc Committee, American Heart Association. Stroke 1995; 26:188–201.

31 Kim SH, Mericle RA, Lanzino G, Qureshi AI, Guterman LR, Hopkins LN: Carotid angioplasty and stent placement in patients with tandem stenosis (abstract). Neurosurgery 1998;43:708A.

32 Villarreal J, Silva J, Eliasziw M, et al: Prognosis of patients with intraluminal thrombus in the internal carotid artery (for the North American Symptomatic Carotid Endarterectomy Trial) (abstract 18). Stroke 1998;29:276.

33 Gasecki AP, Eliasziw M, Ferguson GG, Hachinski V, Barnett HJ: Long-term prognosis and effect of endarterectomy in patients with symptomatic severe carotid stenosis and contralateral carotid stenosis or occlusion: Results from NASCET. North American Symptomatic Carotid Endarterectomy Trial (NASCET) Group. J Neurosurg 1995;83:778–782.

34 Meyer FB, Piepgras DG, Fode NC: Surgical treatment of recurrent carotid artery stenosis. J Neurosurg 1994;80:781–787.

35 AbuRahma AF, Jennings TG, Wulu JT, Tarakji L, Robinson PA: Redo carotid endarterectomy versus primary carotid endarterectomy. Stroke 2001;32:2787–2792.

36 Lanzino G, Mericle RA, Lopes DK, Wakhloo AK, Guterman LR, Hopkins LN: Percutaneous transluminal angioplasty and stent placement for recurrent carotid artery stenosis. J Neurosurg 1999;90:688–694.

37 Wholey M: ARCHeR (Acculink for Revascularization of Carotids in High-Risk Patients) (abstract of presentation at the American College of Cardiology 52nd Annual Scientific Session, Chicago, IL, 2003). Clin Cardiol 2003;26:296.

38 Loftus CM, Biller J, Hart MN, Cornell SH, Hiratzka LF: Management of radiation-induced accelerated carotid atherosclerosis. Arch Neurol 1987;44:711–714.

39 Melliere D, Becquemin JP, Berrahal D, Desgranges P, Cavillon A: Management of radiation-induced occlusive arterial disease: A reassessment. J Cardiovasc Surg (Torino) 1997;38:261–269.

40 Kerber CW, Cromwell LD, Loehden OL: Catheter dilatation of proximal carotid stenosis during distal bifurcation endarterectomy. AJNR Am J Neuroradiol 1980;1:348–349.

41 Mathias K: A new catheter system for percutaneous transluminal angioplasty (PTA) of carotid artery stenoses. Fortschr Med 1977;95:1007–1111.

42 Mullan S, Duda EE, Patronas NJ: Some examples of balloon technology in neurosurgery. J Neurosurg 1980;52:321–329.

43 Kachel R: Results of balloon angioplasty in the carotid arteries. J Endovasc Surg 1996;3:22–30.

44 Phatouros CC, Higashida RT, Malek AM, et al: Carotid artery stent placement for atherosclerotic disease: Rationale, technique, and current status. Radiology 2000;217:26–41.

45 Endovascular versus surgical treatment in patients with carotid stenosis in the Carotid and Vertebral Artery Transluminal Angioplasty Study (CAVATAS): A randomised trial. Lancet 2001; 357:1729–1737.
46 Brown MN: CAVATAS late results: Does carotid balloon angioplasty fare well against endarterectomy? Am J Cardiol 2002;1(14):92.
47 Gil-Peralta A, Mayol A, Marcos JR, et al: Percutaneous transluminal angioplasty of the symptomatic atherosclerotic carotid arteries. Results, complications, and follow-up. Stroke 1996;27: 2271–2273.
48 Hanel RA, Qureshi AI, Saad M, et al: Carotid angioplasty and stent placement for the treatment of carotid stenosis in patients ineligible for the North American Carotid Endarterectomy Trial (abstract 816). Neurosurgery 2002;51:580.
49 Theron JG, Payelle GG, Coskun O, Huet HF, Guimaraens L: Carotid artery stenosis: Treatment with protected balloon angioplasty and stent placement. Radiology 1996;201:627–636.
50 Jaeger HJ, Mathias KD, Hauth E, et al: Cerebral ischemia detected with diffusion-weighted MR imaging after stent implantation in the carotid artery. AJNR Am J Neuroradiol 2002;23:200–207.
51 Mathias K: A vast single center experience from Europe: Immediate and late outcomes in >1400 patients. Am J Cardiol 2002;1(14):96.
52 Whitlow PL, Lylyk P, Londero H, et al: Carotid artery stenting protected with an emboli containment system. Stroke 2002;33:1308–1314.
53 Gruberg L: SAPPHIRE: Stenting and Angioplasty with Protection in Patients at High Risk for Endarterectomy. Medscape, vol 2003. www.medscape.com/viewarticle/445125. November 2002 (accessed July 21, 2003).
54 Yadav J: Stenting and Angioplasty with Protection in Patients at High Risk for Endarterectomy (SAPPHIRE) 30-day complications (American Heart Association, 2002). www.crtonline.org/documents/SAPPHIRE_11.2.ppt (accessed June 2, 2003).
55 Krupski WC, Bass A, Kelly AB, Marzec UM, Hanson SR, Harker LA: Heparin-resistant thrombus formation by endovascular stents in baboons. Interruption by a synthetic antithrombin. Circulation 1990;82:570–577.
56 Yusuf S, Zhao F, Mehta SR, Chrolavicius S, Tognoni G, Fox KK: Clopidogrel in Unstable Angina to Prevent Recurrent Events Trial Investigators: Effects of clopidogrel in addition to aspirin in patients with acute coronary syndromes without ST-segment elevation. N Engl J Med 2001;345: 494–502.
57 Qureshi AI, Suri MF, Ali Z, et al: Carotid angioplasty and stent placement: A prospective analysis of perioperative complications and impact of intravenously administered abciximab. Neurosurgery 2002;50:466–475.
58 Qureshi AI, Luft AR, Sharma M, Guterman LR, Hopkins LN: Prevention and treatment of thromboembolic and ischemic complications associated with endovascular procedures. II. Clinical aspects and recommendations. Neurosurgery 2000;46:1360–1376.
59 Parodi JC, Schonholz C, Ferreira LM, Mendaro E, Ohki T: 'Seat belt and air bag' technique for cerebral protection during carotid stenting. J Endovasc Ther 2002;9:20–24.
60 Levy EI, Kim SH, Bendok BR, Boulos AS, Xavier AR, Yahia AM, Qureshi AI, Guterman LR, Hopkins LN: Interventional neuroradiological therapy; in Mohr JP, Choi D, Grotta JC, Weir B, Wolf PA (eds): Stroke: Pathophysiology, Diagnosis, and Management, ed 4. New York, Elsevier, 2004, chap 78.

L. Nelson Hopkins, MD
University at Buffalo Neurosurgery, Kaleida Health/Millard Gates
3 Gates Circle, Buffalo, NY 14209 (USA)
Tel. +1 716 887 5210, Fax +1 716 887 4378, E-Mail dzbuffns@aol.com

Horowitz MB, Levy EI (eds): Neuroendovascular Surgery.
Prog Neurol Surg. Basel, Karger, 2005, vol 17, pp 54–69

Endovascular Treatment of Acute Ischemic Embolic Stroke

Catalina C. Ionita[a], Stanley H. Kim[b], Andrew R. Xavier[a], Jawad F. Kirmani[c], Amir M. Siddiqui[c], Adnan I. Qureshi[c]

Departments of [a]Neurology and [b]Neurosurgery, School of Medicine and Biomedical Sciences, University at Buffalo, State University of New York, Buffalo, N.Y., and [c]Department of Neurology and Neurosciences, University of Medicine and Dentistry of New Jersey, Newark, N.J., USA

Introduction

Stroke represents a major cause of death and disability worldwide. In the United States, it is the third leading cause of death, surpassed only by heart disease and cancer, and the leading cause of long-term serious disability [1–4]. Approximately 750,000 new cases and 150,000 deaths occur annually in the United States. Embolic strokes, which represent approximately 24% of all strokes, result from occlusion of one of the arteries supplying the brain by fragments of thrombi originating most commonly in a cardiac source. Approximately 80% of cardiogenic emboli travel into the anterior intracranial circulation, with a predisposition for the intracranial bifurcation of the internal carotid artery (ICA), middle cerebral artery (MCA) and its branches, and the anterior cerebral artery (ACA). Animal studies using silicone or autologous blood clots as embolic agents have shown that most emboli localize to the MCA [5, 6]. In the posterior circulation, common sites of emboli include the distal basilar artery (BA) bifurcation (top of the basilar), posterior inferior cerebellar artery, superior cerebellar artery, and posterior cerebral artery [7]. Owing to regional blood flow reduction, the area rendered ischemic by embolic occlusion progresses from initial electrical and metabolic failure to infarction and neuronal death. The neurological deficit depends on the severity and duration of the ischemia. The most important predictor of recovery from stroke is reperfusion of the ischemic brain [8]. Rapid restoration of normal cerebral blood flow and interruption of the ischemic cascade are fundamental goals of intervention.

In this chapter, the authors focus on endovascular approaches for the treatment of embolic stroke. Results of some of the major stroke treatment trials are presented. Intravenous (IV), intra-arterial (IA), and combination pharmacological and mechanical strategies to achieve and maintain vessel patency are discussed. Relevant experimental and clinical research findings providing the foundation of these trials, and the interventions practiced today are described.

Experimental Data

Animal studies in which ligature of the MCA and clot injection were used to create a model of embolic stroke showed maximal ischemic brain injury and ineffective recanalization beyond approximately 6 h [9]. Thrombolysis (IV and IA) was efficient in preserving brain function only if performed within 2 or 3 h of clot injection [10, 11].

Clinical Data

Human studies of embolic stroke have demonstrated that recanalization can occur spontaneously or through mechanical and/or pharmacological thrombolysis. Complete or nearly complete neurological improvement may follow angiographic recanalization [12]. However, an important fact to recognize from the clinical trials that will be discussed in this chapter is that clinical improvement does not always follow angiographic improvement. Moreover, in 15–20% of cases, angiographic studies performed within the first 6 h of the ictus fail to demonstrate an occlusion corresponding to the neurological deficit [13, 14].

Pharmacological IV Thrombolysis

The primary thrombolytic agents used intravenously for acute ischemic stroke in humans are recombinant tissue plasminogen activator (rt-PA), streptokinase, urokinase (UK), recombinant pro-urokinase (rPro-UK), and ancrod. IV streptokinase, the first thrombolytic agent used for the treatment of acute ischemic stroke, was abandoned in the 1990s because of the results of three major studies, the Multicenter Acute Stroke Trial – Italy (MAST-I) [15], Multicenter Acute Stroke Trial – Europe (MAST-E) [16], and the Australian Streptokinase Trial [17]. Each of these studies, besides demonstrating a high case-fatality rate, failed to prove a favorable outcome in the streptokinase arm.

IV rt-PA (alteplase) is the only Food and Drug Administration (FDA)-approved treatment for patients with acute ischemic stroke. In the National Institute of Neurological Disorders and Stroke Study (NINDS), patients treated with 0.9 mg/kg of rt-PA (maximal dose of 90 mg) within 3 h of stroke showed a significant absolute benefit of 11–15% in terms of neurological recovery at 90 days, in spite of a significant increase in the rate of symptomatic intracranial hemorrhage at 36 h (6.4% in the rt-PA group vs. 0.6% in the placebo group) [18]. In a subgroup analysis of NINDS patients, no baseline covariates were identified that could significantly affect response to treatment; rt-PA was found efficient independently of stroke severity or subtype [19]. In a multivariate analysis performed by Chiu et al. [20] in the first year after the FDA had approved IV rt-PA for acute ischemic stroke, the cardioembolic stroke subtype was identified as an independent risk factor for poor prognosis, owing to cardiac comorbid conditions. Moreover, cardioembolic stroke has been considered an independent risk factor for hemorrhagic conversion [20].

The use of IV rt-PA is limited by a long list of exclusion criteria and a short therapeutic window. Because most patients present later than 3 h after symptom onset, IV rt-PA can be used in fewer than 5% of potentially treatable patients [21, 22]. IV thrombolysis administered beyond 3 h of stroke symptom onset has been evaluated in three major studies. The safety and effectiveness of 1.1 mg/kg of IV rt-PA were evaluated in patients treated within 6 h of ischemic stroke occurrence in the European Cooperative Acute Stroke Study (ECASS) I [23]. An increased incidence of major intraparenchymal hemorrhages was found, and no significant treatment benefit was demonstrated. The feasibility and efficacy of 0.9 mg/kg of rt-PA administered within a 3- to 6-hour therapeutic window were evaluated in ECASS II, with an attempt to include patients with computed tomographic (CT) evidence of involvement of less than one third of the MCA territory [24]. No proven benefit was seen in the primary (functional outcome) or secondary [mortality, hemorrhagic transformation, symptomatic intracerebral hemorrhage (ICH)] end points. The safety and efficacy of IV rt-PA administration 3–5 h after symptom onset was assessed in the Alteplase Thrombolysis for Acute Noninterventional Therapy in Ischemic Stroke (ATLANTIS) study [25]. No significant difference was demonstrated in terms of functional outcome at 30 and 90 days between the two groups, and the rates of ICH and death at 90 days were higher among patients receiving rt-PA than those receiving placebo. The risk of hemorrhagic transformation appears to be higher in embolic strokes than in the thrombotic stroke subtype (40 vs. 1.8%) [26]. These clinical trials underscore the importance of timing and selection in the management of patients with acute ischemic stroke.

Alternative agents for IV pharmacological thrombolysis have been proposed, but none of them has received approval from the FDA. Ancrod, a purified fraction of venom from the Malaysian pit viper, is a defibrinogenating agent that enhances local clot thrombolysis and stimulates endogenous plasminogen activators. It has been used prophylactically for thromboembolism and as an alternate anticoagulant. The Stroke Treatment with Ancrod Trial (STAT) demonstrated a favorable benefit-to-risk profile for patients receiving ancrod within 3 h of stroke onset via IV administration of a continuous 72-hour infusion, then by 1-hour infusions at 96 and 120 h [27]. The rate of symptomatic ICH was lower (5.2%) than that for NINDS patients treated with rt-PA (6.4%), but with no statistically significant improvement of functional status.

The success of antiplatelet agent abciximab, a glycoprotein (GP) IIb-IIIa antagonist, in the treatment of acute coronary occlusions, promoted the use of this agent in the setting of acute ischemic stroke. Abciximab has been used to prevent ischemic complications occurring during endovascular procedures. The Abciximab in Ischemic Stroke investigators evaluated the safety and pilot efficacy of a regimen consisting of an escalating dose up to a maximum of 0.25 mg/kg bolus, proceeded by a 12-hour infusion administered within the first 24 h of symptom onset [28]. Better outcomes were obtained in patients receiving abciximab than in those receiving placebo, with a higher rate of asymptomatic ICH among the abciximab group, which was related to high baseline National Institutes of Health Stroke Scale (NIHSS) scores (>14) and not to the antiplatelet agent dose. The 17% (9 of 54 patients) mortality rate in the abciximab group (vs. 15% in the placebo group) was not attributed to the study agent or ICH.

Endovascular Treatment

IA Pharmacological Thrombolysis

IA thrombolysis may offer the following advantages: (1) precision afforded by angiographic detection of the site of occlusion, (2) elimination of the risk of treating those patients in whom spontaneous recanalization has occurred, (3) administration of the smallest effective dose of thrombolytic agent, thus minimizing the risk of local hemorrhagic complications, and (4) recanalization at rates superior to those achieved with IV thrombolysis. The disadvantages include cost and possible delay in treatment [29]. A variety of pharmacological agents have been used to perform IA thrombolysis in clinical studies. These agents include UK, rPro-UK, and two generations of rt-PA (alteplase and reteplase). Early experience with IA UK thrombolysis in embolic stroke suggested a high rate of recanalization (up to 93%) [30]. In a multivariate analysis of predictive factors for outcome at 6 months after IA thrombolysis with UK, cardioembolic stroke was found to be an independent predictor factor for a poor outcome, having a higher rate of hemorrhagic complications compared with thrombotic stroke, especially when it was associated with a baseline severe neurologic deficit and poor residual pretreatment collateral flow evaluated by single photon emission CT [31]. Moreover, when IA thrombolysis with UK was performed, embolic occlusion of the distal ICA, BA, or ACA was found to be associated with a poorer prognosis than MCA occlusion [32].

The Prolyse in Acute Cerebral Thromboembolism (PROACT) I study was the first randomized double-blinded multicenter trial to analyze the recanalization rate and clinical safety and efficacy of 6 mg of IA rPro-UK administered to patients with MCA occlusion within the first 6 h of symptom onset [33]. Patients were randomized to receive either rPro-UK or placebo. All patients received one of two IV heparin regimens: either high-dose (bolus + continuous infusion of 1,000 units/h for 4 h) or low-dose (bolus + 500 units/h for 4 h). The recanalization rate was significantly higher in the rPro-UK group (82% in those who also received high-dose heparin and 40% in those who also received low-dose heparin) than in the placebo group (14%). Hemorrhagic transformation causing neurological deterioration during the first 24 h after treatment occurred in 15.4% of patients receiving rPro-UK versus 7.1% of those receiving placebo. The rates of both recanalization and hemorrhagic complication were directly related to the heparin dose.

In the PROACT II trial, neurological disability at 90 days, assessed using the modified Rankin scale score, was the primary outcome measure [34]. The rate of MCA recanalization, the frequency of ICH with neurological deterioration, and mortality were secondary outcomes. A total of 180 patients with acute occlusion of the M1 or M2 segment of the MCA and symptoms lasting for less than 6 h were included in this trial and were randomized to receive 9 mg of IA rPro-UK plus heparin (n = 121) versus heparin alone (n = 59); all patients received heparin (2,000-unit bolus, then a 500 units/h infusion for 4 h before initiation of the thrombolysis infusion). At the 90-day follow-up, results in patients receiving rPro-UK plus heparin versus those receiving heparin alone were as follows: modified Rankin Scale score of 2 or less: 40 versus 25%, mortality rate: 25 versus 27%, recanalization rate: 66 versus 18%, and ICH with neurological deterioration occurring within 24 h: 10 versus 2%.

After UK was withdrawn from the market and because rPro-UK was not commercially available, rt-PA (alteplase) was introduced as an alternative agent for IA thrombolysis. An accelerating dosing regimen was recommended on the basis of the results of a prospective trial involving 8 patients [35]. Considered poor candidates for IV thrombolysis, these patients received successive doses of IA alteplase (10 mg, up to a maximum of 40 mg) via superselective catheterization within a time window of 1–8 h after stroke symptom onset. The initial NIHSS scores ranged from 16 to 21. Neurological improvement, corresponding with the

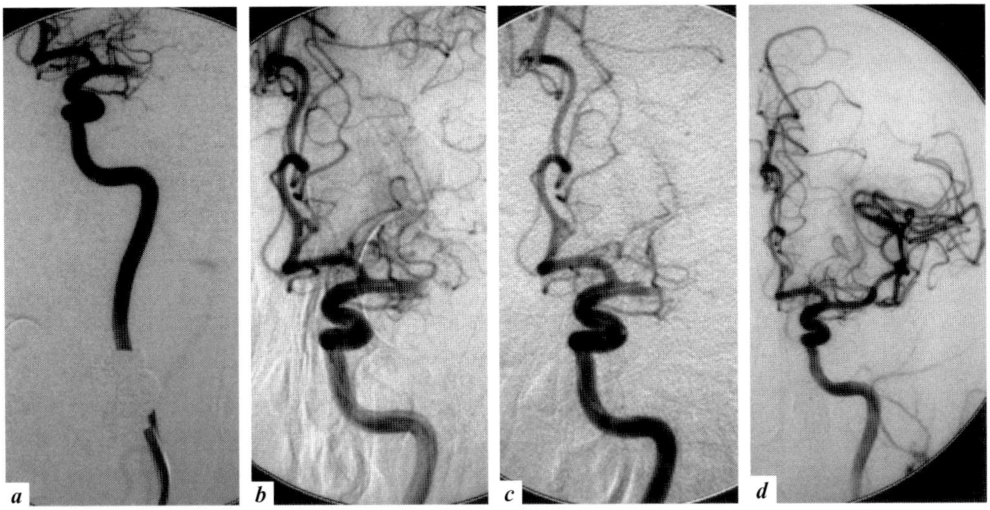

Fig. 1. Left carotid angiogram showing left M1 occlusion in a 57-year-old woman who presented 4 h after symptom onset with an NIHSS score of 24 (***a***). Persistent occlusion of the M1 segment of the left MCA after IA infusion of 1 unit of reteplase (***b***) and mechanical thrombolysis with a 4-mm snare (***c***) in the M1 segment. TIMI 3 recanalization of the left MCA after IA infusion of 2 units of reteplase in the M1 segment (***d***).

dose of rt-PA administered, was observed in 4 of 6 patients. Asymptomatic ICH was observed in 2 patients at 24 h posttreatment. These results prompted the evaluation of newer IA agents.

Encouraging results with the use of IA reteplase, a third-generation rt-PA, have recently been reported [36]. Sixteen patients presenting 2–9 h after the onset of stroke symptoms with NIHSS scores ranging from 10 to 26 underwent IA thrombolysis with maximum total doses of 8 units of reteplase. A high rate of recanalization of 94%, with and without adjunctive angioplasty (used for 7 patients), was reported. An example of recanalization is presented in figure 1. Neurological improvement was observed in 7 patients (44%) at 24 h; ICH occurred in 4 patients (25%; 1 patient had symptomatic ICH; in 3 others, the hemorrhage did not result in neurological worsening). There were nine deaths, of which one was attributed to IA lysis.

Combination IV and IA Thrombolysis

Combination therapy was proposed as a treatment for acute ischemic stroke to test the potential of combining the advantages of IA and IV rt-PA thrombolysis (fast and easy to administer, low cost). The Emergency Management of Stroke (EMS) Bridging Trial [37] included 35 patients presenting within 3 h of symptoms onset; 17 patients received IV and IA rt-PA and 18 patients received IV placebo and IA rt-PA. IV rt-PA or placebo (0.6 mg/kg) was administered, followed by an IA infusion of a maximal dose of 20 mg of rt-PA. A higher Thrombolysis in Myocardial Infarction (TIMI) grade [38] of recanalization was observed in the IV and IA rt-PA group and correlated with the total dose of thrombolytic agent administered, although it was not associated with improved clinical outcomes at 7–10 days or at 90 days posttreatment. The rate of symptomatic ICH was similar in the two groups, suggesting the technical feasibility and safety of this approach.

Hill et al. [39] reported promising results in 6 patients with acute ischemic stroke who received combination therapy (0.9 mg/kg of IV rt-PA, then IA rt-PA up to a maximum of 20 mg), along with IV heparin (administered intraprocedurally). Four patients achieved a good functional and neurological outcome and 2 patients had a poor outcome, but no instances of symptomatic ICH were reported. Ernst et al. [40] obtained better results in terms of recanalization of large proximal occlusions and neurological outcome accompanied by a lower rate of hemorrhagic complications and death, in comparison with other combination therapy studies. They used 0.6 mg/kg of IV rt-PA (initiated within 2 h of stroke onset), followed by a 24-mg IA infusion (median time of administration was 3 h and 30 min). The improved results were attributed to the more rapid initiation of both IV and IA thrombolysis.

More recently, Suarez et al. [41] reported the benefits of combination therapy. Forty-five patients presenting within 3 h after symptom onset received 0.6 mg/kg of IV rt-PA (10% bolus and the remainder via an infusion over the course of 30 min). After magnetic resonance imaging (T2, diffusion and perfusion-weighted) was obtained, the patients underwent cerebral angiography, followed by IA thrombolysis with either UK (up to 750,000 units) or rt-PA (up to 0.3 mg/kg equivalent dose). In terms of efficacy and safety, 77% of survivors had good outcomes (Barthel index >95) at 3 months after treatment; the incidence of symptomatic ICH was 4.4% and the fatality rate 15%, owing to stroke severity or myocardial infarction in the IA rt-PA and IA UK group.

On the basis of the results of these initial pilot studies, NINDS has funded a phase II pilot study, the Interventional Management of Stroke trial [42]. This trial is an open-label phase II study designed to provide preliminary results on the safety and efficacy of combination IV and IA rt-PA thrombolysis initiated within 3 h of symptom onset in 80 patients with ischemic stroke and an NIHSS score of 10 or better. According to the study protocol, patients receive 0.6 mg/kg of IV rt-PA over the course of 30 min (15% as a bolus) followed by a dose of up to 22 mg of IA rt-PA over 2 h if thrombus is evident on the cerebral angiogram. Further studies are needed to evaluate the efficacy of the combination approach.

IA Mechanical Thrombolysis

Mechanical thrombolysis refers to any technique used for mechanical disruption or fragmentation of an IA clot with the goal of rapid reestablishment of blood flow. An obstructive thrombus resulting in a significant neurological deficit is usually large enough to lodge in a proximal, large artery and may be resistant to both IA and IV pharmacological thrombolysis. Such a large clot burden may require large doses of thrombolytic agent, thereby increasing the risk of hemorrhagic complications. Mechanical fragmentation of the thrombus reduces the size of the clot, and the area exposed to the fibrinolytic system will be increased. This approach may completely eliminate the use of the pharmacological agent, reduce the required dose, increase the time window for recanalization, and/or reduce the rate of hemorrhagic complications. Disadvantages of mechanical thrombolysis include distal embolization and the risk of vessel injury or perforation [43].

Snares

Snares are small lassos or loops designed to grasp objects or to retrieve endovascular devices, wires, or coils from blood vessels. Initially, anecdotal individual case reports presented snare retrieval as a potentially efficient method for the removal of a densely fibrotic thrombus [44]. Concerns related to the use of this device include risks of embolization and vessel rupture or dissection. Positive results regarding the safety and effectiveness of mechanical thrombolysis with snares come from a recent study [45]. Five of 19 patients with ischemic stroke received IA reteplase in conjunction with snare maneuvers; 2 of these patients underwent both mechanical angioplasty and snare maneuvers. The mean perfusion grade (evaluated on the basis of the modified TIMI grading system [38]) immediately before snare maneuvers (1.6 ± 2.0) improved (to 2.4 ± 1.8) after snare manipulation. No vascular complications were observed after mechanical disruption of a clot.

Guidewires and Catheters

Microguidewires are the simplest devices that can be used for mechanical fragmentation of a clot. An end-hole microcatheter is navigated to the proximal portion of the thrombus or through the thrombus into the distal vessel. The thrombus may be easily fragmented when it is not well organized, but the procedure carries a high risk of embolization. Microcatheters are advanced into the thrombus and pulled back, fragmenting the clot and improving the efficacy of concomitant chemical thrombolysis. Patients with acute cardioembolic occlusion of the MCA, distal vertebral artery (VA), and BA have been successfully treated by this method [46]. Application of this method can be extended for more difficult situations of artery-to-artery embolic strokes, such as proximal ICA occlusion complicated by embolization of clot within the distal ICA or the

MCA or ACA. In this case, the proximal clot will not allow for efficient thrombolysis of the more distal embolus. The microcatheter can be passed first through the large proximal clot to access and lyse the distal ICA or MCA clot and then into more proximal vessel segments [47]. Positive outcomes have been associated with this approach, with a therapeutic window extended well beyond 6 h (up to 48 h after the onset of stroke symptoms) [48].

Intracranial Angioplasty and Stenting

A significant thrombus burden in an intracranial vessel or a thrombotic occlusion of an atherosclerotic intracranial vessel may be refractory to IA thrombolysis alone. Intracranial angioplasty has been used to fragment the intracranial thrombus in clinical studies. Ringer et al. [49] reported on 9 patients who were treated with balloon angioplasty after inadequate recanalization was observed following IA thrombolytic infusion. Five of these patients had successful recanalization, and 4 had residual distal occlusion after angioplasty. Additionally, Ueda et al. [50] reported positive results of angioplasty within 6 h from symptom onset in 13 acute stroke patients in whom no areas of hypodensity were observed on initial CT scans. No symptomatic complications occurred during or after treatment. In 9 patients who had follow-up angiography 1 month after treatment, no restenosis or reocclusion was demonstrated. The authors performed a modest form of intracranial angioplasty using coronary balloons to treat occlusions in large vessels such as the ICA, proximal M1 segment of the MCA, and BA. Examples of coronary angioplasty balloon catheters used for this application include Cross Sail (Guidant, Advanced Cardiovascular Inc., Temecula, Calif., USA), Open Sail (Guidant, Advanced Cardiovascular Inc.), or Ninja (Cordis Neurovascular, Miami Lakes, Fla., USA). To minimize the risk of vessel rupture or dissection during the angioplasty, the diameter of the balloon was undersized in reference to the diameter of the adjacent portion of the occluded vessel. Other potential complications associated with angioplasty include distal spasm, embolism, and occlusion of perforating branches by forcing plaque or thrombus into the small branches. Intracranial stenting may be required to achieve recanalization in circumstances in which there is a preexistent atherosclerotic stenosis resistant to pharmacological thrombolysis, clot retrieval, or fragmentation devices. The authors have a limited experience with intracranial stenting in the setting of acute ischemic stroke [51]. Similar potential complications exist for intracranial stenting as in angioplasty. Further study is needed to evaluate the safety and efficacy of intracranial stenting in this setting.

Lasers

The most extensive research has focused on the argon ion, neodymium: yttrium aluminum garnet (Nd:YAG), and xenon-chloride lasers [52]. The major advantage of this technique is the ability to vaporize a fresh thrombus without requiring the use of a thrombolytic agent. The possible complications of this procedure in a clinical setting (which have been encountered in animal experiments) are acute vessel rupture as the result of vibration energy and acute vessel perforation [53].

Suction Thrombectomy

Suction thrombectomy involves the aspiration of thrombus through a catheter. Suction thrombectomy is a simple approach that can be tried in cases of acute ICA or VA occlusion. A large-bore (5- or 6-french) guide catheter is navigated over a guidewire into the thrombus, and the clot is aspirated with a 60-ml syringe. This technique is less likely to be efficient for more distal vessel occlusions. When there is distal embolization at the distal segment or bifurcation of the ICA into the MCA or ACA origin, recanalization of the distal occlusion may be performed first, then recanalization of the proximal ICA. The assessment of collateral flow via the circle of Willis and leptomeninges is crucial in selecting the patients who may benefit from this procedure. Suction thrombectomy may be considered within 6 h of neurological deterioration in patients with symptomatic ICA occlusion in whom thrombolytic agents are contraindicated and if no more than one third of the MCA territory is affected [54].

AngioJet

The AngioJet (Possis Medical, Minneapolis, Minn., USA) is an endovascular thrombectomy device that combines local mechanical disruption of the clot with suction of the resultant fragments. The Angioject catheter uses retrograde, high-pressure fluid jets directed to the evacuation lumen to create a hydrodynamic vortex that fragments the thrombus and entraps the debris. This process has been found to be safe and effective in animal models in that most of the thrombus can be removed without significant risk for distal embolization (the major concern in the clinical setting) [55]. At present, the AngioJet is used for recanalization of large extracranial vessels. When more flexible catheters become available, application of this device will potentially be extended to intracranial use, without the need for pharmacological thrombolysis, which confers an important advantage.

Future Directions

A recent meta-analysis of three of the aforementioned major studies, ECASS I and II and NINDS, determined a benefit of IV rt-PA even within a 6-hour window, at the cost of a slight increase in the ICH rate, compared to the

3-hour window (odds ratio 3.23 vs. 2.68) [56]. Thus, a select group of patients may benefit from IV thrombolysis beyond 3 h. Improved patient selection may open new perspectives and lead to additional strategies to achieve or maintain patency of the target vessel.

Efforts are made to identify subgroups of patients who may still benefit from IV thrombolysis beyond the 3-hour therapeutic window. Newer imaging techniques may play a role in improving our ability to identify patients with viable brain tissue who may derive the greatest benefit from therapy. Imaging features including the ratios of relative cerebral blood flow, relative cerebral blood volume, mean transit time, and apparent diffusion coefficient have been proposed [57]. No definite marker for safe and beneficial IV thrombolysis beyond 3 h of the onset has been identified [58, 59]. Further investigations involving magnetic resonance imaging techniques need to be directed toward identifying a marker of ischemia severity and viability thresholds of the ischemic penumbra.

A better understanding of how thrombolytic agents affect coagulation and fibrinolysis may prevent reocclusion during treatment of acute ischemic stroke. Alteplase induces coagulation activation and fibrin formation that peaks within hours of initial IV thrombolysis and persists for up to 72 h thereafter, which can explain, at least partially, the modest recanalization rate and reocclusion associated with this treatment approach. Alexandrov and Grotta [60] demonstrated that reocclusion may occur soon after initial IV rt-PA thrombolysis in 22% of patients with complete recanalization and in 41% of those with partial recanalization. The administration of heparin does not significantly affect the changes in coagulation and fibrinolysis markers induced by rt-PA thrombolysis in patients with acute ischemic stroke [61]. In acute myocardial infarction, adjunctive therapy with heparin improves the patency of initially occluded arteries without providing a better survival rate [62]. Abciximab, in combination with aspirin and an adjusted dose of heparin, has been approved by the FDA for the prevention of reocclusion in patients undergoing percutaneous coronary angioplasty or in those with unstable angina [63–65]. In light of the favorable results obtained in the treatment of myocardial infarction, further studies assessing the efficacy and safety of combination therapy thrombolysis in conjunction with the administration of GP IIb–IIIa receptor inhibitors are in progress [66].

Multiple studies designed to evaluate new thrombolytic agents and mechanical devices are anticipated. To correlate and compare the results, an objective method for angiographic assessment of the site and severity of arterial occlusion is required. The TIMI perfusion grading scheme was used in PROACT I and II [33, 34]. By using a score from 0 to 3, this grading scheme does not account for the site of occlusion and the presence of collateral flow,

Table 1. Grades of increasing severity of arterial occlusion

Grade	Type of occlusion		
0		No occlusion	
1	MCA occlusion (M3 segment)	ACA occlusion (A2 or distal segments)	1 BA and/or VA branch occlusion
2	MCA occlusion (M2 segment)	ACA occlusion (A1 and A2 segments)	≥2BA and/or VA branch occlusions
3		MCA occlusion (M1 segment)	
3A	Lenticulostriate arteries spared and/or leptomeningeal collaterals visualized		
3B	No sparing of lenticulostriate arteries and no leptomeningeal collaterals visualized		
4	ICA occlusion (collaterals present)	BA occlusion (partial filling direct or via collaterals)	
4A	Collaterals fill MCA	Anterograde filling[a]	
4B	Collaterals fill ACA	Retrograde filling[a]	
5	ICA occlusion (no collaterals)	BA occlusion (complete)	

From Qureshi [68] (permission from Lippincott Williams & Wilkins).
[a]Predominant pattern of filling.

both of which are important predictors of outcome. Mori et al. [67] proposed another scheme with a score from 0 to 4 that grades changes in perfusion within the affected area after treatment. This grading system does not provide information regarding the initial site of occlusion and collateral flow. Qureshi [68] recently proposed a six-grade scale, from 0 to 5, incorporating the anatomic site of occlusion and collateral supply (table 1). This scheme demonstrated a higher reliability than preexistent schemes. A significant association between the scheme and functional recovery was found, which can provide a more objective method to assess the various levels of response to treatment strategies.

Conclusions

The endovascular management of acute ischemic embolic stroke has undergone a significant evolution over the past decade. With the availability of potent thrombolytic pharmacological agents and mechanical devices, high recanalization rates have been observed. However, time is still a very critical element in the management of patients with acute ischemic stroke, as demonstrated in all major clinical trials. At institutions with the personnel and resources to provide IV or endovascular therapy, patients with ischemic stroke must be expeditiously transferred and evaluated to determine their eligibility for treatment. Advancement in the area of neuroimaging is essential for improved selection of candidates for thrombolysis or other vascular intervention. We look forward to continuing evolution and advancement in the management of acute ischemic stroke.

Acknowledgment

We thank Paul H. Dressel for preparation of the illustrations.

References

1 2001 Heart and Statistical Update: American Heart Association (Dallas). http://216.185.102.50/statistics/stroke.html (accessed February 8, 2003).

2 Asplund K: Stroke in Europe: Widening the gap between East and West. Cerebrovasc Dis 1996;6:3–6.

3 Broderick J, Brott T, Kothari R, et al: The Greater Cincinnati/Northern Kentucky Stroke Study: Preliminary first-ever and total incidence rates of stroke among blacks. Stroke 1998;29:415–421.

4 Thorvaldsen P, Kuulasmaa K, Rajakangas AM, Rastenyte D, Sarti C, Wilhelmsen L: Stroke trends in the WHO MONICA project. Stroke 1997;28:500–506.

5 Gacs G, Merei FT, Bodosi M: Balloon catheter as a model of cerebral emboli in humans. Stroke 1982;13:39–42.

6 Helgason CM: Cardioembolic stroke: Topography and pathogenesis. Cerebrovasc Brain Metab Rev 1992;4:28–58.

7 Caplan LR: Posterior Circulation Disease, Clinical Findings, Diagnosis and Management. Boston, Blackwell, 1996.

8 Caplan LR: Stroke, a Clinical Approach. Boston, Butterworth-Heinemann, 2000, chap 9, pp 247–282.

9 Zivin JA: Factors determining the therapeutic window for stroke. Neurology 1998;50:599–603.

10 Overgaard K: Thrombolytic therapy in experimental embolic stroke. Cerebrovasc Brain Metab Rev 1994;6:257–286.

11 Overgaard K, Sereghy T, Pedersen H, Boysen G: Effect of delayed thrombolysis with rt-PA in a rat embolic stroke model. J Cereb Blood Flow Metab 1994;14:472–477.

12 Minematsu K, Yamaguchi T, Omae T: 'Spectacular shrinking deficit': Rapid recovery from a major hemispheric syndrome by migration of an embolus. Neurology 1992;42:157–162.

13 Fieschi C, Argentino C, Lenzi GL, Sacchetti ML, Toni D, Bozzao L: Clinical and instrumental evaluation of patients with ischemic stroke within the first six hours. J Neurol Sci 1989;91:311–321.

14 Wolpert SM, Bruckmann H, Greenlee R, Wechsler L, Pessin MS, del Zoppo GJ: Neuroradiologic evaluation of patients with acute stroke treated with recombinant tissue plasminogen activator. The rt-PA Acute Stroke Study Group. AJNR Am J Neuroradiol 1993;14:3–13.

15 Randomised controlled trial of streptokinase, aspirin, and combination of both in treatment of acute ischaemic stroke. Multicentre Acute Stroke Trial – Italy (MAST-I) Group. Lancet 1995;346:1509–1514.

16 Thrombolytic therapy with streptokinase in acute ischemic stroke. The Multicenter Acute Stroke Trial – Europe Study Group. N Engl J Med 1996;335:145–150.

17 Donnan GA, Davis SM, Chambers BR, et al: Streptokinase for acute ischemic stroke with relationship to time of administration: Australian Streptokinase (ASK) Trial Study Group. JAMA 1996;276:961–966.

18 Tissue plasminogen activator for acute ischemic stroke. The National Institute of Neurological Disorders and Stroke rt-PA Stroke Study Group. N Engl J Med 1995;333:1581–1587.

19 Generalized efficacy of t-PA for acute stroke. Subgroup analysis of the NINDS t-PA Stroke Trial. Stroke 1997;28:2119–2125.

20 Chiu D, Krieger D, Villar-Cordova C, et al: Intravenous tissue plasminogen activator for acute ischemic stroke: Feasibility, safety, and efficacy in the first year of clinical practice. Stroke 1998; 29:18–22.

21 Hanson S, Brauer D, Anderson D, Koller R, Davenport R: Stroke treatment in the community (STIC) – Intravenous rt-PA in clinical practice. Neurology 1998;50(suppl 4):A155–A156.

22 Tanne D, Macsback H, Verro P: Intravenous rt-PA therapy for stroke in clinical practice: A multicenter evaluation of outcome (abstract). Stroke 1998;29:288.

23 Hacke W, Kaste M, Fieschi C, et al: Intravenous thrombolysis with recombinant tissue plasminogen activator for acute hemispheric stroke. The European Cooperative Acute Stroke Study (ECASS). JAMA 1995;274:1017–1025.

24 Hacke W, Kaste M, Fieschi C, et al: Randomised double-blind placebo-controlled trial of thrombolytic therapy with intravenous alteplase in acute ischaemic stroke (ECASS II). Second European-Australasian Acute Stroke Study Investigators. Lancet 1998;352:1245–1251.

25 Clark WM, Wissman S, Albers GW, Jhamandas JH, Madden KP, Hamilton S: Recombinant tissue-type plasminogen activator (Alteplase) for ischemic stroke 3 to 5 hours after symptom onset. The ATLANTIS Study: A randomized controlled trial. Alteplase Thrombolysis for Acute Noninterventional Therapy in Ischemic Stroke. JAMA 1999;282:2019–2026.

26 Okada Y, Yamaguchi T, Minematsu K, et al: Hemorrhagic transformation in cerebral embolism. Stroke 1989;20:598–603.

27 Sherman DG, Atkinson RP, Chippendale T, et al: Intravenous ancrod for treatment of acute ischemic stroke: The STAT study: A randomized controlled trial. Stroke Treatment with Ancrod Trial. JAMA 2000;283:2395–2403.

28 Abciximab in acute ischemic stroke: A randomized, double-blind, placebo-controlled, dose-escalation study. The Abciximab in Ischemic Stroke Investigators. Stroke 2000;31:601–609.

29 Suarez JI, Sunshine JL, Tarr R, et al: Predictors of clinical improvement, angiographic recanalization, and intracranial hemorrhage after intra-arterial thrombolysis for acute ischemic stroke. Stroke 1999;30:2094–2100.

30 Ueda T, Hatakeyama T, Kohno K, Kumon Y, Sakaki S: Endovascular treatment for acute thrombotic occlusion of the middle cerebral artery: Local intra-arterial thrombolysis combined with percutaneous transluminal angioplasty. Neuroradiology 1997;39:99–104.

31 Ueda T, Hatakeyama T, Kumon Y, Sakaki S, Uraoka T: Evaluation of risk of hemorrhagic transformation in local intra-arterial thrombolysis in acute ischemic stroke by initial SPECT. Stroke 1994;25:298–303.

32 Ueda T, Sakaki S, Kumon Y, Ohta S: Multivariable analysis of predictive factors related to outcome at 6 months after intra-arterial thrombolysis for acute ischemic stroke. Stroke 1999;30:2360–2365.

33 del Zoppo GJ, Higashida RT, Furlan AJ, Pessin MS, Rowley HA, Gent M: PROACT: A phase II randomized trial of recombinant pro-urokinase by direct arterial delivery in acute middle cerebral artery stroke. PROACT Investigators. Prolyse in Acute Cerebral Thromboembolism. Stroke 1998; 29:4–11.

34 Furlan A, Higashida R, Wechsler L, et al: Intra-arterial prourokinase for acute ischemic stroke. The PROACT II study: A randomized controlled trial. Prolyse in Acute Cerebral Thromboembolism. JAMA 1999;282:2003–2011.

35 Qureshi AI, Suri MF, Shatla AA, et al: Intraarterial recombinant tissue plasminogen activator for ischemic stroke: An accelerating dosing regimen. Neurosurgery 2000;47:473–479.

36 Qureshi AI, Ali Z, Suri MF, et al: Intra-arterial third-generation recombinant tissue plasminogen activator (reteplase) for acute ischemic stroke. Neurosurgery 2001;49:41–50.

37 Lewandowski CA, Frankel M, Tomsick TA, et al: Combined intravenous and intra-arterial r-TPA versus intra-arterial therapy of acute ischemic stroke: Emergency Management of Stroke (EMS) Bridging Trial. Stroke 1999;30:2598–2605.

38 Anderson HV, Willerson JT: Thrombolysis in acute myocardial infarction. N Engl J Med 1993; 329:703–709.

39 Hill MD, Barber PA, Demchuk AM, et al: Acute intravenous-intra-arterial revascularization therapy for severe ischemic stroke. Stroke 2002;33:279–282.
40 Ernst R, Pancioli A, Tomsick T, et al: Combined intravenous and intra-arterial recombinant tissue plasminogen activator in acute ischemic stroke. Stroke 2000;31:2552–2557.
41 Suarez JI, Zaidat OO, Sunshine JL, Tarr R, Selman WR, Landis DM: Endovascular administration after intravenous infusion of thrombolytic agents for the treatment of patients with acute ischemic strokes. Neurosurgery 2002;50:251–260.
42 Broderick J: The Interventional Management of Stroke (IMS) Study: Preliminary results. 7th International Symposium on Thrombolysis and Acute Stroke Therapy, Lyon, 2002.
43 Kuether TA, Nesbit GM, Barnwell SL: Other endovascular treatment strategies for acute ischemic stroke. Neuroimaging Clin N Am 1999;9:509–525.
44 Chopko BW, Kerber C, Wong W, Georgy B: Transcatheter snare removal of acute middle cerebral artery thromboembolism: Technical case report. Neurosurgery 2000;46:1529–1531.
45 Qureshi AI, Siddiqui AM, Suri MF, et al: Aggressive mechanical clot disruption and low-dose intra-arterial third-generation thrombolytic agent for ischemic stroke: A prospective study. Neurosurgery 2002;51:1319–1329.
46 Higashida RT, Tsai FY, Halbach VV, Barnwell SL, Dowd CF, Hieshima GB: Interventional neurovascular techniques in the treatment of stroke – State-of-the-art therapy. J Intern Med 1995;237:105–115.
47 Nesbit GM, Clark WM, O'Neill OR, Barnwell SL: Intracranial intraarterial thrombolysis facilitated by microcatheter navigation through an occluded cervical internal carotid artery. J Neurosurg 1996;84:387–392.
48 Barnwell SL, Clark WM, Nguyen TT, O'Neill OR, Wynn ML, Coull BM: Safety and efficacy of delayed intraarterial urokinase therapy with mechanical clot disruption for thromboembolic stroke. AJNR Am J Neuroradiol 1994;15:1817–1822.
49 Ringer AJ, Qureshi AI, Fessler RD, Guterman LR, Hopkins LN: Angioplasty of intracranial occlusion resistant to thrombolysis in acute ischemic stroke. Neurosurgery 2001;48:1282–1290.
50 Ueda T, Sakaki S, Nochide I, Kumon Y, Kohno K, Ohta S: Angioplasty after intra-arterial thrombolysis for acute occlusion of intracranial arteries. Stroke 1998;29:2568–2574.
51 Kim SH, Yahia AM, Boulos AS, Kirmani JF, Siddiqui AM, Hopkins LN: Balloon-expandable stents for intracranial occlusion in patients with ischemic stroke. 7th International Symposium on Thrombolysis and Acute Stroke Therapy, Lyon, 2002.
52 Watson BD, Prado R, Veloso A, Brunschwig JP, Dietrich WD: Cerebral blood flow restoration and reperfusion injury after ultraviolet laser-facilitated middle cerebral artery recanalization in rat thrombotic stroke. Stroke 2002;33:428–434.
53 Lee G, Ikeda RM, Theis JH, et al: Acute and chronic complications of laser angioplasty: Vascular wall damage and formation of aneurysms in the atherosclerotic rabbit. Am J Cardiol 1984;53:290–293.
54 Lutsep HL, Clark WM, Nesbit GM, Kuether TA, Barnwell SL: Intraarterial suction thrombectomy in acute stroke. AJNR Am J Neuroradiol 2002;23:783–786.
55 Sharafuddin MJ, Hicks ME, Jenson ML, Morris JE, Drasler WJ, Wilson GJ: Rheolytic thrombectomy with use of the AngioJet-F105 catheter: Preclinical evaluation of safety. J Vasc Interv Radiol 1997;8:939–945.
56 Ringleb PA, Schellinger PD, Schranz C, Hacke W: Thrombolytic therapy within 3 to 6 hours after onset of ischemic stroke: Useful or harmful? Stroke 2002;33:1437–1441.
57 Rohl L, Ostergaard L, Simonsen CZ, et al: Viability thresholds of ischemic penumbra of hyperacute stroke defined by perfusion-weighted MRI and apparent diffusion coefficient. Stroke 2001;32:1140–1146.
58 Fiehler J, Foth M, Kucinski T, et al: Severe ADC decreases do not predict irreversible tissue damage in humans. Stroke 2002;33:79–86.
59 Fink JN, Kumar S, Horkan C, et al: The stroke patient who woke up: Clinical and radiological features, including diffusion and perfusion MRI. Stroke 2002;33:988–993.
60 Alexandrov AV, Grotta JC: Arterial reocclusion in stroke patients treated with intravenous tissue plasminogen activator. Neurology 2002;59:862–867.

61 Fassbender K, Dempfle CE, Mielke O, et al: Changes in coagulation and fibrinolysis markers in acute ischemic stroke treated with recombinant tissue plasminogen activator. Stroke 1999;30: 2101–2104.
62 Mahaffey KW, Granger CB, Collins R, et al: Overview of randomized trials of intravenous heparin in patients with acute myocardial infarction treated with thrombolytic therapy. Am J Cardiol 1996; 77:551–556.
63 Randomised placebo-controlled trial of abciximab before and during coronary intervention in refractory unstable angina: The CAPTURE Study. Lancet 1997;349:1429–1435.
64 Platelet glycoprotein IIb/IIIa receptor blockade and low-dose heparin during percutaneous coronary revascularization. The EPILOG Investigators. N Engl J Med 1997;336:1689–1696.
65 Use of a monoclonal antibody directed against the platelet glycoprotein IIb/IIIa receptor in high-risk coronary angioplasty. The EPIC Investigation. N Engl J Med 1994;330:956–961.
66 Qureshi AI, Suri MFK, Ali Z, et al: Intraarterial reteplase and intravenous abciximab for treatment of acute ischemic stroke. A preliminary feasibility and safety study in a nonhuman primate model (Paper 17) (abstract). J Neurosurg 2003;98:717.
67 Mori E, Tabuchi M, Yoshida T, Yamadori A: Intracarotid urokinase with thromboembolic occlusion of the middle cerebral artery. Stroke 1988;19:802–812.
68 Qureshi AI: New grading system for angiographic evaluation of arterial occlusions and recanalization response to intra-arterial thrombolysis in acute ischemic stroke. Neurosurgery 2002;50: 1405–1415.

Adnan I. Qureshi, MD
Department of Neurology and Neurosciences
University of Medicine and Dentistry of New Jersey
H-506, 185 South Orange Avenue, Newark, NJ 07103 (USA)
Tel. +1 973 972 5208, Fax +1 973 972 5059, E-Mail aiqureshi@hotmail.com

Horowitz MB, Levy EI (eds): Neuroendovascular Surgery.
Prog Neurol Surg. Basel, Karger, 2005, vol 17, pp 70–84

Intracranial Stenting

Mark R. Harrigan, Elad I. Levy, Lee R. Guterman,
L. Nelson Hopkins

Department of Neurosurgery and Toshiba Stroke Research Center,
School of Medicine and Biomedical Sciences, University at Buffalo,
State University of New York, Buffalo, N.Y., USA

The use of endovascular stents in the intracranial circulation has been made possible by rapid developments in stent technology in recent years. Improvements in stent design, delivery devices, and technique have expanded the use of stenting for the treatment of a wide variety of intracranial disorders, including atherosclerosis, aneurysms, and arterial dissections. In this chapter, the authors briefly review the history of endovascular stent placement, describe the periprocedure management and stenting technique used, review the indications for intracranial stenting, and discuss topics for future investigation.

Historical Background

The term 'stent' originated with Charles Stent (1845–1901), an English dentist who developed a mold to form an impression of the teeth and oral cavity [1]. The term later came to indicate a device used to hold a skin graft in position and has been defined as an 'expandable coil or mesh tube prosthesis that can be introduced into the body through a catheter' [2].

The concept of intravascular stenting was introduced in 1912 by Nobel laureate Alexis Carrel, who described experiments in which glass and metal tubes covered with paraffin were introduced into the canine thoracic aorta [1]. Intravascular stenting as a treatment for peripheral arteriosclerosis was proposed by Charles Dotter and Melvin Judkins [3] in 1964. Dotter went on to report intravascular placement of a coil-spring tube graft in the canine popliteal artery [4]. These early stents were relatively small, and although they remained patent after placement, dislocation and subsequent narrowing within the stents occurred. In the early 1980s, Dotter et al. [5] reported further work with a canine model in which nickel-titanium alloy (nitinol) stents, sized to match the adjacent vessel, remained patent 4 weeks after placement.

Clinical development of stenting was driven by a need for improvement in coronary balloon angioplasty, in which acute occlusion and restenosis are problematic. Palmaz et al. [6] introduced the concept of balloon-mounted stents in 1985. Experimental work in a canine model in which expandable stents were mounted on angioplasty balloon catheters laid the groundwork for later clinical trials [7]. Reports of numerous case series and registries preceded two landmark randomized trials, the Benestent Study in Europe [8] and the Stent Restenosis Study in North America [9]. Both trials reported a lower incidence of coronary artery restenosis after angioplasty and stent placement as compared with angioplasty alone. These findings led to US Food and Drug Administration approval of the first two stents for the treatment of select coronary artery lesions to prevent restenosis and to manage acute or impending artery closure. Since that time, experimental and clinical data has accumulated rapidly, and stents are now used in most percutaneous coronary revascularization procedures [10]. Endovascular stents are also currently being used in a wide variety of noncardiac settings, such as for aortic and carotid disorders and peripheral vascular occlusive disease.

Technique

Medical Management

All endovascular procedures carry some risk of intimal injury and subsequent thrombosis and vessel occlusion. Stenting may elevate this risk: angioplasty produces deep arterial injury [11] and stents are thrombogenic [12]. Therefore, patient preparation for stenting hinges on adequate antiplatelet and anticoagulation therapy. However, selection and dosing of antithrombotic medications must also minimize the risk of hemorrhagic complications. Most information about antithrombotic treatment must be gleaned from the cardiac literature because clinical data in the neurosurgical literature is limited.

Aspirin is a cyclooxygenase-1 inhibitor that irreversibly inhibits platelet aggregation but does not impede platelet adhesion or platelet-activated mitogenic activity. Ticlopidine and clopidogrel are thienopyridine derivatives with potent antiplatelet action that inhibits adenosine phosphate-induced platelet aggregation. These drugs work synergistically with aspirin, and evidence from the cardiac literature supports the use of combination antiplatelet regimens [13, 14]. Clopidogrel has a more favorable safety profile than ticlopidine and, in combination with aspirin, has become the standard treatment for patients undergoing coronary angioplasty and stenting [15]. When possible, patients are placed on aspirin

(325 mg daily) and clopidogrel (75 mg daily) administered orally for at least 3 days before the procedure; otherwise, the patient is given a loading dose of clopidogrel (300 mg orally) and aspirin (325 mg orally) early on the day of the procedure.

Platelet glycoprotein (GP) IIb-IIIa inhibitors block the final common pathway of platelet aggregation by preventing the binding of fibrinogen to platelets and are the most potent of the antiplatelet drugs. Three intravenous GP IIb-IIIa inhibitors are abciximab (a monoclonal antibody), eptifibatide (a cyclic heptapeptide), and tirofiban (a nonpeptide mimetic). All three of these drugs have a rapid onset of antiplatelet activity and have been found to provide similar benefits in the setting of ischemic heart disease [16]. However, reversal of platelet inhibition after discontinuing the drug infusion is more rapid with eptifibatide and tirofiban, and both agents are more specific GP IIb-IIIa receptor antagonists than abciximab [17]. Preliminary data from the Department of Neurosurgery at the University at Buffalo suggests that GP IIb-IIIa inhibitor administration places patients with chronically ischemic brain at an elevated risk of intracranial hemorrhage; therefore, these drugs should be reserved for patients at high risk of thrombosis without evidence of cerebral infarction [18]. Abciximab can be given as an intravenous loading dose of 0.25 mg/kg 10–60 min before the procedure, followed by a 12-hour infusion at a rate of 10 μg/min. Alternatively, eptifibatide may be administered as an intravenous loading dose of 135 μg/kg prior to the procedure, followed by a 20- to 24-hour infusion of 0.5 μg/kg. Heparin is infused during the procedure only to maintain the activated coagulation time at approximately 200 s. When GP IIb-IIIa inhibitors are used, we recommend obtaining a computed tomography scan immediately after the procedure as continuing the drug infusion would be contraindicated in the presence of intracerebral hemorrhage.

For most intracranial stent procedures, an intra-arterial or intravenous bolus dose of heparin (70 U/kg) is administered after catheterization of the common carotid artery. In addition, all saline solutions used for irrigation should be prepared with heparin (5 U/ml). The activated coagulation time should be maintained between 250 and 300 s for the duration of the procedure.

Following stent placement, heparin therapy is usually discontinued but not actively reversed. In some situations, such as when an angiographically visible dissection or thrombosis is present, the heparin infusion is continued to maintain the activated prothrombin time at 1.5–2.3 times the baseline value. Clopidogrel (75 mg daily) should be administered for at least 4 weeks and aspirin (325 mg daily) for life [19].

Endovascular Technique

The technique of stent placement varies from case to case, depending on the clinical situation. The following is a general outline of the procedure used by the authors for most indications.

The procedure is performed in an angiography suite with biplane digital subtraction and fluoroscopic imaging capabilities. Sedative and analgesic agents are administered (rather than general anesthesia) to permit continuous neurological assessment of the patient in an awake state. A 6-french sheath is inserted into the femoral artery, and a 5-french catheter is advanced over a 0.035-inch hydrophilic wire into the aortic arch. The intracranial artery of interest is catheterized. The sheath and catheter are then removed with the wire left in place, and a 6-french guide catheter is placed into the vessel. An angiogram is obtained and the road-mapping technique is used. A 3-french catheter is then advanced coaxially over a 0.014-inch microwire into the vessel. The catheter and wire system should be advanced a sufficient distance beyond the portion of the artery to be stented to provide enough scaffolding to support deployment of the stent, particularly if the vessel is tortuous. The microwire is removed, and a stiffer 300-cm, 0.014-inch exchange wire is then placed through the microcatheter. The microcatheter is withdrawn and a balloon-mounted, over-the-wire stent is navigated across the area of interest where it is deployed at 6–8 atm of pressure. An angiogram is obtained following balloon deflation and withdrawal.

Stents

A variety of stents are becoming available for intracranial application. They fall into three general categories [20]. Balloon-expandable stents (e.g., Express; Boston Scientific, Natick, Mass., USA) are constructed of a malleable metal such as annealed stainless steel. These stents are deployed in the target vessel after they have been expanded beyond their elastic limit by inflation of a coaxial balloon. Self-expanding stents (e.g., the Wallstent; Schneider, Minneapolis, Minn., USA) are generally made from stainless steel filaments woven into a flexible mesh cylinder. They are preloaded into a constraining sheath, and are deployed by retracting the sheath. Shape-memory stents are composed of nitinol. They change shape when warmed to body temperature to adopt a predetermined configuration. Nitinol stents can be preset to expand to a specific diameter after deployment and compressed into delivery sheaths. They usually have a higher outward radial force than their stainless-steel counterparts.

Numerous stent characteristics can influence stent performance [1]. Precise sizing of stents is important. The stent must be sized to match the diameter of the nondiseased portion of the vessel and correspond to the length of the lesion [21]. The term profile refers to the diameter of the stent. The stent should be long enough to overlap the lesion. Trackability refers to the ease of negotiating the stent through the tortuosities of the intracranial vessels before deployment at the target site, whereas flexibility is a measure of the plasticity of the stent itself. Porosity indicates the percentage of total stent wall area that is fenestrated. Low-porosity stents (meaning stents with a low ratio of the area of all pores in the material to the area of the whole stent) are useful when the diversion of flow is necessary, whereas higher porosity is necessary when the region of the vessel being stented has important branches, such as brainstem perforators, that must remain patent. Experimental evidence from a canine model suggests that small carotid branches remain patent if less than 50% of the ostial diameter is covered by the stent struts [22]. A biocompatible stent is nonthrombogenic, promotes rapid endothelialization, and impedes myointimal hyperplasia. Different vessels and different kinds of lesions require different stent characteristics. Stenting for arteriosclerosis, for instance, calls for a low-profile stent with a high degree of trackability to permit passage of the stent past narrow, potentially friable lesions, with relatively high outward radial force to counter lesion recoil and, possibly, low porosity to stabilize the plaque (i.e., prevent embolization of plaque fragments). Stent-assisted aneurysm treatment, on the other hand, requires stents with low porosity to minimize flow into the aneurysm.

Stent-Assisted Angioplasty

Some 5–10% of all ischemic strokes are directly attributable to intracranial atherosclerotic lesions [23]. The risk of stroke for patients with symptomatic intracranial atherosclerosis is significant, despite antithrombotic therapy [24]. For instance, patients with middle cerebral artery stenosis have an annual risk of stroke ipsilateral to the stenosis of 7.8% per patient-year [25].

Endovascular balloon angioplasty can be useful for patients with intracranial atherosclerosis who remain symptomatic despite aggressive antithrombotic therapy. However, complication rates with intracranial angioplasty have ranged as high as 20% [26]. Intracranial angioplasty without stenting can lead to vessel dissection, vasospasm, distal embolization, or acute occlusion [27]. Adjunctive use of a stent has been shown to increase the safety and effectiveness of angioplasty in cervical carotid disease [28]. Another drawback to angioplasty alone is recurrent stenosis, which can occur from fibrosis caused by injury to the intima. Mori et al. [29] found that eccentric intracranial atherosclerotic lesions that are 5–10 mm in length have a 31% rate of restenosis at 3 months, and lesions that are tortuous, angulated, or longer than 10 mm have a 67% rate of restenosis at 3 months. Evidence from the cardiology literature has shown that stent use in combination with angioplasty may reduce the rate of restenosis by approximately two thirds [30].

Intracranial vessels have features that are unique in comparison to the coronary or peripheral vessels, making them a challenge for achieving a technically successful result with angioplasty alone. Cerebral vessels have less adventitia and are surrounded by cerebrospinal fluid, which may increase the risk of dissection or rupture. Moreover, the bone surrounding the tortuous petrous portion of the internal carotid artery makes this vessel segment difficult to traverse [31].

Published experience with intracranial angioplasty and stenting so far has been limited to case reports and retrospective series [32–38]. Most authors reserve angioplasty and stenting for patients with at least 50% stenosis who are symptomatic despite antithrombotic therapy. In a study reported by Mori et al. [39], 10 patients with cerebral ischemia in whom neurological symptoms persisted despite antithrombotic therapy and intracranial stenosis of at least 60% underwent treatment with balloon-expandable coronary stents. The procedures were unsuccessful in 2 patients because the site of arterial stenosis could not be accessed. In the 8 patients (10 lesions) who underwent angioplasty and stenting, the amount of stenosis was reduced from an average of 80% before treatment to 7% after treatment. No complications occurred during or after the procedures. No recurrent stenosis was evident on angiographic follow-up at 3 months, and no neurological ischemic events were observed during an average follow-up period of 10 months.

Lylyk et al. [21] reported a series of 34 patients with symptomatic intracranial atherosclerosis or dissections. The lesions were located in the anterior circulation (53%) and the vertebrobasilar system (47%), with at least 50% stenosis (mean 75%). One patient died after the procedure because of hemorrhagic transformation as a result of reperfusion, and another died of a myocardial infarction, for a mortality rate of 6%. The transient procedural morbidity rate was 12%, and the transient neurological morbidity rate was 6%; however, no patients had ongoing medical or neurological problems because of the procedures. Twenty patients underwent follow-up angiography within 6 months. There was an average residual stenosis of 18%, but no evidence of recurrent stenosis.

In a series reported by Gomez et al. [40], 12 patients with persistent episodes of vertebrobasilar ischemia, despite anticoagulation, underwent basilar artery stenting without the occurrence of periprocedure mortality, stent thrombosis, vessel perforation, rupture, or myocardial infarction. The basilar artery stenosis was reduced from an average of 71% before stenting to 10% after stenting. One patient required a repeat angioplasty for stenosis proximal to the stent; all others remained asymptomatic during an average follow-up period of 6 months.

In a series of 11 patients treated with stent-assisted vertebrobasilar angioplasty, Levy et al. [41] reported three periprocedural deaths and one delayed death from a procedure-related brainstem infarction. Another patient had a pontine infarction after stenting with subsequent residual diplopia. The remaining 7 patients were symptom-free at an average of 4 months. Follow-up angiography at an average of 4 months showed improved patency of the stented lesions for 5 (71%) of 7 survivors; 1 patient exhibited minimal intrastent intimal hyperplasia, and another patient developed a new stenosis proximal to the stent as well as an aneurysm within the stented portion of the basilar artery.

Rasmussen et al. [42] reported on 8 patients treated with stent-assisted vertebrobasilar angioplasty. The average prestent stenosis was 84%, and the average postprocedure stenosis was 17%. One patient died after the procedure from a subarachnoid hemorrhage. Four other patients had procedure-related complications (2 developed groin hematomas; 1 had congestive heart failure, and 1 had a transient episode of encephalopathy).

Intracranial atherosclerotic lesions usually cause neurological symptoms by reducing regional cerebral blood flow, in contrast to extracranial carotid atherosclerosis, in which embolic ischemic injury is more common than hemodynamic failure. The primary goal of intracranial stenting for atherosclerosis is to enhance blood flow through the affected artery. A poor technical result may increase the risk of acute stent thrombosis or restenosis. An important factor associated with restenosis after coronary angioplasty and stenting is the degree of residual stenosis after the procedure [43]. However, significant improvement in flow in intracranial vessels can be attained with moderate improvements in luminal diameter [44]. Moreover, recanalization of a clinically significant, high-grade intracranial stenosis can cause a reperfusion hemorrhage [45]. Thus, it may not be necessary, or even desirable, to achieve a poststent vessel diameter equivalent to that of the parent vessel.

Staged angioplasty and stenting may be associated with lower neurological morbidity. The rationale of the staged approach is to minimally dilate a high-grade stenosis, thus increasing flow and minimizing the risk of a dissection or embolic shower. By crossing the lesion with a small angioplasty balloon, the risk of dislodging plaque is lower than if the lesion were to be crossed with a higher profile device, such as a balloon-mounted stent. In a series of 8 patients treated with staged procedures for vertebrobasilar artery stenosis, there were no permanent neurological complications [46]. By staging the angioplasty and stenting over a 1-month period, a fibrous healing response induced by the angioplasty may lessen the risk of embolic shower or snowplowing (plaque forced into perforator ostia by stent struts, resulting in perforator occlusion). Although direct stenting has been shown to be safe in the coronary circulation [47], this technique may result in snowplowing and resultant perforator occlusion (fig. 1). In addition to staged and direct stenting, conventional stenting (predilation of the lesion followed by stenting during the same sitting) is most commonly used for intracranial stent deployment (fig. 2).

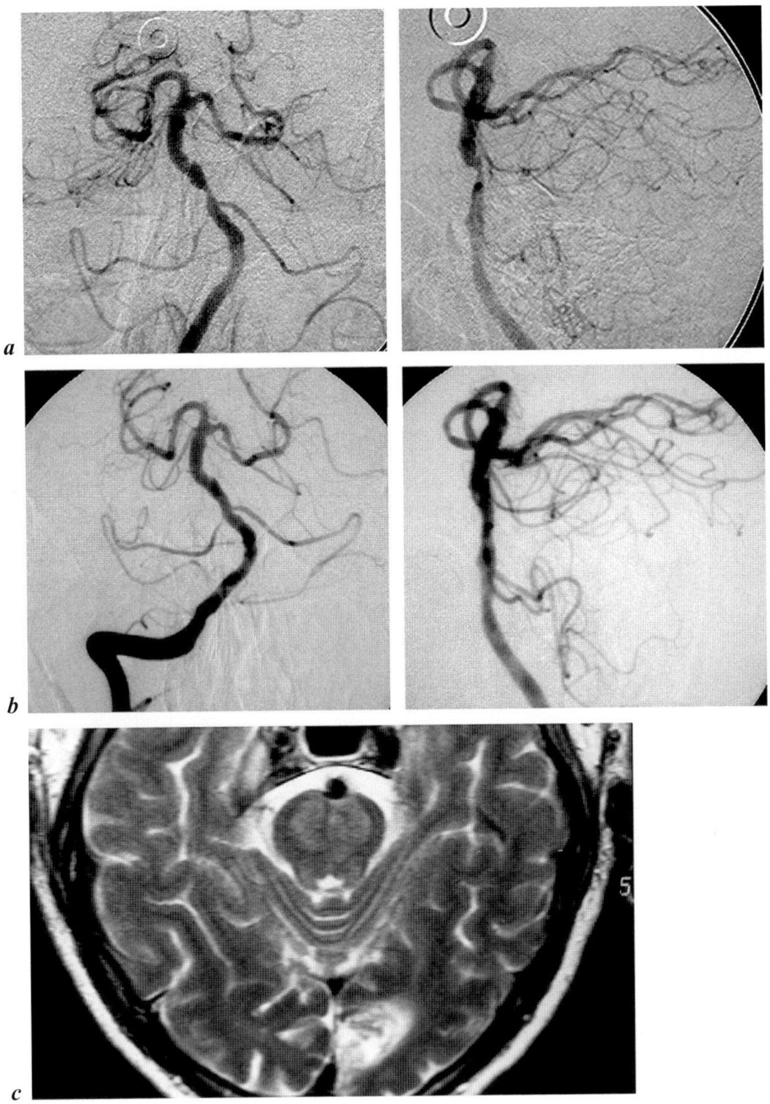

Fig. 1. ***a*** Anteroposterior (left) and lateral (right) angiographic images demonstrating a high-grade stenosis of the midbasilar artery. ***b*** Anteroposterior (left) and lateral (right) angiographic images demonstrating stent-assisted endoluminal revascularization of the basilar artery. ***c*** T2-weighted magnetic resonance imaging demonstrating acute pontine infarction likely resulting from perforator occlusion.

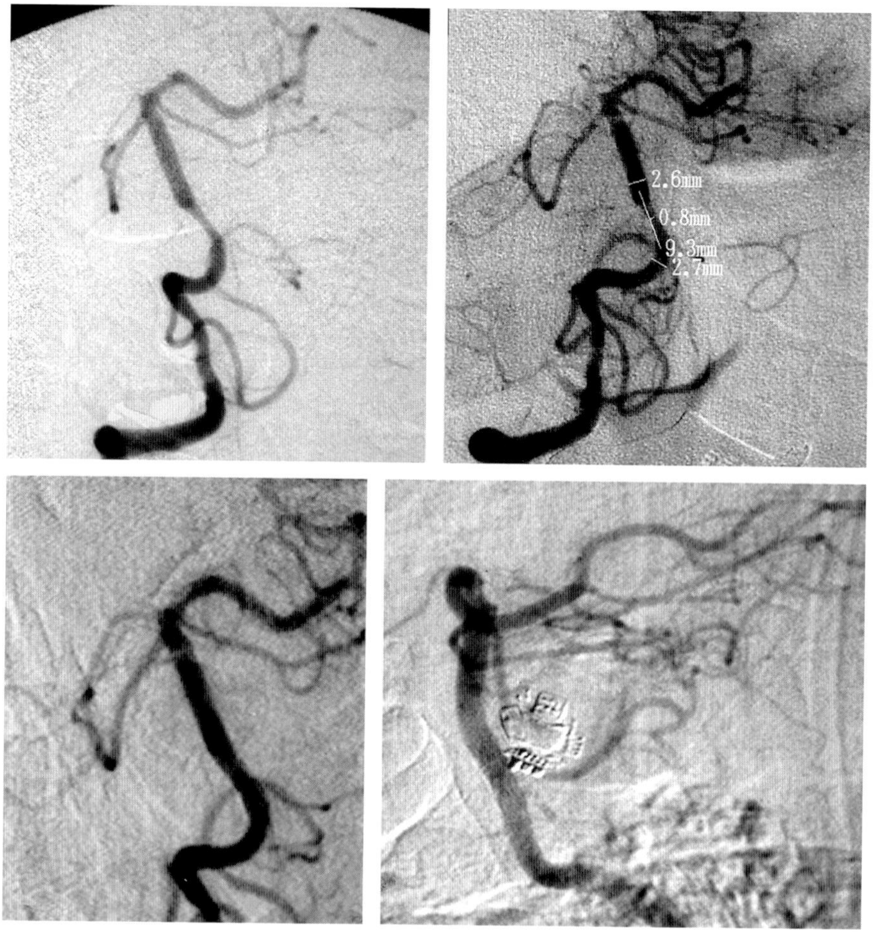

Fig. 2. ***a*** Anteroposterior angiographic images (left, right with measurements) showing a high-grade stenosis at the proximal third of the basilar artery. ***b*** Anteroposterior (left) and lateral (right) views demonstrating excellent endoluminal revascularization after conventional stent-assisted angioplasty.

Stent-Assisted Aneurysm Management

Endovascular treatment of wide-neck and fusiform aneurysms is problematic. Wide-neck aneurysms are difficult to treat with detachable coils because of coil herniation into the parent artery. Endovascular treatment of fusiform aneurysms is often limited to partial coil embolization or parent vessel occlusion. For these lesions, stents can be a useful adjunct to embolization. The technique consists of stent deployment within the parent artery across the neck of the aneurysm. A microcatheter is then navigated through the metallic mesh into the aneurysm lumen, and coil embolization is undertaken. Alternatively, the microcatheter can be positioned in the aneurysm before stent placement, then withdrawn following stent and coil placement. The use of stent-supported coil embolization for the treatment of experimental wide-neck aneurysms was first reported in 1994 [48–50] and for experimental fusiform aneurysms in 1995 [51]. Stents may serve as a scaffold for coils or other embolic agents [49–56]. Hemodynamic alterations within the aneurysm after stenting of the parent artery may promote stasis and thrombosis within the aneurysm [48]. A stent can also serve as an endovascular bypass by creating a new flow conduit in the diseased parent vessel [57], which can be particularly useful in the treatment of giant aneurysms [58].

Lanzino et al. [59] reported on 10 patients with surgically challenging intracranial aneurysms for whom coil treatment alone was considered to be inadequate. The aneurysms in 8 patients were treated with stent-supported coil embolization or stenting alone. No permanent complications occurred, and more than 90% coil occlusion was accomplished in the aneurysms treated with stent-supported coil embolization.

Phatouros et al. [60] reported on stent-supported coil embolization of wide-neck aneurysms in 7 patients. Successful coiling of the aneurysm was performed in 6 patients; in 1 patient, entanglement of the coil with the stent struts prevented coiling of the aneurysm. There were no neurological complications. Three patients underwent follow-up angiography an average of 6 months after the procedure, and each had complete aneurysm occlusion with normal appearance of the parent artery.

Using liquid polymer injection rather than coil embolization, Mawad et al. [58] treated 11 patients with symptomatic large or giant aneurysms that were felt to be inoperable. After positioning a balloon-expandable stent in the parent vessel, a microcatheter was guided through the stent mesh, and the aneurysm was obliterated with ethyl vinyl alcohol. One patient died as the result of overinflation of the balloon and dissection of the parent artery, and another patient developed watershed ischemia from prolonged balloon occlusion of the parent artery. The remaining patients were free of complications, and all but one follow-up angiogram at 6 months showed complete obliteration of the aneurysm.

Other Applications

Stenting of arterial dissections has resulted in recanalization of the vessel and exclusion and stabilization of the endothelial defect. Intracranial stents have been used for the repair of spontaneous arterial dissections [21, 53, 60], treatment of an iatrogenic basilar artery dissection following stent placement [61], and management of a pseudoaneurysm caused by injury to the internal carotid artery during middle ear surgery [62]. In a similar manner, Pride et al. [63] used stents to provide stabilization of irretrievable intravascular devices in 2 patients, an unraveled coil fragment in 1 case, and a partially deployed coronary stent in the other. Likewise, Fessler et al. [64] used a stent to secure an extruded coil loop during endovascular treatment of a superior hypophyseal artery aneurysm.

In the setting of acute stroke, significant stenosis of a recanalized vessel may remain after intra-arterial thrombolysis. Angioplasty and stent placement can be used to improve flow through the affected vessel [65]. The authors use this approach only as a last resort.

Stents have also been used to treat intracranial venous disease. Murphy et al. [66] reported on a patient with transverse sinus thrombosis related to a dural arteriovenous fistula. Mechanical thrombolysis was followed by placement of stents within the transverse sinus to reestablish normal drainage and obliterate the fistula. Malek et al. [67] described a patient with chronic sinus thrombosis treated with angioplasty and stenting of the occipital sinus.

Future Developments

Intracranial stenting is often limited by the tortuous anatomy of the cerebral circulation, calling for stents with improved flexibility and trackability. A generation of stents designed specifically for intracranial use is now undergoing development and clinical testing. One such stent is the Neurolink stent (Guidant, Menlo Park, Calif., USA), which is being used by the Stenting of Symptomatic Atherosclerotic Lesions in the Vertebral or Intracranial Arteries (SSYLVIA) trial. This industry-sponsored, nonrandomized, multicenter, phase I study is the first prospective clinical trial to evaluate a stent designed specifically for intracranial atherosclerosis [68].

Another drawback to intravascular stenting is the threat of acute thrombosis or recurrent stenosis. Stents coated with drugs to inhibit restenosis have generated interest in the coronary literature. Rapamycin, an antifungal and immunosuppressive agent that induces cell cycle arrest, reduces neointima formation in animal models. In a clinical trial of rapamycin-coated coronary artery stents, vessels in the coated stent group showed significantly less evidence of restenosis and neointimal volume at 6 months than those in the noncoated stent group [69]. Paclitaxel, another inhibitor of neointimal proliferation, leads to diminished cellular migration and proliferation by altering microtubule formation. Preliminary clinical data indicates that paclitaxel-coated coronary stents may reduce neointimal hyperplasia [70]. To date, no clinical trials of drug-coated stents in the intracranial circulation are underway. Recently, the use of intracranial drug-coated stents in vivo has been investigated using a canine model [71]. Preliminary results have indicated that a lower percentage of occlusion occurs after stenting with heparin-coated versus uncoated (control) stents. With this model, it may be possible to test the vascular response of other drug-eluting stents in cerebral vessels.

References

1 Ruygrok P, Serruys P: Intracoronary stenting: From concept to custom. Circulation 1996;94: 882–890.
2 Palmaz JC: Intravascular stenting: From basic research to clinical application. Cardiovasc Intervent Radiol 1992;15:279–284.
3 Dotter C, Judkins M: Transluminal treatment of arteriosclerotic obstruction: Description of a new technique and a preliminary report of its application. Circulation 1964;30:654–670.
4 Dotter CT: Transluminally-placed coilspring endarterial tube grafts. Long-term patency in canine popliteal artery. Invest Radiol 1969;4:329–332.
5 Dotter CT, Buschmann RW, McKinney MK, Rosch J: Transluminal expandable nitinol coil stent grafting: Preliminary report. Radiology 1983;147:259–260.
6 Palmaz J, Sibbitt R, Reuter S, Tio F, Rice W: Expandable intraluminal graft: A preliminary study. Radiology 1985;156:73–77.
7 Palmaz J, Sibbitt R, Tio F, Reuter S, Peters J, Garcia F: Expandable intraluminal vascular graft: A feasibility study. Surgery 1986;99:199–205.
8 Serruys P, de Jaegere P, Kiemeneij F, et al: A comparison of balloon-expandable stent implantation with balloon angioplasty in patients with coronary artery disease. N Engl J Med 1994;331: 489–495.
9 Fischman D, Leon M, Baim D, et al: A randomized comparison of coronary stent placement and balloon angioplasty in the treatment of coronary artery disease. N Engl J Med 1994;331:496–501.
10 Al Suwaidi J, Berger PB, Holmes DR Jr: Coronary artery stents. JAMA 2000;284:1828–1836.
11 Lam JY, Chesebro JH, Steele PM, Dewanjee MK, Badimon L, Fuster V: Deep arterial injury during experimental angioplasty: Relation to a positive indium-111-labeled platelet scintigram, quantitative platelet deposition and mural thrombosis. J Am Coll Cardiol 1986;8:1380–1386.
12 Krupski WC, Bass A, Kelly AB, Marzec UM, Hanson SR, Harker LA: Heparin-resistant thrombus formation by endovascular stents in baboons. Interruption by a synthetic antithrombin. Circulation 1990;82:570–577.
13 Mehta SR, Yusuf S, Peters RJ, et al: Effects of pretreatment with clopidogrel and aspirin followed by long-term therapy in patients undergoing percutaneous coronary intervention: The PCI-CURE study. Lancet 2001;358:527–533.
14 Yusuf S, Zhao F, Mehta SR, et al: Effects of clopidogrel in addition to aspirin in patients with acute coronary syndromes without ST-segment elevation. N Engl J Med 2001;345:494–502.
15 Gruberg L, Beyar R: Optimized combination of antiplatelet treatment and anticoagulation for percutaneous coronary intervention: The final word is not out yet! J Invasive Cardiol 2002;14:251–253.
16 Topol E: Toward a new frontier in myocardial reperfusion therapy: Emerging platelet preeminence. Circulation 1998;97:211–218.
17 Gibson CM: Primary angioplasty compared with thrombolysis: New issues in the era of glycoprotein IIb/IIIa inhibition and intracoronary stenting. Ann Intern Med 1999;130:841–847.
18 Qureshi AI, Saad M, Zaidat OO, et al: Intracerebral hemorrhages associated with neurointerventional procedures using a combination of antithrombotic agents including abciximab. Stroke 2002;33:1916–1919.

19 Qureshi AI, Luft AR, Sharma M, Guterman LR, Hopkins LN: Prevention and treatment of thromboembolic and ischemic complications associated with endovascular procedures. II. Clinical aspects and recommendations. Neurosurgery 2000;46:1360–1375.

20 Sullivan TM: Endovascular stenting. Am J Surg 1997;173:27–29.

21 Lylyk P, Cohen JE, Ceratto R, Ferrario A, Miranda C: Angioplasty and stent placement in intracranial atherosclerotic stenoses and dissections. AJNR Am J Neuroradiol 2002;23:430–436.

22 Wakhloo AK, Tio FO, Lieber BB, Schellhammer F, Graf M, Hopkins LN: Self-expanding nitinol stents in canine vertebral arteries: Hemodynamics and tissue response. AJNR Am J Neuroradiol 1995;16:1043–1051.

23 Sacco RL, Roberts JK, Boden-Albala B, et al: Race-ethnicity and determinants of carotid atherosclerosis in a multiethnic population. The Northern Manhattan Stroke Study. Stroke 1997;28: 929–935.

24 Thijs V, Albers G: Symptomatic intracranial atherosclerosis: Outcome of patients who fail antithrombotic therapy. Neurology 2000;55:490–498.

25 Bogousslavsky J, Barnett HJ, Fox AJ, Hachinski VC, Taylor W: Atherosclerotic disease of the middle cerebral artery. Stroke 1986;17:1112–1120.

26 Takis C, Kwan ES, Pessin MS, Jacobs DH, Caplan LR: Intracranial angioplasty: Experience and complications. AJNR Am J Neuroradiol 1997;18:1661–1668.

27 Clark WM, Barnwell SL, Nesbit G, O'Neill OR, Wynn ML, Coull BM: Safety and efficacy of percutaneous transluminal angioplasty for intracranial atherosclerotic stenosis. Stroke 1995;26: 1200–1204.

28 Yadav JS, Roubin GS, Iyer S, et al: Elective stenting of the extracranial carotid arteries. Circulation 1997;95:376–381.

29 Mori T, Mori K, Fukuoka M, Arisawa M, Honda S: Percutaneous transluminal cerebral angioplasty: Serial angiographic follow-up after successful dilatation. Neuroradiology 1997;39: 111–116.

30 Erbel R, Haude M, Hopp HW, et al: Coronary-artery stenting compared with balloon angioplasty for restenosis after initial balloon angioplasty. Restenosis Stent Study Group. N Engl J Med 1998;339:1672–1678.

31 Fessler RD, Lanzino G, Guterman LR, Miletich RS, Lopes DK, Hopkins LN: Improved cerebral perfusion after stenting of a petrous carotid stenosis: Technical case report. Neurosurgery 1999; 45:638–642.

32 Al-Mubarak N, Gomez CR, Vitek JJ, Roubin GS: Stenting of symptomatic stenosis of the intracranial internal carotid artery. AJNR Am J Neuroradiol 1998;19:1949–1951.

33 Dorros G, Cohn JM, Palmer LE: Stent deployment resolves a petrous carotid artery angioplasty dissection. AJNR Am J Neuroradiol 1998;19:392–394.

34 Feldman RL, Trigg L, Gaudier J, Galat J: Use of coronary Palmaz-Schatz stent in the percutaneous treatment of an intracranial carotid artery stenosis. Catheter Cardiovasc Diagn 1996;38:316–319.

35 Gomez CR, Misra VK, Campbell MS, Soto RD: Elective stenting of symptomatic middle cerebral artery stenosis. AJNR Am J Neuroradiol 2000;21:971–973.

36 Horowitz MB, Pride GL, Graybeal DF, Purdy PD: Percutaneous transluminal angioplasty and stenting of midbasilar stenoses: Three technical case reports and literature review. Neurosurgery 1999;45:925–930.

37 Mori T, Kazita K, Mori K: Cerebral angioplasty and stenting for intracranial vertebral atherosclerotic stenosis. AJNR Am J Neuroradiol 1999;20:787–789.

38 Phatouros CC, Lefler JE, Higashida RT, et al: Primary stenting for high-grade basilar artery stenosis. AJNR Am J Neuroradiol 2000;21:1744–1749.

39 Mori T, Kazita K, Chokyu K, Mima T, Mori K: Short-term arteriographic and clinical outcome after cerebral angioplasty and stenting for intracranial vertebrobasilar and carotid atherosclerotic occlusive disease. AJNR Am J Neuroradiol 2000;21:249–254.

40 Gomez CR, Misra VK, Liu MW, et al: Elective stenting of symptomatic basilar artery stenosis. Stroke 2000;31:95–99.

41 Levy EI, Horowitz MB, Koebbe CJ, et al: Transluminal stent-assisted angiplasty of the intracranial vertebrobasilar system for medically refractory, posterior circulation ischemia: Early results. Neurosurgery 2001;48:1215–1221.

42 Rasmussen PA, Perl J II, Barr JD, et al: Stent-assisted angioplasty of intracranial vertebrobasilar atherosclerosis: An initial experience. J Neurosurg 2000;92:771–778.
43 Kishi K, Hiasa Y, Suzuki N, et al: Predictors of recurrent restenosis after coronary stenting: An analysis of 197 patients. J Invasive Cardiol 2002;14:187–191.
44 Derdeyn CP, Cross DT III, Moran CJ, Dacey RG Jr: Reversal of focal misery perfusion after intracranial angioplasty: Case report. Neurosurgery 2001;48:436–439.
45 Liu AY, Do HM, Albers GW, Lopez JR, Steinberg GK, Marks MP: Hyperperfusion syndrome with hemorrhage after angioplasty for middle cerebral artery stenosis. AJNR Am J Neuroradiol 2001; 22:1597–1601.
46 Levy EI, Hanel RA, Bendok BR, et al: Staged stent-assisted angioplasty for symptomatic intracranial vertebrobasilar artery stenosis. J Neurosurg 2002;97:1294–1301.
47 Baim DS, Flatley M, Caputo R, et al: Comparison of PRE-dilatation vs direct stenting in coronary treatment using the Medtronic AVE S670 Coronary Stent System (the PREDICT trial). Am J Cardiol 2001;88:1364–1369.
48 Geremia G, Haklin M, Brennecke L: Embolization of experimentally created aneurysms with intravascular stent devices. AJNR Am J Neuroradiol 1994;15:1223–1231.
49 Szikora I, Guterman LR, Wells KM, Hopkins LN: Combined use of stents and coils to treat experimental wide-necked carotid aneurysms: Preliminary results. AJNR Am J Neuroradiol 1994;15: 1091–1102.
50 Turjman F, Massoud TF, Ji C, Guglielmi G, Vinuela F, Robert J: Combined stent implantation and endosaccular coil placement for treatment of experimental wide-necked aneurysms: A feasibility study in swine. AJNR Am J Neuroradiol 1994;15:1087–1090.
51 Massoud TF, Turjman F, Ji C, et al: Endovascular treatment of fusiform aneurysms with stents and coils: Technical feasibility in a swine model. AJNR Am J Neuroradiol 1995;16:1953–1963.
52 Higashida RT, Smith W, Gress D, et al: Intravascular stent and endovascular coil placement for a ruptured fusiform aneurysm of the basilar artery. Case report and review of the literature. J Neurosurg 1997;87:944–949.
53 Lylyk P, Ceratto R, Hurvitz D, Basso A: Treatment of a vertebral dissecting aneurysm with stents and coils: Technical case report. Neurosurgery 1998;43:385–388.
54 Perez-Cruet MJ, Patwardhan RV, Mawad ME, Rose JE: Treatment of dissecting pseudoaneurysm of the cervical internal carotid artery using a wall stent and detachable coils: Case report. Neurosurgery 1997;40:622–626.
55 Sekhon LH, Morgan MK, Sorby W, Grinnell V: Combined endovascular stent implantation and endosaccular coil placement for the treatment of a wide-necked vertebral artery aneurysm: Technical case report. Neurosurgery 1998;43:380–383.
56 Szikora I, Guterman LR, Standard SC, Wakhloo AK, Hopkins LN: Endovascular treatment of experimental aneurysms with liquid polymers: The protective potential of stents. Neurosurgery 1996;38:339–347.
57 Wakhloo AK, Lanzino G, Lieber BB, Hopkins LN: Stents for intracranial aneurysms: The beginning of a new endovascular era? Neurosurgery 1998;43:377–379.
58 Mawad ME, Cekirge S, Ciceri E, Saatci I: Endovascular treatment of giant and large intracranial aneurysms by using a combination of stent placement and liquid polymer injection. J Neurosurg 2002;96:474–482.
59 Lanzino G, Wakhloo AK, Fessler RD, Hartney ML, Guterman LR, Hopkins LN: Efficacy and current limitations of intravascular stents for intracranial internal carotid, vertebral, and basilar artery aneurysms. J Neurosurg 1999;91:538–546.
60 Phatouros CC, Sasaki TY, Higashida RT, et al: Stent-supported coil embolization: The treatment of fusiform and wide-neck aneurysms and pseudoaneurysms. Neurosurgery 2000;47:107–113.
61 Malek AM, Higashida RT, Halbach VV, Phatouros CC, Meyers PM, Dowd CF: Tandem intracranial stent deployment for treatment of an iatrogenic, flow-limiting, basilar artery dissection: Technical case report. Neurosurgery 1999;45:919–924.
62 Alexander MJ, Smith TP, Tucci DL: Treatment of an iatrogenic petrous carotid artery pseudoaneurysm with a Symbiot covered stent: Technical case report. Neurosurgery 2002;50:658–662.
63 Pride GL Jr, Horowitz MB, Purdy PD: Endovascular problem solving with intravascular stents. AJNR Am J Neuroradiol 2000;21:532–540.

64 Fessler RD, Ringer AJ, Qureshi AI, Guterman LR, Hopkins LN: Intracranial stent placement to trap an extruded coil during endovascular aneurysm treatment: Technical note. Neurosurgery 2000;46:248–253.
65 Phatouros CC, Higashida RT, Malek AM, et al: Endovascular stenting of an acutely thrombosed basilar artery: Technical case report and review of the literature. Neurosurgery 1999;44:667–673.
66 Murphy KJ, Gailloud P, Venbrux A, Deramond H, Hanley D, Rigamonti D: Endovascular treatment of a grade IV transverse sinus dural arteriovenous fistula by sinus recanalization, angioplasty, and stent placement: Technical case report. Neurosurgery 2000;46:497–500.
67 Malek AM, Higashida RT, Balousek PA, et al: Endovascular recanalization with balloon angioplasty and stenting of an occluded occipital sinus for treatment of intracranial venous hypertension: Technical case report. Neurosurgery 1999;44:896–901.
68 Chimowitz MI: Angioplasty or stenting is not appropriate as first-line treatment of intracranial stenosis. Arch Neurol 2001;58:1690–1692.
69 Morice MC, Serruys PW, Sousa JE, et al: A randomized comparison of a sirolimus-eluting stent with a standard stent for coronary revascularization. N Engl J Med 2002;346:1773–1780.
70 Liistro F, Stankovic G, Di Mario C, et al: First clinical experience with a paclitaxel derivate-eluting polymer stent system implantation for in-stent restenosis: Immediate and long-term clinical and angiographic outcome. Circulation 2002;105:1883–1886.
71 Levy EI, Boulos AS, Hanel RA, et al: In vivo model of intracranial stent implantation: A pilot study examining the histological response of cerebral vessels after randomized implantation of heparin-coated and uncoated endoluminal stents in a blinded fashion. J Neurosurg 2003;98: 532–541.

L. Nelson Hopkins, MD
University at Buffalo Neurosurgery
Kaleida Gates Hospital, 3 Gates Circle
Buffalo, NY 14209 (USA)
Tel. +1 716 887 5200, Fax +1 716 887 4378, E-Mail dzbuffns@aol.com

Horowitz MB, Levy EI (eds): Neuroendovascular Surgery.
Prog Neurol Surg. Basel, Karger, 2005, vol 17, pp 85–100

Angioplasty for Repair of Intracranial Arterial Stenosis

Andrew J. Ringer

Department of Neurosurgery and Mayfield Clinic, The Neuroscience Institute, University of Cincinnati College of Medicine, Cincinnati, Ohio, USA

Introduction

The treatment of intracranial arterial stenosis has long been a matter of considerable debate. Treatment options have ranged from simple medical management to complex surgical repair with unclear benefits to virtually all available options. When a prospective, randomized trial comparing aspirin therapy to extracranial-intracranial (ECIC) bypass failed to demonstrate a benefit for bypass surgery [1], the search for an effective treatment continued. Despite the limitations cited regarding patient selection in the ECIC bypass trial, such as the failure to identify patients with hypoperfusion prior to bypass [2], two conclusions were proposed: ECIC bypass does little to reduce the thromboembolic complications of intracranial stenosis and the risk of stroke during aspirin therapy remains high. With these findings in hand, clinicians have explored the option of endovascular revascularization.

This chapter will explore the indications for intracranial angioplasty, technique, and complication avoidance and management.

Natural History

The risk of stroke related to intracranial stenosis was probably unrecognized and underreported in the past. Focus on the more easily treatable extracranial carotid and cardiac or aortic sources of stroke may, in fact, detract attention from coexistent concomitant intracranial disease. Although atherosclerosis of the extracranial cerebral arteries is more common, intracranial stenosis occurs in more than 30% of patients with atherosclerotic disease. In 1968, Hass et al. [3] identified intracranial stenosis in 22.6% of the 4,748 consecutive patients evaluated with cerebral angiography. In another consecutive series of 3,788 patients with angiographic evidence of cerebrovascular stenosis Connors [4] reported that 39.4% had evidence of significant intracranial disease. The most common sites of intracranial disease included the intracranial internal carotid artery (ICA), the main trunk, or M1 segment, of the middle cerebral artery (MCA), the distal vertebral artery or vertebrobasilar junction, and the midbasilar artery. Considering these frequencies, intracranial stenosis should be considered in patients with cerebral ischemic signs and symptoms. Population studies suggesting that intracranial stenoses occur more often in African-Americans than in Caucasians necessitate a higher index of suspicion when symptoms are found.

After identification of intracranial stenosis, estimation of the risk of the lesion is difficult; the extent of stenosis cannot be as accurately estimated as it can be for stenosis of the extracranial ICA. Normal intracranial arteries may have a diameter of only 2.5 mm. If stenoses were 80%, the residual lumen would be only 0.5 mm – a diameter that is difficult to measure accurately. Accordingly, most clinicians consider stenosis exceeding 50% as significant intracranial stenosis and group patients with this extent of stenosis together for clinical studies. Significant intracranial stenosis by this measure poses a high risk of stroke in virtually all locations. Intracranial ICA stenosis has a risk of ipsilateral stroke that ranges between 3.2 and 7.6% per year and an overall stroke risk that ranges between 4 and 11% per year [5–7].

In the medical arm of the ECIC bypass study, the annual risk of stroke with ICA siphon or MCA stenosis ranged from 8 to 10% [1]. The posterior circulation disease risk may be even higher. In the Warfarin Aspirin Symptomatic Intracranial Disease (WASID) study, patients with significant basilar artery stenosis treated with aspirin had an annual stroke risk exceeding 10% despite medical therapy [8]. Perhaps even more concerning is the manner in which patients present with symptoms. In 1984, Borozan et al. [9] reported that in patients with 115 stenotic intracranial arteries, 93 of which were symptomatic, the stroke-free survival was no different between symptomatic and asymptomatic patients. Equally disturbing at the time of new symptoms was that mean stenosis ($\pm$ standard deviation) was $35.4 \pm 14.4\%$ [9]. In the ECIC bypass trial, only one third of all major strokes were preceded by transient ischemic attacks (TIAs) [1]. In another review of patients presenting with symptoms while on antithrombotic therapy, the mean time to recurrent symptoms was 36 days [10]. These results collectively imply that clinicians may have difficulty predicting the patients at highest risk for stroke.

Medical Therapy

Appropriate medical therapy for intracranial stenosis remains a matter of debate. Several retrospective studies including the prospective, observational arm of the WASID trial [8] have suggested a reduced risk of stroke with warfarin therapy versus aspirin [10, 11]. In the WASID report, annual stroke risk declined from 10.4% with aspirin to 3.6% with warfarin [11]. Subsequently many clinicians considered warfarin a more aggressive therapy for patients symptomatic on aspirin. However, more recent, prospective trials, failed to demonstrate the benefit of warfarin and found a higher risk of hemorrhagic complications than with aspirin. In the initial WASID trial, two of three major hemorrhagic complications were fatal, for a rate of 7.8/100 patient years associated with warfarin versus only 1.4/100 patient years associated with aspirin.

Surgical Therapy

The failure of the ECIC bypass trial to show benefits for patients treated with surgical bypass all but halted the use of this procedure. Since publication of these results, some detractors of the ECIC bypass trial have argued that patient selection may have doomed the study: that is, no efforts were made to differentiate patients symptomatic from either embolic events or hypoperfusion. New imaging techniques, including xenon computed tomography (CT), single photon emission computed tomography (SPECT), and positron emission tomography provide valuable data regarding brain perfusion and metabolism in specific vascular territories.

Using cerebral oxygen extraction ratios to augment cerebral blood flow data, researchers at the Washington University identified patients with cervical ICA occlusion and cerebral hypoperfusion ranging from stage 1 (vasodilatory compensation) to stage 2 (maximized vasodilatation with increased cerebral oxygen extraction) to stage 3 (exceeding compensatory mechanisms). Grubb et al. [12] reported that patients with stage 2 hypoperfusion were at a dramatically higher risk of stroke. Buoyed by these findings, a new, prospective, randomized trial will reexamine ECIC bypass for the treatment of cerebral hypoperfusion called the Carotid Occlusion Surgery Study (COSS). Perhaps a similar selection from patients with intracranial stenosis will yield surgical indications in the future.

Intracranial Angioplasty

Because the stroke risk remains high after the best medical therapy, many endovascular surgeons now consider angioplasty for the repair of intracranial stenosis. Angioplasty as primary treatment of arterial atherosclerotic disease became widely accepted for the coronary artery disease in the 1980s [13]. Its application to intracranial disease first gained popularity in the treatment of arterial vasospasm after aneurysmal subarachnoid hemorrhage [14–20]. However, the popularity of angioplasty for intracranial atherosclerosis waned because of the high risk associated with the procedure; in initial studies, the periprocedural neurological event rate ranged from 8 to 33% [21–24]. However, in four later series with more than 10 patients, the complication rates were less than 10% [25–28]. In another series, 20 patients with intracranial vertebrobasilar stenosis who were treated with angioplasty alone developed a 5% complication rate [26]. In a series of 23 patients [27], Marks et al. reported a 5% periprocedural risk by using an undersized balloon relative to the target artery and by accepting residual stenosis. Clearly selection bias remains in these series as only patients with the highest risk lesions were referred for angioplasty after medical therapy failed. Therefore, clinicians must carefully evaluate the risk of angioplasty when considering candidates for therapy.

In addition to the severity of stenosis, several factors that may affect the risk of angioplasty should be considered before treatment. First, the angiographic appearance of the lesion (i.e., location, length, eccentricity) rather than severity of stenosis may influence procedural success. Mori et al. [29] described their experience with procedural results and angiographic follow-up of intracranial angioplasty based on the length and eccentricity of the lesions. In patients with short (<5 mm) mildly eccentric or concentric lesions called type A lesions, Mori et al. reported periprocedural complication rates of 8% (i.e., one stroke in 12). In patients with type B lesions (between 5 and 10 mm or totally occluded lesions) less than 3 months old, the success rate of intracranial angioplasty was 86%. Angiographic restenosis occurred in 33% of patients during a 2-year follow-up. In 2 of the 21 patients, attempts to perform angioplasty were unsuccessful. In 9 patients with type C lesions, chronic occlusions more than 3 months old or highly angular, long (>10 mm) lesions fared the worst with a 33% initial success rate and 100% restenosis at 1 year. These findings suggest that angiographic characteristics may help determine feasibility and periprocedural risks. Mori et al. [29] reported a higher incidence of restenosis or procedural failure with long, eccentric lesions than with short, concentric lesions; in long lesions, the restenosis was 29.6% at 3 months and no additional restenosis at 12 months. The cumulative risk of ipsilateral stroke was 12% in patients with type B lesions and 56% in those with type C lesions.

Lesion accessibility is another important factor. Highly tortuous proximal anatomy makes navigation of endovascular devices difficult and creates risks of proximal dissection. In a review (unpubl. data) of attempted intracranial stent placements at the University of Buffalo, 8 of 27 consecutive attempts were

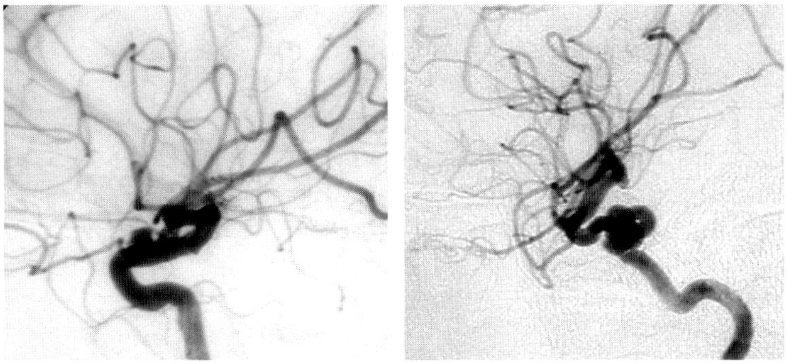

Fig. 1. Digital subtraction angiogram shows successful versus unsuccessful attempts of intracranial carotid stent placement in 2 patients. ***a*** Successful attempt shows the large radius of curvature through the carotid siphon. ***b*** Unsuccessful attempt shows the smaller radius of curvature through the carotid siphon; this patient suffered an asymptomatic carotid dissection during attempted stent advancement (with permission from Mayfield Clinic).

aborted because of a failure to deliver the stent; comparison of successful and unsuccessful cases revealed significant differences in the proximal anatomy. In measurement of the curvature radius of the proximal vascular loop (carotid siphon or vertebral C1 loop), we noted significantly smaller radii in the unsuccessful cases (unpubl. data) (fig. 1). While stent devices are more difficult to navigate through tortuous arteries than angioplasty balloons, the more tortuous the vasculature, the relatively greater degree of difficulty may occur with any device.

Technique

The steps necessary to successful angioplasty may be divided into perioperative, intraoperative, and postoperative.

Perioperative Management

Preoperative preparation specific to intracranial angioplasty primarily concerns the management of anticoagulant medication. Although many patients are being treated with warfarin when referred for angioplasty, many interventionalists rely on aggressive antiplatelet therapy to prevent perioperative complications. In my practice, warfarin is discontinued 3 days before intracranial angioplasty when patients begin combination therapy with aspirin (325 mg/day) and clopidogrel (75 mg/day) concomitantly to allow adequate time for the natural, gradual reversal of warfarin anticoagulation with simultaneous 'loading' of clopidogrel. For patients taking aspirin only, clopidogrel is added 3 days before angioplasty. For urgent cases without time to use either protocol, glycoprotein (GP) IIb/IIIa inhibitors are given followed by clopidogrel loaded postoperatively via a single 300-mg dose.

Other preoperative steps are typical of all surgical or interventional procedures. A complete neurological examination before the neuroendovascular procedure is paramount; it not only familiarizes the examiner with the patient but also permits rapid identification of neurological compromise. Additionally, in patients with preexisting neurological deficits, documentation before the procedure ensures that no additional deficits have accrued. Peripheral pulses should be noted, and if diminished, should be marked for easy identification during angiography. Review of any previous studies and an in-depth knowledge of the medical history are important to develop an appropriate plan and complete a diagnostic study for each patient. Incomplete reviews of either available studies or histories may result in the need for additional invasive procedures. A history of significant peripheral vascular occlusive disease or coronary artery disease signals an increased risk for arterial access complications, periprocedural myocardial infarction, or stroke [30]. Congestive heart failure requires judicious use of periprocedural fluid intake and contrast load. Necessary lab work includes at least the following: a baseline hemoglobin and hematocrit, platelet count, partial thromboplastin time, prothrombin time, blood urea nitrogen, serum creatinine, and blood glucose.

Certain issues (e.g., contrast load, anesthesia) bear consideration before performing any endovascular procedure. For patients with impaired renal function and for all patients who will undergo spinal angiographic studies, the maximum potential contrast load for each should be calculated. For an assumed nonionic iodine contrast preparation, the maximum contrast volume calculated is: patient weight (kg) $\times$ 5 $\div$ serum creatinine levels. Example: a 90-kg patient with a 1.5 serum creatinine level could receive $90 \times 5 \div 1.5 = 300$ ml of contrast.

For longer procedures that require large contrast loads, assumptions are that patients with adequate hydration and normal renal function will have excreted approximately 50% of the administered contrast load and that dosing can be recalculated. For patients with a history of allergic reaction to contrast material, the administration of prednisone, diphenhydramine, and acetaminophen before the procedure typically prevents unwanted contrast reactions and their sequelae [25]. Generally, prednisone (10 mg 3 times daily) is administered orally beginning 1 day before the procedure and as a single dose on the morning of the procedure. Diphenhydramine (25–50 mg orally) and acetaminophen (10 mg) are given about 1–2 h before the procedure. Additionally, the mode of sedation or anesthesia should be addressed before the procedure. I typically perform all spinal angiography and interventional procedures by administration of intravenous local anesthesia with sedative hypnotics and narcotic analgesics before and throughout the procedure. During the procedure, the patient is awake so that the angiographer can note changes in neurological function on serial neurological examination. We reserve general anesthesia for patients unable to tolerate recumbency for long periods.

Operative Technique

Intracranial angioplasty is typically performed via the transfemoral route using standard angiographic techniques. Patients are positioned supine on the neuroangiography table, with the knees slightly bent; support under the knees is used for patients with a history of low back pain. The maximum contrast load is calculated; venous access obtained well in advance of the procedure permits intravenous hydration. For lengthy procedures, such as intracranial interventions, a Foley catheter is placed. Access to the common femoral artery is procured under sterile conditions, with two- to three-finger breadths below the ilioinguinal ligament using the modified Seldinger technique. We prefer the single-wall puncture technique because of the need for anticoagulation perioperatively. A 6-french sheath is placed followed by administration of anticoagulant medications. In most of our cases, heparin anticoagulation and GP IIb/IIIa blockade are administered for antiplatelet effect. GP IIb/IIIa blockade is withheld only in cases of chronic, severe hypoperfusion or recent infarction due to the risk of hemorrhage [34]. After confirmation of appropriate anticoagulation, selective catheterization of the appropriate vascular tree (i.e., carotid or vertebral artery) with a 6-french guide catheter is performed. An activated clotting time of 220–250 s is targeted when using GP IIb/IIIa agents in conjunction with heparin or an activated clotting time longer than 300 s with heparin alone; this can frequently be achieved with a heparin bolus of 40–50 IU/kg with GP IIb/IIIa or 60–70 IU/kg with heparin alone.

After proximal access is secured, angiographic images are obtained to measure the lesion and determine the optimal view for visualization. For this purpose, the lesion is best viewed from a position perpendicular to the arterial course. When viewed from a more acute angle, the lesion appears shorter than it really is, which may affect the surgeon's choice of balloon size. The artery diameter is measured; biplanar angiographic units are typically supported by software that calculates the diameter, taking magnification into account. The diameter can also be measured by comparison to an object of known size; for example, the diameter of an indwelling catheter or two washers affixed to either side of the patient's head might be used for magnification control. The artery diameter proximal to the lesion is the basis for the selection of the appropriately sized balloon for angioplasty (fig. 2a). This and all subsequent interventional images are performed under high magnification to improve visualization.

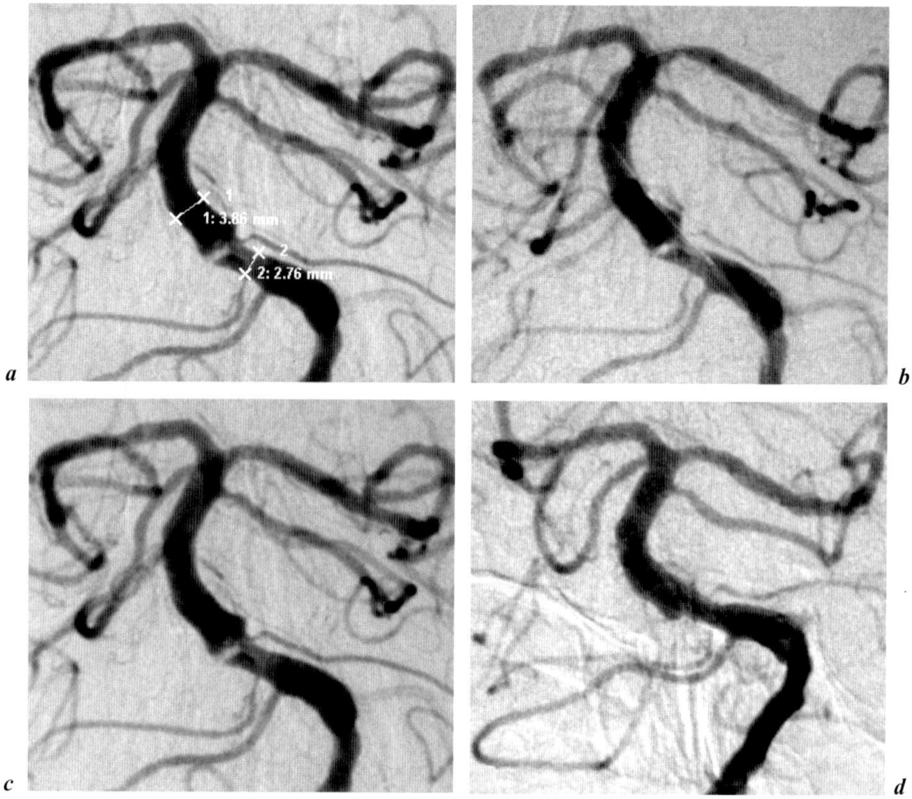

Fig. 2. Typical steps during intracranial angioplasty as seen on digital subtraction angiography. ***a*** Measurement of the parent artery determines the size of the native lumen proximal and distal to the stenotic lesion to aid in selection of an appropriately sized balloon. ***b*** Angiography confirms the position of the balloon. Despite advancing the balloon catheter using roadmap guidance, inaccuracies can result if the artery straightens or the patient changes position. Centering the balloon on the lesion is necessary to prevent 'watermelon seeding' or its migration during inflation. ***c*** After initial angioplasty attempts, angiograms may reveal significant residual stenosis. For this reason, it is paramount to maintain wire position across the lesion to prevent the need to recross the lesion and risk dissection. ***d*** Final angiogram after angioplasty shows the lesion is completely resolved and all distal branches fill normally. High-magnification or 'coned-down' views may fail to fully evaluate these branches and may miss distal emboli (with permission from Mayfield Clinic).

Access is then secured across the lesion. Access across the target lesion can be difficult in cases of severe stenosis or with distal lesions [e.g., posterior cerebral artery (PCA) or distal MCA lesions]. In these cases, I prefer to cross the lesion with a microcatheter before inserting of the balloon catheter. A 175-cm-long (0.014-inch) wire with a soft, shapable tip will typically cross with reasonable ease, allowing the advancement of a microcatheter across the lesion. With the wire removed, the position is confirmed angiographically by injecting through the microcatheter to ensure that no dissection has resulted in an extraluminal catheter position. Subsequently, an exchange length wire (300 cm long; 0.014 inch) with a stiff proximal segment and short, soft tip is advanced for the exchange of the balloon catheter with the microcatheter. The balloon position is confirmed angiographically prior to inflation. The balloon is inflated with diluted contrast (2:1 contrast:saline) via an indeflator device; this device offers fine control of inflation pressure, permitting the interventionalist to slowly inflate the balloon to a diameter slightly less than the arterial diameter. After slow deflation, an angiogram is performed (through the guide catheter) to assess the result; although the balloon catheter may have to be withdrawn slightly to permit better visualization of the treated segment, the wire should always remain across the lesion. Additional angioplasty may be performed as necessary (fig. 2b, c). Neurological exams are obtained before and after all balloon inflations for conscious patients.

After satisfactory results are attained, a standard magnification angiogram viewing the patient's full head can rule out distal branch occlusion from emboli before withdrawing the wire. This permits thrombolysis of distal occlusions if necessary or deemed appropriate. Upon completion, we fully withdraw the balloon catheter and wire, and remove the guide catheter. The femoral artery access sheath may be left in place and later removed after reversal of anticoagulation, or the arteriotomy may be closed by one of several devices available for this purpose that permits early mobilization of the patient.

Strict adherence to careful technique contributes greatly to the safety of intracranial angioplasty. Nowhere is this principle more eloquently discussed than in the series report by Connors and Wojak [28] that covers their experiences from 1989 to 1998 into three periods. The early and middle periods from 1989 to 1993 have higher complications including angiographic evidence of dissection in 82%, stroke in 6%, and death in 6% of the 17 patients. Since 1993, the authors have reported rates of 14% dissection, 8% neurological events (4% TIAs), and 2% mortalities. They attribute these improvements to smaller balloon diameters, acceptance of residual stenosis, a slow (2–5 min) inflation of the balloon, and routine use of GP IIb/IIIa receptor inhibitors (e.g., abciximab) during angioplasty. In the latter period, there were two hemorrhages (included in the strokes). They also advocate not recrossing the lesion because of a higher likelihood of raising an intimal flap and occluding the vessel. One intrinsic advantage endovascular approaches have versus surgical approaches is the ability to return for repair of a suboptimal result. Because the approach itself is rarely difficult, endovascular surgeons may initially choose to treat the lesions less aggressively knowing that they can return to improve the result if necessary. The authors also discovered that the use of shorter angioplasty balloons prevented the straightening of the intracranial vessels with balloon inflation, making injury or dissection less likely.

Postoperatively, GP IIb/IIIa blockade is maintained for 12–24 h. The patient is observed in the intensive care unit undergoing continuous blood pressure monitoring and hourly nursing evaluations. If no untoward events occur during the ensuing 24 h, the patient may be discharged on aspirin (325 mg/day) and clopidogrel (75 mg/day).

Postoperative Follow-Up

Early and continuous follow-up is paramount to ensure early identification of delayed complications of angioplasty (see below). One to 2 weeks after discharge, patients are typically seen for clinical follow-up to ensure compliance with medications and identify any potential ischemic symptoms that may have developed after discharge. Clinical follow-up is coupled with radiographic imaging, typically magnetic resonance angiography, at 3, 6, 12, 18 and 24 months. Transcranial Doppler studies, which may be used in addition to or in place of magnetic resonance angiography, are most useful if baseline studies are obtained immediately after angioplasty. Any evidence of restenosis should be evaluated angiographically. After 2 years of uneventful follow-up, annual or biannual follow-up may be sufficient.

Complications and Management

Thromboembolus

The most feared complication of intracranial angioplasty is thromboembolism that causes downstream vascular occlusion. As with any complication of treatment, the best management is prevention. As described previously, judicious administration and monitoring of anticoagulation and antiplatelet therapies can reduce the risk of thromboembolism. New clot formation at the angioplasty site can occur by several mechanisms [31]. Local endothelial injury causes the release of thromboxane A_2 and adenosine diphosphate, which stimulate platelet aggregation; exposure of the subendothelium stimulates the production of thrombin via the coagulation cascade. However, these events can prevent the platelet aggregation and thrombin production with the use of antiplatelet (aspirin and clopidogrel) and heparin, respectively. The binding of fibrin to platelets, the final common pathway in thrombus formation, is mediated by GP IIb/IIIa receptors, which are blocked by the GP IIb/IIIa inhibitors abciximab and Integrilin.

If thromboembolism occurs, however, revascularization should be attempted. In the absence of established infarction, a thrombolytic agent (e.g., tissue-type plasminogen activator) may be administered locally via intra-arterial injection. However, administration of a thrombolytic agent after cerebral ischemia is associated with intracranial hemorrhage, thus leading to an increased risk for postangioplasty thromboembolism [32]. Abciximab, by either intra-arterial or intravenous administration, has also demonstrated thrombolytic properties and appears effective in the resolution of thromboembolism after angioplasty. When administered intravenously within 6 h of acute stroke in doses typically used for acute coronary syndrome, there appears to be no increased risks of intracerebral hemorrhage [33]. However, fatal intracerebral hemorrhage has been reported after carotid artery angioplasty, particularly in patients with evidence of hypoperfusion before treatment [34]. Accordingly, GP IIb/IIIa inhibitors must be used in carefully selected patients, cautiously for a limited time perioperatively and with the intent of minimizing the dose administered. An alternative is intra-arterial injection of papaverine. Because acute arterial occlusion may be associated with vasospasm, resolution of the spasm may permit reperfusion in some cases. Local thrombotic occlusion at the angioplasty site may also be treated by any measure described above. In addition, mechanical clot disruption with angioplasty or snare manipulation at the thrombus site has been effective in the treatment of acute intracranial occlusion resistant to thrombolysis [35, 36]. Angioplasty may reestablish flow through the occluded segment, augmenting the delivery of thrombolytic agents and increasing the surface area of the thrombus available for binding of these agents.

Arterial Dissection

The risk of arterial dissection with intracranial angioplasty appears to be higher than in other vascular territories, including the carotid and coronary arteries. Although dissection after intracranial angioplasty occurs in approximately 20% of cases [24, 37, 38], dissection after coronary angioplasty occurs in 2–10% of cases [39]. The reason for this difference is unclear. However, one explanation may be the relatively fixed position of the coronary artery in cardiac muscle versus the mobile cerebral artery in the subarachnoid space. Another anatomical factor unique to the cerebral vasculature is the tortuous course of the arteries. As mentioned above, highly tortuous proximal vascular anatomy or a distal target location (distal MCA, PCA) increases the difficulty of reaching the target lesion with an angioplasty balloon. Dissections may occur during attempts to navigate these proximal segments. Finally, the surgical technique influences the risk of dissection. Slow, gentle inflation and deflation, without inflation beyond the normal diameter of the target artery, may reduce the risk of dissection [28].

Restenosis

The risk of restenosis after successful intracranial angioplasty has dissuaded some clinicians from recommending angioplasty for stroke prevention; reported restenosis rates range from 0 to 50% in numerous small series [21, 23, 28, 29, 40–42]. Several factors may influence the risk of restenosis.

Mori et al. [29] described an increased risk of restenosis in long, eccentric lesions. Restenosis may also be more common after procedures complicated by dissection (fig. 2). Accordingly, factors that increase the dissection risk may increase the risk of restenosis. Some authors have advocated the use of antioxidant medications to reduce the restenosis risk. A major prospective, randomized trial demonstrated a statistically significant reduction in restenosis after coronary angioplasty with the use of probucol [43]. However, the manufacturer discontinued its production when its intended use as an anticholesterolemic proved less effective than other agents and the FDA denied approval because the QT interval may be prolonged. This trial also demonstrated no clear benefit with the use of antioxidant vitamins alone. Cilostazol alone and in combination with probucol has also been shown to have some benefit over placebo when administered for 6 months after coronary angioplasty [44]. However, no medication has been adequately tested to determine efficacy in the prevention of intracranial restenosis.

Vascular Perforation or Rupture

Vascular perforation can occur when angioplasty causes target artery rupture or with guidewire perforation of a more distal artery. Target artery rupture is uncommon [27, 42, 45]; it is avoidable by using a balloon diameter smaller than the expected normal diameter of the target artery and avoiding overdilatation. Wire perforation of distal arteries may be less often fatal, but nonetheless devastating. The roadmap technique aids in positioning the wire in a large distal branch; during balloon advancement, careful attention to wire stability minimizes movement of its tip in narrow, easily perforated segments. Complications of artery rupture and perforation are particularly troublesome when full anticoagulation with heparin and GP IIB/IIIA blockades are used. In such cases, rapid reversal of anticoagulation and transfusion of platelets is paramount. Standard procedures of emergency resuscitation are required that include securing a safe airway, monitoring or providing adequate ventilation, controlling blood pressure, and correcting coagulopathy. After emergency CT scanning, the patient should be monitored in an intensive care unit until near normal coagulation has returned. Attempts at surgical evacuation prior to reversal are unlikely to prove successful. With appropriate reversal of pharmacological coagulopathy and supportive care, however, an excellent recovery may be possible (fig. 3).

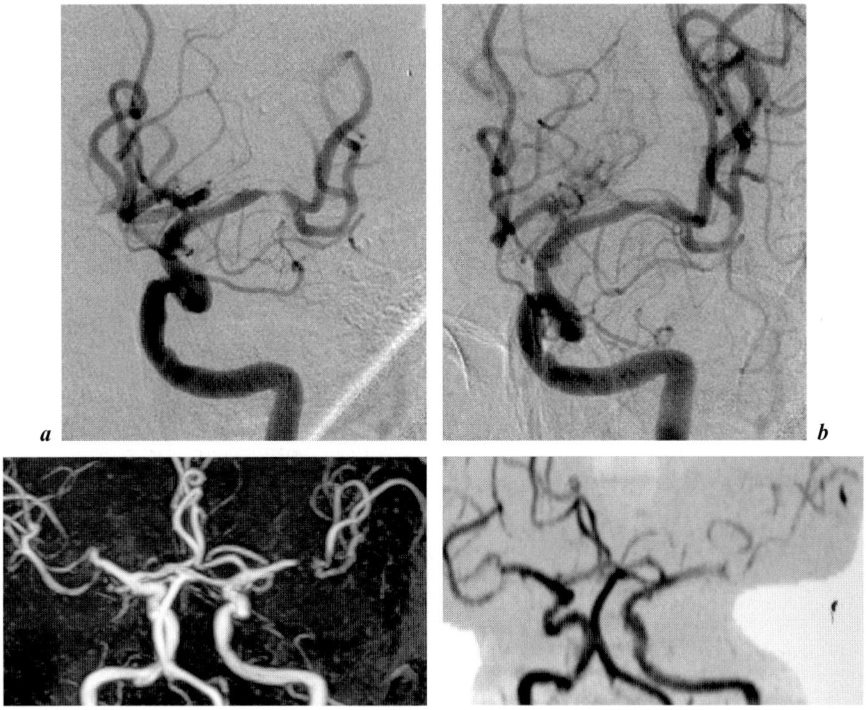

a b c d

Fig. 3. Dissection resulting in restenosis. ***a*** Digital subtraction angiogram of a patient who presented with recurrent left MCA TIAs while on warfarin. ***b*** When we could not navigate a stent into the lesion, we used angioplasty with a balloon matched to the artery size that caused dissection within the plaque (arrow) shown on this angiogram. Initially, the patient's symptoms resolved. ***c*** Three months later, the patient developed recurring TIAs that resolved with recumbency. Magnetic resonance angiography (MRA) reveals recurrent stenosis at the angioplasty sight. ***d*** After confirming hypoperfusion with a SPECT scan, the patient underwent an ECIC bypass and symptoms resolved. Six months later, he remains symptom free, with a patent graft shown by this MRA scan and on examination.

Long-Term Results

Procedural success, which is defined as stenosis reduction to less than 30%, can be achieved in 60–80% of patients with currently available devices [25–28]. Periprocedural neurological complication rates in recent series have been approximately 10%. Among those who are successfully treated, about 90% remain clinically stable or improve at 6 months to 1 year follow-up [23, 46], and few patients require additional treatment.

References

1 Failure of extracranial-intracranial arterial bypass to reduce the risk of ischemic stroke. Results of an international randomized trial. The EC/IC Bypass Study Group. N Engl J Med 1985;313: 1191–1200.

2 Ausman JI, Diaz FG: Critique of the extracranial-intracranial bypass study. Surg Neurol 1986; 26:218–221.

3 Haas WK, Fields WS, North RR, et al: Joint study of extracranial arterial occlusion. II. Arteriography, techniques, sites and complications. JAMA 1968;203:961–968.

4 Connors JJ III: Intracranial angioplasty; in Connors JJ III, Wojak JC (eds): Interventional Neuroradiology: Strategies and Practical Techniques. Philadelphia, Saunders, 1999, pp 500–555.

5 Craig DR, Meguro K, Watridge C, Robertson JT, Barnett HJ, Fox AJ: Intracranial internal carotid artery stenosis. Stroke 1982;13:825–828.

6 Moufarrij NA, Little JR, Furlan AJ, Williams G, Marzewski DJ: Vertebral artery stenosis: Long-term follow-up. Stroke 1984;15:260–263.

7 Marzewski DJ, Furlan AJ, St Louis P, Little JR, Modic MT, Williams G: Intracranial internal carotid artery stenosis: Long-term prognosis. Stroke 1982;13:821–824.

8 Prognosis of patients with symptomatic vertebral or basilar artery stenosis. The Warfarin-Aspirin Symptomatic Intracranial Disease (WASID) Study Group. Stroke 1998;29:1389–1392.

9 Borozan PG, Schuler JJ, LaRosa MP, Ware MS, Flanigan DP: The natural history of isolated carotid siphon stenosis. J Vasc Surg 1984;1:744–749.

10 Thijs VN, Albers GW: Symptomatic intracranial atherosclerosis: Outcome of patients who fail antithrombotic therapy. Neurology 2000;55:490–497.

11 Chimowitz MI, Kokkinos J, Strong J, Brown MB, Levine SR, Silliman S, Pessin MS, Weichel E, Sila CA, Furlan AJ, et al: The Warfarin-Aspirin Symptomatic Intracranial Disease Study. Neurology 1995;45:1488–1493.

12 Grubb RL Jr, Derdeyn CP, Fritsch SM, Carpenter DA, Yundt KD, Videen TO, Spitznagel EL, Powers WJ: Importance of hemodynamic factors in the prognosis of symptomatic carotid occlusion. JAMA 1998;280:1055–1060.

13 Gruntzig A, Schneider HJ: The percutaneous dilatation of chronic coronary stenoses – Experiments and morphology. Schweiz Med Wochenschr 1977;107:1588.

14 Higashida RT, Halbach VV, Cahan LD, Brant-Zawadzki M, Barnwell S, Dowd C, Hieshima GB: Transluminal angioplasty for treatment of intracranial arterial vasospasm. J Neurosurg 1989;71: 648–653.

15 Konishi Y, Maemura E, Sato E, Hara M, Takeuchi K: A therapy against vasospasm after subarachnoidal haemorrhage: Clinical experience of balloon angioplasty. Neurol Res 1990;12: 103–105.

16 Eskridge JM, Newell DW, Pendleton GA: Transluminal angioplasty for treatment of vasospasm. Neurosurg Clin N Am 1990;1:387–399.

17 Dion JE, Duckwiler GR, Vinuela F, Martin N, Bentson J: Pre-operative micro-angioplasty of refractory vasospasm secondary to subarachnoid hemorrhage. Neuroradiology 1990;32:232–236.

18 Cook HA: Cerebral angioplasty: A new treatment for vasospasm secondary to subarachnoid hemorrhage. J Neurosci Nurs 1990;22:319–321.

19 Brothers MF, Holgate RC: Intracranial angioplasty for treatment of vasospasm after subarachnoid hemorrhage: Technique and modifications to improve branch access. AJNR Am J Neuroradiol 1990;11:239–247.

20 Bracard S, Picard L, Marchal JC, Ducrocq X, Per A, Czorny A, Islak C, Roy D, Roland J, Lepoire J: Role of angioplasty in the treatment of symptomatic vascular spasm occurring in the post-operative course of intracranial ruptured aneurysms. J Neuroradiol 1990;17:6–19.

21 Clark WM, Barnwell SL, Nesbit G, O'Neill OR, Wynn ML, Coull BM: Safety and efficacy of percutaneous transluminal angioplasty for intracranial atherosclerotic stenosis. Stroke 1995;26: 1200–1204.

22 Higashida RT, Tsai FY, Halbach VV, Dowd CF, Hieshima GB: Cerebral percutaneous transluminal angioplasty. Heart Dis Stroke 1993;2:497–502.

23 Terada T, Higashida RT, Halbach VV, Dowd CF, Nakai E, Yokote H, Itakura T, Hieshima GB: Transluminal angioplasty for arteriosclerotic disease of the distal vertebral and basilar arteries. J Neurol Neurosurg Psychiatry 1996;60:377–381.
24 Takis C, Kwan ES, Pessin MS, Jacobs DH, Caplan LR: Intracranial angioplasty: Experience and complications. AJNR Am J Neuroradiol 1997;18:1661–1668.
25 Mori T, Fukuoka M, Kazita K, Mori K: Follow-up study after intracranial percutaneous transluminal cerebral balloon angioplasty. AJNR Am J Neuroradiol 1998;19:1525–1533.
26 Nahser HC, Henkes H, Weber W, Berg-Dammer E, Yousry TA, Kuhne D: Intracranial vertebrobasilar stenosis: Angioplasty and follow-up. AJNR Am J Neuroradiol 2000;21:1293–1301.
27 Marks MP, Marcellus M, Norbash AM, Steinberg GK, Tong D, Albers GW: Outcome of angioplasty for atherosclerotic intracranial stenosis. Stroke 1999;30:1065–1069.
28 Connors JJ III, Wojak JC: Percutaneous transluminal angioplasty for intracranial atherosclerotic lesions: Evolution of technique and short-term results. J Neurosurg 1999;91:415–423.
29 Mori T, Mori K, Fukuoka M, Arisawa M, Honda S: Percutaneous transluminal cerebral angioplasty: Serial angiographic follow-up after successful dilatation. Neuroradiology 1997;39: 111–116.
30 Chimowitz MI: Angioplasty or stenting is not appropriate as first-line treatment of intracranial stenosis. Arch Neurol 2001;58:1690–1692.
31 Qureshi AI, Luft AR, Sharma M, Guterman LR, Hopkins LN: Prevention and treatment of thromboembolic and ischemic complications associated with endovascular procedures. I. Pathophysiological and pharmacological features. Neurosurgery 2000;46:1344–1359.
32 Cross DT III, Derdeyn CP, Moran CJ: Bleeding complications after basilar artery fibrinolysis with tissue plasminogen activator. AJNR Am J Neuroradiol 2001;22:521–525.
33 Sherman DG: Antithrombotic therapy in the acute phase: New approaches. Cerebrovasc Dis 2001;11(suppl 1):49–54.
34 Qureshi AI, Saad M, Zaidat OO, Suarez JI, Alexander MJ, Fareed M, Suri K, Ali Z, Hopkins LN: Intracerebral hemorrhages associated with neurointerventional procedures using a combination of antithrombotic agents including abciximab. Stroke 2002;33:1916–1919.
35 Ringer AJ, Qureshi AI, Fessler RD, Guterman LR, Hopkins LN: Angioplasty of intracranial occlusion resistant to thrombolysis in acute ischemic stroke. Neurosurgery 2001;48:1282–1290.
36 Qureshi AI, Siddiqui AM, Suri MF, Kim SH, Ali Z, Yahia AM, Lopes DK, Boulos AS, Ringer AJ, Saad M, Guterman LR, Hopkins LN: Aggressive mechanical clot disruption and low-dose intraarterial third-generation thrombolytic agent for ischemic stroke: A prospective study. Neurosurgery 2002;51:1319–1329.
37 Alazzaz A, Thornton J, Aletich VA, Debrun GM, Ausman JI, Charbel F: Intracranial percutaneous transluminal angioplasty for arteriosclerotic stenosis. Arch Neurol 2000;57:1625–1630.
38 Barakate MS, Snook KL, Harrington TJ, Sorby W, Pik J, Morgan MK: Angioplasty and stenting in the posterior cerebral circulation. J Endovasc Ther 2001;8:558–565.
39 Stauffer JC, Eeckhout E, Goy JJ, Nacht CA, Vogt P, Kappenberger L: Major dissection during coronary angioplasty: Outcome using prolonged balloon inflation versus coronary stenting. J Invasive Cardiol 1995;7:221–227.
40 Lee JH, Kwon SU, Suh DC, Kim JS: Percutaneous transluminal angioplasty for symptomatic middle cerebral artery stenosis: Long-term follow-up. Cerebrovasc Dis 2003;15:90–97.
41 Suh DC, Sung KB, Cho YS, Choi CG, Lee HK, Lee JH, Kim JS, Lee MC: Transluminal angioplasty for middle cerebral artery stenosis in patients with acute ischemic stroke. AJNR Am J Neuroradiol 1999;20:553–558.
42 Callahan AS III, Berger BL: Balloon angioplasty of intracranial arteries for stroke prevention. J Neuroimaging 1997;7:232–235.
43 Tardif JC, Cote G, Lesperance J, Bourassa M, Lambert J, Doucet S, Bilodeau L, Nattel S, de Guise P: Probucol and multivitamins in the prevention of restenosis after coronary angioplasty. Multivitamins and Probucol Study Group. N Engl J Med 1997;337:365–372.
44 Sekiya M, Funada J, Watanabe K, Miyagawa M, Akutsu H: Effects of probucol and cilostazol alone and in combination on frequency of poststenting restenosis. Am J Cardiol 1998;82: 144–147.

45 Volk EE, Prayson RA, Perl J II: Autopsy findings of fatal complication of posterior cerebral circulation angioplasty. Arch Pathol Lab Med 1997;121:738–740.
46 Lylyk P, Cohen JE, Ceratto R, Ferrario A, Miranda C: Angioplasty and stent placement in intracranial atherosclerotic stenoses and dissections. AJNR Am J Neuroradiol 2002;23:430–436.

Andrew Ringer, MD
c/o Editorial Office, Department of Neurosurgery, Neuroscience Institute
ML 0515, 231 Albert Sabin Way
Cincinnati, Ohio 45267-0515 (USA)
Tel. +1 513 558 3563, Fax +1 513 558 7702, E-Mail editor@mayfieldclinic.com

Horowitz MB, Levy EI (eds): Neuroendovascular Surgery.
Prog Neurol Surg. Basel, Karger, 2005, vol 17, pp 101–121

Endovascular Therapy for Intracranial Aneurysms: A Historical and Present Perspective

Michael B. Horowitz[a], *Elad I. Levy*[b], *Amin Kassam*[a], *Phillip D. Purdy*[a]

[a] Center for Cranial Nerve Disorders, UPMC Presbyterian, Pittsburgh, Pa., USA
[b] Millard Filmore Hospital, Dept. of Neurosurgery, Buffalo, N.Y., USA

As we enter the new millennium and exit the Decade of the Brain neurosurgeons treating neurovascular disease must be acutely aware of the changing landscape with regard to aneurysm therapy. As new interventional procedures develop, traditional concepts concerning aneurysm treatment are being challenged by a group of radiologists and neurosurgeons who seek to occlude these lesions through endovascular routes. Cognizance of prior works relating to endovascular and nontraditional exovascular aneurysm therapy is important if we are to understand the foundation on which the growing specialty of endovascular neurosurgery is built. Such knowledge also provides practitioners with a new view on past ideas that may become pertinent in the future. The goal of this review is not to be inclusive of all papers published on the topic of endovascular aneurysm therapy, but rather to provide the reader with a chronological framework for understanding the field's evolution to its current status so that future treatment can be anticipated and proposed.

Pre-20th Century

During the 19th century innovative endovascular techniques emerged for the treatment of peripheral aneurysms. These techniques included the use of both heated needles and large pins to incite clot formation in these lesions. This technique was abandoned due to the unpredictable degree and time course of clot formation. During this same time period Moore introduced 26 yards of metallic coil into a thoracic aorta aneurysm. Though this patient died of sepsis the autopsy demonstrated that the aneurysm 'was filled, for the most part, with a fibrinous coagulum'. This technique was replicated by others over the ensuing years. Modifications included the use of metal watch springs, steel wire, silvered copper, and gold wire. By 1907 Boinet reported 34 cases of aortic aneurysms treated with wire insertion of which 30 patients died within 12 months of therapy. The concept of providing denser coil packing of aneurysms using trocars, cannulas, and ram rods is credited to Sir D'Arcy Power and G.H. Colt. Electrothrombosis was also developed in this century to induce dense coagulum in experimental models. In 1879, Corradi postulated that a combination of electrical current and permanent metallic coil deposition would provide the greatest chance for aneurysm thrombosis. This technique was referred to as the Moore-Corradi method. Following Barwell's report of a similar technique in 1886 this method also became known as the Barwell method [69a].

1960s

In 1964 Luessenhop and Velasquez [44] tried to occlude an aneurysm by advancing a silicon balloon into a supraclinoid carotid lesion. Although this treatment was unsuccessful it represented the first attempt by a neurosurgeon to treat an intracranial aneurysm using endovascular technique. In 1965 Alksne and Fingerhut [2] reported their experimental findings using a magnet and 3-μm-diameter carbonyl iron spheres suspended in 25% polyvinylpyrolidine to occlude arteries and aneurysms. Using a magnet applied to the external surface of a dog femoral artery and an aneurysm pouch made on a dog femoral artery these authors injected their iron particle suspension into the descending aorta via a catheter and occluded the vessel beneath the magnet in one experiment and the aneurysm pouch in another. In 1969, Alksne and Rand [3] published their results relating to metallic thrombosis of aneurysms in 9 patients. Three patients had partial aneurysm occlusion, 1 of whom reruptured and the other of whom suffered a middle cerebral artery (MCA) occlusion secondary to an embolus. Six patients had complete aneurysm occlusion. Three Hunt and Hess grade 1 patients did well. One Hunt and Hess grade 3 patient failed to recover and two Hunt and Hess grade 4 patients suffered anterior cerebral artery strokes secondary to vessel thrombosis after aneurysm occlusion. While Alksne and Rand experimented with iron as an embolic agent to occlude aneurysms, Mullan et al. [51, 52] in Chicago concentrated on the concept of aneurysm thrombosis using electric current. In 1964 and 1965 Mullan and others in his group reported their initial work involving the direct and stereotactic insertion of needles and copper wires transfundally into ruptured and unruptured aneurysms. Once the aneurysm was punctured, 200–2,000 mA would be applied to the electrode for 1–2 h. Arteriograms performed every 30 min charted the progress of thrombus formation within the fundus. Of 12 patients reported in the 1965 paper, 1 worsened following the procedure (8.3%). No rebleeding occurred at 6- to 14-month follow-up although 3 patients required surgical clipping due to aneurysm recurrence. While this therapy offered an alternative to surgical clipping, the authors felt that control of the degree of thrombosis was exceedingly difficult.

1970s

In 1973 Serbinenko [68] expanded the concept of Luessenhop and Velasquez and selectively obliterated an aneurysm using a latex balloon. In 1974 he reported two additional cases of aneurysm treatment using detachable balloons [68]. While Serbinenko continued his pioneering balloon work in Russia, Mullan [53] in 1974 reported his additional experience using electrothrombosis to treat 61 aneurysms. This series reported a 6.5% procedural death rate secondary to bleeding or excessive thrombosis and a 3.2% stroke rate. In 1977, Alksne and Smith [4] described their experience embolizing an anterior communicating artery aneurysm with carbonyl iron and methymethacrylate introduced stereotactically into the aneurysm fundus. This report provided no details regarding the procedure itself or the patient outcome. While Alksne [2, 3, 4] used iron as an embolic agent, Sheptak et al. [69] reported a series of 20 patients whose aneurysms were treated by injecting isobytyl-2-cyanoacrylate into the fundus under direct visualization or using a stereotactic technique. Sixteen patients achieved good to excellent results, 2 worsened and 2 died (one death occurred 3 years following the procedure). Eighteen patients had follow-up arteriography 10–14 days after the procedure. Seven had complete occlusion and 11 had incomplete occlusion. Two patients rehemorrhaged within 1 month of treatment and were found at surgery to have bled from an unoccluded portion of the lesion. Both recovered in good to excellent condition. In 1978, Debrun et al. [13] described his results using balloons to treat 14 carotid siphon aneurysms. Eight lesions were successfully treated, with parent vessel preservation in five. Three patients died and 2 suffered postprocedural hemiplegia.

1980s

In 1981, Debrun et al. [15] reported nine cases of aneurysms treated using detachable balloons placed in proximal parent vessels. In 1982 Romodanov and Shcheglov [25] reported 137 intravascular occlusions of saccular aneurysms using detachable balloons [25]. Fifteen patients had parent vessel occlusion and

93 had selective fundal obliteration with parent vessel preservation. Three patients were reported to have aneurysm recanalization and 3 patients died from vessel thrombosis. In 1984 Berenstein et al. [7] described nine cavernous aneurysms, one vertebral aneurysm and one posterior inferior cerebellar artery aneurysm that were treated with proximal vessel balloon occlusion. One embolic complication was listed. Hieshima and Higashida [25] reported cases of balloon embolization of aneurysms in 1987 and 1988 [25]. In 1989 Higashida et al. [27] published their group's experience with 26 aneurysms treated using balloon embolization. Sixty-five percent of the cases had selective aneurysm occlusion with parent vessel sparing while the remainder had parent vessel sacrifice. Complications included an 11% incidence of transient ischemic events, 11% incidence of stroke, and 20% incidence of death secondary to immediate or delayed aneurysm rupture.

1990s

The use of balloons for aneurysms was again reported by Higashida et al. [28] in 1990. In this paper the author described his group's use of balloons to manage 87 cavernous carotid artery aneurysms between 1981 and 1989. Seventy-eight percent of these patients had their internal carotid artery occluded across or just proximal to the aneurysm neck while 22% had selective aneurysm occlusion and vessel preservation. All patients that had vessel sacrifice had partial or complete symptom alleviation and aneurysm thrombosis. Sixty-three percent of selectively embolized aneurysms were occluded at follow-up and 37% had greater than 85% thrombosis. Stroke rate was 4.6%. Other reports from the 1990s regarding the use of detachable balloons included Scheglov's 725 cases [25], Serbinenko's 267 cases [25], George's 92 cases [25], and Hodes' 16 cases [25]. Good results from these series ranged from 43 to 80%. Mortality rates were 5–8% and neurological morbidity was less than 10%. In 1991 Moret et al. [49] also reported his results with attempted balloon treatment of 128 aneurysms. Of 101 treated lesions 91 had selective placement of the balloon within the fundus and 10 had aneurysm and parent vessel occlusion. Eighteen recurrences were recorded in the selective group (20%). Six of these were successfully retreated. Four patients died from postprocedural hemorrhage and 10 patients suffered neurological deficits secondary to thrombi and emboli [49].

Endovascular therapy for aneurysms shifted focus in the 1990s from balloon occlusion to platinum coil occlusion. This shift grew out of dissatisfaction with the ability of balloons to adequately fill a complex geometrical shape without either leaving unprotected fundus or creating a ball valve system of aneurysm refilling. It was also spurred on by the development of catheters and guidewires that allowed safe, selective catheterization of the neck and fundus, thus permitting delivery of highly pliable coils that easily and atraumatically assumed the shape of the aneurysm thus permitting more complete occlusion. In 1990 and 1991 Dowd et al. [16], Arnaud [in 25] and Higashida et al. [29] selectively embolized intracranial aneurysms using platinum coils. The single greatest problem with platinum minicoil insertion, however, remained the inability to control the embolic agent once it was pushed out of the catheter and into the aneurysm. Inadvertent migration of these highly thrombogenic devices into distal vasculature made their use for embolization of aneurysms a dangerous procedure.

In 1991 Guglielmi et al. [22], an Italian neurosurgeon, revolutionized the endovascular treatment of aneurysms by introducing a device that permitted introduction of platinum coils into the aneurysm fundus with relative security. Guglielmi's invention of the Guglielmi detachable coils (GDC) permitted the interventionalist to place a coil attached to a stainless steel guide wire into an aneurysm and consider its position and effectiveness. Once the physician was satisfied with the coil's position an electric current was applied to the portion of the guide wire that remained in the operator's hand outside the femoral sheath. The electric current would electrolytically dissolve the connection between the guide wire and the platinum coil thus ultimately separating the two and releasing the coil from its tether. Once this was achieved the guide wire was removed and another coil advanced into the aneurysm fundus. The process was repeated until the aneurysm no longer opacified on follow-up arteriograms. In addition to electrolytically releasing the coil, Guglielmi felt that the positive current promoted thrombosis within the fundus by attracting negatively charged blood elements such as red blood cells, white blood cells, platelets, and fibrinogen. He based this belief on earlier work by Mullan [51, 52, 53] (see previous section) and Araki [in 29]. In the same journal issue where Guglielmi published his experimental work on GDC he published his group's results in 15 patients treated in 1990 [22]. The new system achieved immediate 70–100% intra-aneurysmal occlusion. There were no periprocedural strokes or deaths and only one transient aphasia. In 1992 Guglielmi's group [23] published the first multicenter results with GDC. The results in 43 posterior fossa aneurysms with 1- to 18-month follow-up showed 81% immediate complete occlusion in small-necked lesions and 15% immediate complete occlusion in wide-necked aneurysms. Eighty-five percent of wide-necked aneurysms and 19% of small-necked aneurysms demonstrated 70–98% thrombosis. Procedure-related morbidity and mortality was 4.8 and 2.4%, respectively.

While Guglielmi and others focused on GDC, other individuals continued to work with alternative methods. In 1992 and again in 1994 Kinugasa et al.

[33, 34] published preliminary experience with the embolization agent cellulose acetate polymer. Nine aneurysms were filled with this agent. One patient suffered a transient neurological deficit and 1 patient bled 3 months following treatment. In 1993 Casasco et al. [11] reported results with nonretrievable fibered platinum coils in 71 aneurysms. With mean angiographic follow-up of 13 months, immediate complete occlusion was achieved in 84.5% of cases with the remainder achieving greater than 90% occlusion. Clinical follow-up at 6 months revealed 85% good outcome. A 3% procedural subarachnoid hemorrhage (SAH) rate, 3% delayed bleed rate, and 6% procedural stroke rate were recorded. In 1994 Halbach et al. [26] investigated the role of embolization in alleviating the effects of mass effect from large aneurysms compressing brain parenchyma and cranial nerves. Of 26 aneurysms located both inside and outside the cavernous sinus presenting with symptoms from mass effect, 50% had symptom resolution, 43.3% improved and 7.7% demonstrated no change. The authors felt that the improved group tended to have less calcium in the aneurysm wall and had symptoms for a shorter duration of time.

Since 1994 the vast majority of published work regarding endovascular aneurysm therapy has centered on the GDC system. In 1994 Zubillaga et al. [77] reported 79 GDC cases with 85% complete occlusion in small-necked aneurysms and 15% complete occlusion in wide-necked aneurysms. This paper pointed out the difficulty of achieving compete obliteration of wide-necked aneurysms with GDC alone. In 1995 Byrne et al. [9] reported two GDC series. The first involved 50 GDC embolized aneurysms. Immediate complete obliteration was achieved in 100, 95, and 85% of small, large, and giant aneurysms, respectively. Follow-up in 42 aneurysms at 6 months demonstrated recanalization of 17% of small aneurysms, 19% of large aneurysms, and 50% of giant aneurysms. Procedure-related morbidity and mortality was 18 and 4%, respectively. The second series involved 69 lesions. Morbidity and mortality in that study was 4.3 and 1.4% [10]. Richling et al. [64] also published a series of 74 GDC cases in 1995 with a 76% greater than 90% occlusion rate at 8 months in 40 patients eligible for follow-up. In 1996 the series McDougall et al. [47] of 33 coiled basilar apex aneurysms demonstrated 84% greater than 90% obliteration at a mean follow-up of 12 months with a 3% stroke rate and 3% delayed rebleed rate. The 1996 series of Pierot et al. [59] of 35 basilar aneurysms noted a 74% immediate complete occlusion rate and 27% greater than 90% occlusion rate [47]. There was a 3% procedure-related death rate and no delayed hemorrhages although the follow-up period was less than 2 years [59].

1997 was a banner year for publications of case series relating to GDC aneurysm embolization. The 6-month results of Nichols et al. [57] of 28 ruptured posterior circulation aneurysms showed 90% incidence of 99–100% obliteration and 5% incidence of 90% obliteration. Treatment-related mortality was 3.8%, and serious procedure-related morbidity was 0%. Roy's group [65] reported their results with 28 ophthalmic segment aneurysms. At a mean follow-up of 15 months 50% complete occlusion was achieved while 39% of cases were classified as having small residual necks. Procedural stroke rate was 3.5%. There were no deaths and no cases of rebleeding. Vinuela et al. [74], in 1997, reported the results of an 8-center series of 403 coiled aneurysms treated between 1990 and 1995. Small-necked small aneurysms achieved 71% complete occlusion, large aneurysms achieved 35% complete occlusion and giant aneurysms achieved 50% complete occlusion. Complications included aneurysm perforation (2.7%), unintended parent vessel occlusion (3%), embolization (2.48%), and procedure-related death (1.74%). Because this series included patients treated from the initial use of first generation GDC to more current use of improved coils in more experienced hands it is difficult to determine the true current status of GDC procedures from such an extended study. The UCLA group in this same year published their midterm clinical results in 100 consecutive patients [46]. Seventy-five percent of patients achieved excellent clinical status and 11% achieved good status at a mean follow-up of 3.5 years. Rehemorrhage rate was 0% with small aneurysms, 4% with large aneurysms, and 33% with giant aneurysms. Of note, 20 of the 100 coiled cases were referred for interventional therapy because of initial failed surgical clipping. In 1997 Raymond et al. [61] added to his group's reporting of location-specific results with aneurysm coiling by publishing findings in 31 embolized basilar apex lesions. Forty-two percent of cases had immediate complete obliteration while 52% had small residual necks or dog ears. There were no incidences of post-coiling SAH over a short follow-up period. Repeat angiography at 6 months in 27 cases revealed 30% complete obliteration and 59% residual neck. Seven recurrences over 42 months required retreatment. Death and stroke rate related to therapy were each 3%. Raymond and Roy [62] in this same year described a series of 75 treated ruptured aneurysms (likely including cases from their two previous series on ophthalmic and basilar lesions) in which 40% had complete occlusion, 37% had residual neck or dog ear and 16% had fundal opacification. Follow-up angiography in 50 cases at 6 months demonstrated 46% complete occlusion and 42% residual neck or dog ear. Good to excellent outcomes were achieved in 72% of cases. Klein et al. [35] also contributed to the 1997 literature with a series of 21 basilar aneurysms. Immediate complete and greater than 90% occlusion was achieved in 67 and 33% of patients, respectively. Fourteen patients underwent repeat arteriography after 6 months. Three patients with partially occluded wide-necked aneurysms recanalized. All 3 were retreated without incident. No episodes of rebleeding occurred. While 24% of patients had one posterior cerebral artery occluded only 1 patient suffered a permanent neurological deficit. Overall morbidity and mortality was 5% each.

Beginning in 1997 papers began to be published about the management of wide-necked aneurysms. It was clear from previous reports that larger aneurysms with larger necks were not being satisfactorily obliterated over the short or long term. The difficulty in managing these lesions was devising a means of keeping the coils within the aneurysm fundus and neck during and after deployment. In 1997 and 1998 Moret et al. [50], Levy [41, 42], Mericle et al. [48], and Sanders et al. [66] each published their experiences using Moret's balloon remodeling technique. These authors demonstrated excellent short-term results with lesions that were previously untreatable using endovascular methods. Surprisingly, the morbidity and mortality rates in this small number of cases was no higher than with routine GDC embolization. Taking advantage of the availability of new, highly flexible coronary stents Higashida et al. [30] in 1997 took an alternative approach to the treatment of previously endovascularly unapproachable fusiform aneurysms. The author's group placed a stent across the lesion and then advanced coils through the stent's walls to thrombose the aneurysm outside the stent while maintaining a patent lumen. The use of stents to maintain a parent vessel lumen while at the same time to provide a buttress that keeps coils within the aneurysm was expanded upon by Lanzino et al. [37] and Sekhon et al. [67] in 1998. Five lesions were treated in all, four of which were combined with GDC embolization. Results over the short term have been favorable.

Some of the first medium-term outcome studies began to surface in 1998. In a series by Leber et al. [38], the medium-term results of endovascular treatment of intracranial aneurysms were compared to open surgery. These authors examined the results of 162 aneurysms treated microsurgically and 134 aneurysms treated by endovascular embolization with GDC. The mean follow-up was 2.6 years (range 1.5–4.5 years). Each group was well matched for age, sex and location of aneurysms. These authors reported no significant difference between the patient outcomes of surgically or endovascularly treated aneurysms. Most importantly, they concluded that endovascular surgery was not associated with a higher risk of morbidity and mortality than surgical clipping of aneurysms, but cautioned that the results have to be confirmed by a longer follow-up.

Collice et al. [12] attempted to develop a multidisciplinary approach to aneurysm management. Using a team of neurosurgeons, neuroradiologists, and neurointerventionalists, aneurysms were selected for either endovascular coiling or surgical clipping. Their analysis was stratified into four groups: group 1 consisting of 104 surgically treated patients with ruptured aneurysms, group 2 with 27 patients with ruptured aneurysms treated with GDC, group 3 had 7 patients who were untreated, and group 4 had 26 patients with unruptured aneurysms treated with either modality. These authors suggested that aneurysms should be surgically clipped if they occur in patients less than 65 years old, in good condition, and Hunt and Hess grade 1–3, except if it is a basilar apex aneurysm. Patients in poor health or older than 65 should be treated endovascularly regardless of the Hunt and Hess grade, except if the aneurysm is in the MCA distribution. Giant aneurysms should be treated on a case-by-case basis. Though the number of cases treated with coiling were too small to derive statistical significance for their proposed management scheme, patient outcomes were comparable with many purely surgical series.

In 1998 additional series were published regarding longer-term GDC results. The series of Debrun et al. [14] of 152 aneurysms contained two important observations. The first was that when a coiled aneurysm had a dome-to-neck ratio greater than or equal to two there was a 72–80% incidence of complete occlusion. The second was that operator experience counted. In their last 123 cases there was no procedural mortality, 1% morbidity and 2.5% incidence of procedure-related transient ischemic events. While the authors describe using balloon remodeling in selected cases it is not clear how often this technique was utilized with those aneurysms having a dome:neck <2. Turjman et al. [72] seconded Debrun's statement concerning the importance of experience in achieving better results with GDC embolization. In their paper factors predicting incomplete occlusion were larger aneurysm size, more direct direction of inflow, and earlier chronological treatment. The 1998 series of Keuther et al. [36] of 77 aneurysms also provided some additional longer-term evaluation of the GDC technology. Average angiographic and clinical follow-up in this study was 1.4 and 2.2 years, respectively. Initial angiographic results demonstrated 40% complete occlusion, 52% near complete occlusion (90–99%) and 8% incomplete occlusion (less than 90%). Procedure-related morbidity was 9.1%. No completely occluded lesions hemorrhaged over 1.9 years of follow-up while 2.6% of incompletely occluded lesions bled in a delayed fashion (1.4%/year). Follow-up angiograms in 45 patients revealed 41% complete occlusion, 46% near complete occlusion, and 13% incomplete occlusion. For those patients presenting with mass effect, 35% had complete resolution of their symptoms following embolization, 40% improved and 25% were either unchanged or worsened. The report of Eskridge and Song [17] relating to basilar apex aneurysms in the Food and Drug Administration's multicenter trial revealed greater than 90% occlusion in 75% of cases. Mortality, however, in the unruptured group was 12% while rebleeding rates for unruptured and ruptured aneurysms ranged from 3.3 to 4.1%. Permanent neurological deficits in unruptured aneurysms was 9%. Why unruptured aneurysms did so poorly in this study requires further investigation. In 1999 Murayama et al. [54] reported results with GDC embolization of 120 incidental aneurysms. Initial complete or near compete occlusion was achieved in 91% of cases. Ninety-five percent of patients had no neurological change following their procedure. Delayed bleed rate was 0.8% and the average hospital stay was 3.3 days.

In 1999 Byrne et al. [10] published their results over the past 5 years in 317 GDC-treated patients followed for a median of 22.3 months (6- to 65-month range). Stable occlusion was found in 86 and 85% of small and large aneurysms, respectively, while recurrent filling was identified in 14.7%. Rebleeding secondary to recurrence was 0.8% in year 1, 0.6% in year 2, and 2.4% in year 3. Excellent or good outcomes at 6 months were achieved in 87.8% of patients with Hunt and Hess 1 and 2, 71.4% of patients with Hunt and Hess 3, and 48.5% of patients with Hunt and Hess 4 and 5.

In 1999, Vanninen et al. [73] published their group's 3-month results in the first prospective, randomized study comparing GDC to surgery. Aneurysms felt by a group of neurosurgeons and radiologists to be good candidates for either therapy were randomized to one treatment arm and matched for age, Hunt and Hess score, Fischer grade, site, and size. With the exception of anterior communicating artery aneurysms, angiographic results were equivalent between the two modalities with better results in the endovascular group for posterior circulation lesions. One rebleed occurred in an incompletely coiled lesion. Technique-related mortality was 4 and 2% for the surgical and endovascular groups, respectively. The 3-month angiograms demonstrated 95% of coiled aneurysms to be 95% or more occluded (67% complete occlusion, 28% small-neck remnant). Immediate postsurgical angiograms demonstrated 74% complete ligation. Small-neck remnants were visible in 16% and fundal filling was visible in 9%. Follow-up studies for the surgical group were not performed. Functional outcome in the two groups was not revealed in the paper of Vanninen et al. but will, according to the authors, be disclosed after 1 year's follow-up.

Gruber et al. [21] revealed their 1999 findings relating to basilar apex aneurysms and demonstrated what they felt were comparable if not better results with endovascular therapy. Forty-one patients with equivalent aneurysms (from an anatomical standpoint) were compared retrospectively. Overall outcomes, while better for GDC, are difficult to interpret because more patients in the surgical group were treated following SAH. However, when the SAH group was looked at separately the authors found the following trends. Despite a mean Hunt and Hess score of 3 in the GDC group and 1 in the surgical group, Glasgow Outcome Scale (GOS) at discharge was identical, mean length of stay was 60% shorter in the GDC group, and hospital charges were on average 36% lower for embolized patients. Initial anatomical outcomes were better in the surgical group with a 20% incidence of aneurysm remnant in the exovascular group and 34% incidence of less than 95% obliteration in the endovascular group. Shortcomings of this paper include no long-term follow-up, and poor angiographic follow-up. Despite lower initial hospital costs, the authors fail to take into consideration the expense of repeat imaging studies in both groups. Another report by Steiger et al. [71] compared surgical versus endovascular management of 100 posterior circulation aneurysms. The authors utilized surgical clipping as treatment of choice in good grade patients, while endovascular therapy was preferred for patients in poor clinical grade or if the aneurysm was judged difficult to be accessed surgically. Complications resulting in significant morbidity or mortality occurred following 5 surgical and 1 endovascular procedures. These authors concluded that decision making regarding treatment modalities should be based on aneurysm location, rather than size and shape. Additionally, it was the authors' opinion that endovascular treatment for small, narrow-necked aneurysms on proximal arteries of the posterior circulation should be considered, whereas large, distal, and broad-necked aneurysms should be managed with surgery.

In a larger series of 395 aneurysms, Lot et al. [43] attempted to compare results of endovascular and microsurgical aneurysm management. One hundred and two aneurysms were surgically clipped, and 293 were coiled. Management decisions were based on the shape of the aneurysm as follows: aneurysms with a narrow neck and a ratio of neck diameter by sac diameter of less than one third were selected for coiling. Satisfactory results with complete or subtotal obliteration and no recanalization were obtained in 92% before retreatment and in 98.8% after retreatment. For both clipped or coiled aneurysms, good and excellent clinical outcomes were achieved in 90% of small aneurysms and in 86.5% of larger ones. These authors' results are comparable to large series reported for microsurgical management alone. Hence, with appropriate patient selection, Lot et al. demonstrated that endovascular management is an excellent alternative for many aneurysms with suitable anatomy.

Additional 1999 manuscripts by Bavinzski et al. [6], Solander et al. [70] and Yamaura et al. [76] point out the utility of using GDC in the management of basilar aneurysms, multiple intracranial aneurysms, and dissecting aneurysms. Each of these works documents the excellent short-term clinical outcomes following endovascular therapy. As with all recent publications longer-term results relating to rebleeding are yet to be available.

In 1999, Kahara et al. [32] examined an often overlooked aspect of aneurysm management, that of postoperative psychosocial sequelae. Postprocedural clinical, emotional and social outcome on a disability scale was reported for 44 GDC-treated patients and 106 surgically treated patients. In 75% of the embolized aneurysms successful occlusion was achieved, procedural mortality was 2.3% and morbidity 18.2%. The clinical status of all 15 patients with unruptured aneurysms was preserved. Of the surviving 29 patients with ruptured aneurysms 12 improved and the rest preserved their clinical status. In 91% of the embolized patients and in 85% of the operated patients clinical, emotional and social outcome was categorized as good or excellent (not statistically significant).

An earlier paper by Bavinzski et al. [6] during the same year reported 4 patients, 3 with recurrent and 1 with residual aneurysm after surgical clipping. Each was retreated using GDCs. Three aneurysms were totally occluded and the other had greater than 90% occlusion, suggesting that treatment with GDC is a viable alternative to reoperation in all patients with recurrent or residual aneurysms following a failed attempt at surgical obliteration [7].

Also during 1999 Regli et al. [63] examined the angiographic and anatomical features that determine whether a patient with an unruptured MCA aneurysm is treated using endovascular coil placement or surgical clipping. They attempted prospective management of their patients, with endovascular management as the first-line treatment, and surgical clipping reserved only for those aneurysms that could not be coiled. Thirty consecutive patients harboring 34 unruptured MCA aneurysms were evaluated. Of 34 unruptured MCA aneurysms, only 2 (6%) were successfully embolized and 32 (94%) were clipped. Of these 32 surgically treated aneurysms, in 11 (34%) an attempt at GDC embolization had failed, whereas in 21 (66%) primary clipping was performed because of unfavorable anatomy. GDC treatment failed in 11 (85%). An unfavorable dome/neck ratio (<2) and an arterial branch originating at the aneurysm base were the reasons for embolization failure. These authors concluded that for unruptured MCA aneurysms, surgical clipping appears to be the most efficient treatment option. It is clear that larger studies in centers with significant endovascular and surgical experience need to conduct similar studies.

In 1999, Gruber et al. [20] reported their experience with the coiling of giant and very large wide-necked aneurysms. To evaluate prevention of aneurysmal rebleeding, relief of aneurysmal mass effect, and prevention of embolic complications, they studied 30 patients with 31 giant or very large aneurysms that were considered unacceptable risk/benefit ratios for open surgery and were treated with GDCs. With GDC treatment, 73.3% of the population experienced excellent to good recoveries (GOS scores of 4 or 5), with a 13.3% procedure-related morbidity rate and a 6.7% procedure-related mortality rate. Two hemorrhaging episodes occurred after GDC treatment (annual bleeding rate, 2.5%; 2 hemorrhaging episodes/79.2 patient-year). Symptoms related to aneurysmal mass effect were improved in 45.5% of the patients presenting with signs of neural compression. Among 23 patients with 24 aneurysms with angiographic follow-up, complete or nearly complete occlusion was observed for 17 aneurysms (71%) over an angiographic follow-up period of 24.3 ± 19.6 months. A single total embolization served as definitive treatment for only 12.5% of the giant aneurysms and 31% of the very large aneurysms, with the remaining aneurysms requiring repeat coiling. The report of Gruber et al. demonstrates that endovascular treatment of giant aneurysms may be an attractive option with procedure-related morbidity and mortality rates comparable to (or less than) those for open surgery. Retreatment, however, should be anticipated.

The evolution of stent technology now allows for the endovascular treatment of previously untreatable aneurysms. Wilms et al. [75] described a case of a superior hypophyseal aneurysm of the left supraclinoid carotid artery that could not be treated with GDC, even in combination with a supporting non-detachable balloon. Following unsuccessful surgical clipping, treatment consisted of the placement of a stent over the neck of the aneurysm, advancement of a microcatheter through the stent mesh, and subsequent embolization with a GDC resulting in an excellent outcome. Additional recently reported applications of stent technology include rescue from procedural complications and the solving of complex clinical problems. Pride et al. [60] described 3 patients who underwent unplanned placement of intravascular stents. In 2 patients a stent was used to provide stabilization of irretrievable included unraveled fragments of a GDC and a partially deployed coronary stent. No periprocedural neurological complications were encountered and a 6-month follow-up angiography in 1 patient showed only minimal myointimal hyperplasia induced by stent-stabilized GDC fragments adjacent to the internal carotid vessel wall. Similarly, Fessler et al. [18] described the use of a low profile, navigable stent to trap an extruded GDC during treatment of an internal carotid artery cavernous segment aneurysm. A paper by Johnston et al. [31] in 1999 retrospectively compared matched groups of coiled and clipped unruptured aneurysms treated at university hospitals. This paper demonstrated a significant reduction in adverse outcomes, in-patient deaths, length of stay, and mean charges when aneurysms were treated with endovascular techniques.

2000s

In 2000, an excellent retrospective analysis of 112 patients with ruptured posterior circulation aneurysms was reported by Lempert et al. [40]. The Hunt and Hess grade at presentation of treated patients was I in 26 patients (24%), II in 24 (22%), III in 27 (25%), IV in 24 (22%), and V in 8 (7%). Clinical follow-up for the total population was achieved in 104 of 109 patients (96%), with a mean duration of 13.1 months. Angiographic follow-up for the subset excluding parent vessel occlusion cases was obtained in 93% of cases, with a mean duration of 7.2 months. One hundred and nine of 112 of cases (97%) were successfully embolized. The mean projected area of the aneurysm occlusion was 94.6%. At the latest clinical follow-up, 81 of 109 patients (74%) achieved a good recovery with a GOS score of I, 10 of 109 (9%) were moderately (GOS II) and 5 of 109 (5%) were severely (GOS III) disabled, 1 of 109 (1%) remained in a vegetative state (GOS IV), and 12 of 109 (11%) were dead. Of the subset of 77 patients with Hunt and Hess grades 1–3, 68 (88%) achieved good clinical outcomes (GOS I). Procedure-related permanent morbidity was 2.8%, and 1 patient had a second SAH following a partial coiling [40]. The observed favorable outcome and low morbidity in this group of high-risk patients suggest that GDC embolization may be a first-line intervention for the management of patients with ruptured posterior circulation aneurysms.

With the recent development and refinement of catheter-delivered stent technology there has been a paradigm shift in the treatment of wide-necked aneurysms. Catheter-delivered stents facilitate the delivery of stents through tortuous anatomy without the added risks of vessel injury or aneurysmal rupture following balloon inflation (as is required with balloon-mounted stents). Early work by Wanke et al. [74a] demonstrated the ability of such stents to provide a permanent buttress that can contain coils within the aneurysm and achieve satisfactory lesion packing. As next generation technology becomes available the use of such stents may replace the use of balloon remodeling for wide-necked or complex aneurysms.

International Subarachnoid Aneurysm Trial (ISAT)

International Subarachnoid Aneurysm Trial (ISAT) was the first prospective, randomized study comparing aneurysm coiling and clipping. Randomization commenced in 1994 with a pilot phase. This study, published in 2002, studied clinical outcomes at 2 and 12 months and reported primary outcome with a modified Rankin scale. The trial was prematurely stopped by the oversight committee following planned interim analysis due to overwhelming evidence demonstrating increased morbidity following aneurysm clipping as compared to endovascular therapy. Twenty-four percent of patients treated with endovascular coiling were dependent or dead at 12 months as compared to 31% of those patients who underwent clipping. The relative and absolute risk reductions in death and dependency following treatment with endovascular versus surgical intervention were 22.6 and 7%, respectively. The risk of rebleeding following endovascular therapy was 2/1,276 patient-years [30a].

Future Directions

As we embark on the new millennium, we will appreciate novel advances in basic science as it directly enhances our surgical devices. One example is the report by Murayama et al. [56]. This study describes a porcine model in which ion-implanted surface modification technology creates a borderless surface on protein-coated platinum GDCs. GDCs were coated with either type I collagen, fibronectin, vitronectin, laminin, or fibrinogen. A total of 56 experimental aneurysms were constructed microsurgically in the common carotid arteries of 28 swine. These experimental aneurysms were embolized with standard GDCs ($n = 23$), collagen GDC-Is ($n = 11$), vitronectin GDC-Is ($n = 6$), laminin GDC-Is ($n = 4$), fibrinogen GDC-Is ($n = 6$), and fibronectin GDC-Is ($n = 6$). They found no evidence of increased coil friction/stiffness was observed during delivery of GDC-Is through microcatheters in this aneurysm model. Interestingly, more scar formation and neoendothelium at the neck of aneurysms were observed macroscopically when treated with GDC-Is. Perhaps most importantly, differences in the proportion of neck coverage between standard GDCs (48.3 ± 20.5%) and all GDC-I groups were observed (collagen GDC-I 89.4 ± 14.9%, $p < 0.01$; vitronectin GDC-I 71.5 ± 7.0%, $p < 0.05$; laminin GDC-I 76.5 ± 11.0%, $p < 0.05$; fibrinogen GDC-I 74.8 ± 13.9%, $p < 0.05$; fibronectin GDC-I 87.5 ± 15.0%, $p < 0.01$). Histopathology demonstrated well-organized fibrous tissue bridging the aneurysms' necks when using GDC-Is, whereas only a fibrin-like thin layer covered the standard GDC surfaces. Another article by Murayama et al. [55] in 2001 demonstrated the efficacy of treating experimental porcine aneurysms with a coil coated with bioabsorbable polymeric material. These coils led to improved formation of neointima across aneurysm necks when compared to standard platinum coils. This promising data may decrease the chances of coil compaction and aneurysm recanalization in future years.

Summary and Conclusion

Endovascular therapy for cerebral aneurysms has grown exponentially over the last few years owing to the development of new technologies that have made aneurysm occlusion safer and more effective. With the advent of new catheters, wires, balloons, flexible stents, aneurysm neck occlusion devices, and embolic agents the field of endovascular neurosurgery will continue to make inroads into aneurysm treatment.

We continually look towards past series to compare the results of open surgical and endovascular aneurysm therapy. Comparisons, however, are difficult for a number of reasons. Many surgical series have poor angiographic follow-up thus making it hard to ascertain the true complete occlusion rate of open surgical clipping. Those studies that do provide follow-up have often depended upon low-resolution limited-view intraoperative angiography. Nevertheless, studies that have specifically examined the role of postsurgical angiography have pointed out the relatively high incidence of unexpected findings. Macdonald et al. [45] found unexpected residual aneurysms, unexpected completely unclipped aneurysms, and unexpected major vessel occlusions in 4, 4 and 12% of his group's cases, respectively. The same investigator in another study found unexpected arterial occlusions in 6% of cases and unexpected persistently filling aneurysms in 10% of cases studied following clipping [1]. A study of 597 clipped aneurysms by Le Roux revealed 5.7% incidence of aneurysm remnants and 5.7% incidence of vessel occlusion [39]. Payner et al. [58], likewise, identified 3.2% incidence of unexpected residual aneurysm and 1.9% incidence of parent vessel stenosis. In all of these series the operant word is 'unexpected'. The postsurgery angiography papers and other surgical series do not take into consideration and rarely report the cases of expected and accepted residual aneurysm neck or fundus opacification following clipping. While residual neck is not necessarily reported as a failure of surgical treatment in cases of wide-necked, calcified, or atherosclerotic aneurysms located throughout the cerebral arterial tree it is invariably viewed as an example of technical failure in endovascular series. All neurosurgeons that care for aneurysms are aware that preservation of afferent and efferent vessels often necessitates incomplete aneurysm clipping. Nevertheless, such remnants are rightfully viewed as surgical necessity rather than failure. A second reason why comparisons are difficult is the duration of time it will take to determine rehemorrhage rates from coiled lesions. Perhaps the best paper relating to the topic of rerupture of aneurysm is by Feuerberg et al. [19]. The author followed 28 residual aneurysms following clipping and found a rebleed rate of 0.38–0.79%/year during the observation period (4–13 years). It is difficult to conceive of a study involving endovascular cases that will be able to follow patients with residual necks and small dog ears long enough to determine the rebleed rate in view of the small rebleed rate observed by Feuerberg et al. While we know from past experience that continued fundal filling puts patients at high risk for rebleeding, as endovascular devices improve fundal filling will become a rare entity. As a result, comparisons between exo- and endovascular surgery will rest on the true incidence of and risk posed by residual aneurysm neck. Having viewed the extent of retrospective literature available on endovascular aneurysm treatment many will propose a large, multicenter prospective randomized trial comparing embolization with open surgery. The limitations of such a study, however, are obvious. We already know from most published papers that the short-term (less than 5-year) rehemorrhage rate, stroke rate, procedural death rate and 1-year clinical outcomes of endovascular therapy compare favorably with open surgical clipping. What we do not know is the long-term durability of endovascular aneurysm occlusion. In an ever-changing field with new devices being released on an almost monthly basis at what point do we feel comparisons are justified?

Likewise, what group will fund a study that runs long enough to detect the true rebleed rate from residual necks and dog ears? By the time such a study was completed, the technology used to conduct its endovascular arm would be obsolete thus depreciating the study's value. Such questions and dilemmas are ones endo-/exovascular neurosurgeons will face for years to come. Only with continued observation can we hope to come up with an ultimate answer.

References

1 Alexander TD, Macdonald RL, Weir B, Kowalczuk A: Intraoperative angiograpphy in cerebral aneurysms surgery: A prospective study of 100 craniotomies. Neurosurgery 1996;39:10–18.

2 Alksne JF, Fingerhut AG: Magnetically controlled metallic thrombosis of intracranial aneurysms: A preliminary report. Bull Los Angeles Neurol Soc 1965;3:154–155.

3 Alksne JF, Rand RN: Current status of metallic thrombosis of intracranial aneurysms. Prog Neurol Surg 1969;2:212–274.

4 Alksne JF, Smith RW: Iron-acrylic compound for stereotactic aneurysm thrombosis. J Neurosurg 1977;47:137–141.

5 Bavinski G, Killer M, Gruber A, Reinprecht A, Gross CE, Richling B: Treatment of basilar artery bifurcation aneurysms by using Guglielmi detachable coils: A 6-year experience. J Neurousrg 1999;90:843–852.

6 Bavinzski G, Talazoglu V, Killer M, Gruber A, Richling B, al-Shameri R: Coiling of recurrent and residual cerebral aneurysms after unsuccessful clipping. Minim Invasive Neurosurg 1999;42/1: 22–26.

7 Berenstein A, Ransohoff J, Kupersmith M, Flamm E, Graeb D: Transvascular treatment of giant aneurysms of the cavernous and vertebral arteries. Surg Neurol 1984;21:3–12.

8 Byrne JV, Adams CBT, Kerr RSC, Molyneux AJ: Endosaccular treatment of inoperable intracranial aneurysms with platinum coils. Br J Neurosurg 1995;9:585–592.

9 Byrne JV, Molyneux AJ, Brennan RP, Renowden SA: Embolization of recently ruptured intracranial aneurysms. J Neurol Neurosurg Psychiatry 1995;59:616–620.

10 Byrne JV, Sohn MJ, Molyneux AJ: Five-year experience using coil embolization for ruptured intracranial aneurysms: Outcomes and incidence of late rebleeding. J Neurosurg 1999;90: 656–663.

11 Casasco AE, Aymard A, Gobin P, Houdart E, Rogopoulos A, George B, Hodes JE, Cophignon J, Merland JJ: Selective endovascular treatment of 71 intracranial aneurysms with platinum coils. J Neurosurg 1993;79:3–10.

12 Collice M, D'Aliberti G, Arena O, Fontana RA, Bizzozero L, Solaini C, Villa F, Talamonti G, Levati A, Scialfa G, Boccardi E, Branca V: Multidisciplinary (surgical and endovascular) approach to intracranial aneurysms. J Neurosurg Sci 1998;42(1 suppl 1):131–140.

13 Debrun G, Lacour P, Caron JP, Hurth M, Comoy J, Keravel Y: Detachable balloon and calibrated-leak balloon techniques in the treatment of cerebral vascular lesions. J Neurosurg 1978;49: 635–649.

14 Debrun GM, Aletich VA, Kehrli P, Misra M, Ausman, Charbel F: Selection of cerebral aneurysms for treatment using Guglielmi detachable coils: The preliminary University of Illinois at Chicago experience. Neurosurgery 1998;43:1281–1297.

15 Debrun GM, Fox AJ, Drake C: Giant unclippable aneurysms: Treatment with balloons. AJNR Am J Neuroradiol 1981;2:167–173.

16 Dowd CF, Halbach VV, Higashida RT: Endovascular coil embolization of unusual posterior inferior cerebellar artery aneurysms. Neurosurgery 1990;27:954–961.

17 Eskridge JM, Song JK: Endovascular embolization of 150 basilar tip aneurysms with Guglielmi detachable coils: Results of the Food and Drug Administration multicenter clinical trial. J Neurosurg 1998;89:81–86.

18 Fessler RD, Ringer AJ, Qureshi AI, Guterman LR, Hopkins LN: Intracranial stent placement to trap an extruded coil during endovascular aneurysm treatment: Technical note. Neurosurgery 2000; 46/1:248–253.
19 Feuerberg I, Lindquist C, Lindqvist M, Steiner L: Natural history of postoperative aneurysm rests. J Neurosurg 1987;66:30–34.
20 Gruber A, Killer M, Bavinzski G, Richling B: Clinical and angiographic results of endosaccular coiling treatment of giant and very large intracranial aneurysms: A 7-year, single-center experience. Neurosurgery 1999;45:793–804.
21 Gruber DP, Zimmerman GA, Tomsick TA, van Loveren HR, Link MJ, Tew JM: A comparison between endovascular and surgical management of basilar artery apex aneurysms. J Neurosurg 1999;90:868–874.
22 Guglielmi G, Vinuela F, Dion J, Duckwiler G: Electrothrombosis of saccular aneurysms via endovascular approach. 2. Preliminary clinical experience. J Neurosurg 1991;75:8–14.
23 Guglielmi G, Vinuela F, Duckwiler G, Dion J, Lylyk P, Berenstein A, Strother C, Graves V, Halbach V, Nichols D, Hopkins N, Ferguson R, Sepetka I: Endovascular treatment of posterior circulation aneurysms by electrothrombosis using electrically detachable coils. J Neurosurg 1992; 77:515–524.
24 Guglielmi G, Vinuela F, Sepetka I, Macellari V: Electrothrombosis of saccular aneurysms via endovascular approach. 1. Electrical basis, technique, and experimental results. J Neurosurg 1991; 75:1–7.
25 Guterman LR, Hopkins LN: Endovascular treatment of cerebral aneurysms. Diagnosis and treatment; in Selman W (ed): Clinical Neurosurgery. The Congress of Neurological Surgeons, 1993, vol 40, pp 56–83.
26 Halbach VV, Higashida RT, Dowd CF, Barnwell SL, Fraser KW, Smith T, Teitelbaum GP, Jieshima GB: The efficacy of endovascular aneurysms occlusion in alleviating neurological deficits produced by mass effect. J Neurosurg 1994;80:659–666.
27 Higashida RT, Halbach VV, Cahan LD, Hieshima GB, Konishi Y: Detachable balloon embolization therapy of posterior circulation intracranial aneurysms. J Neurosurg 1989;71:512–519.
28 Higashida RT, Halbach VV, Dowd C, Barnwell SL, Dormandy B, Bell J, Hieshima GB: Endovascular detachable balloon embolization therapy of cavernous carotid artery aneurysms: Results in 87 cases. J Neurosurg 1990;72:857–863.
29 Higashida RT, Halbach VV, Dowd DF: Interventional neurovascular treatment of a giant intracranial aneurysms using platinum microcoils. Surg Neurol 1991;35:64–68.
30 Higashida RT, Smith W, Gress D, Urwin R, Dowd CF, Balousek PA, Halbach VV: Intravascular stent and endovascular coil placement for a ruptured fusiform aneurysm of the basilar artery: Case report and review of the literature. J Neurosurg 1997;87:944–949.
30a Molyneux A, Kerr R, Stratton I, Sandercock P, Clarke M, Shrimpton J, Holman R: International Subarachnoid Aneurysm Trial (ISAT) Collaborative Group: International Subarachnoid Aneurysm Trial (ISAT) of neurosurgical clipping versus endovascular coiling in 2143 patients with ruptured intracranial aneurysms: A randomised trial. Lancet 2002;360:1267–1274.
31 Johnston SC, Dudley RA, Gress DR, Ono L: Surgical and endovascular treatment of unruptured cerebral aneurysms at university hospitals. Neurology 1999;52:1799–1805.
32 Kahara VJ, Seppanen SK, Kuurne T, Laasonen EM: Patient outcome after endovascular treatment of intracranial aneurysms with reference to microsurgical clipping. Acta Neurol Scand 1999; 99/5:284–290.
33 Kinugasa K, Mandai S, Terai Y, Kamata I, Sugiu K, Ohmoto T, Nishimoto A: Direct thrombosis of aneurysms with cellulose acetate polymer. 2. Preliminary clinical experience. J Neurosurg 1992;77:501–507.
34 Kinugasa K, Mandai S, Tsuchida S, Sugiu K, Kamata I, Tokunaga K, Ohmoto T, Taguchi K: Cellulose acetate polymer thrombosis for the emergency treatment of aneurysms: Angiographic findings, clinical experience, and histopathological study. Neurosurgery 1994;34:694–701.
35 Klein GE, Szolar DH, Leber KA, Karaic R, Hausegger KA: Basilar tip aneurysm: Endovascular treatment with Guglielmi detachable coils – Midterm results. Radiology 1997;205: 191–196.

36 Kuether TA, Nesbit GM, Barnwell SL: Clinical and angiographic outcomes, with treatment data, for patients with cerebral aneurysms treated with Guglielmi detachable coils: A single-center experience. Neurosurgery 1998;43:1016–1025.

37 Lanzino G, Wakhloo AK, Fessler RD, Mericle RA, Guterman LR, Hopkins LN: Intravascular stents for intracranial internal carotid and vertebral artery aneurysms: Preliminary clinical experience. Neurosurg Focus 1998;5:1–8.

38 Leber KA, Klein GE, Trummer M, Eder HG: Intracranial aneurysms: A review of endovascular and surgical treatment in 248 patients. Minim Invasive Neurosurg 1998;41/2:81–85.

39 Le Roux PD, Elliott JP, Eskridge JM, Cohen W, Winn HR: Risks and benefits of diagnostic angiography after aneurysm surgery: A retrospective analysis of 597 studies. Neurosurgery 1998; 42:1248–1255.

40 Lempert TE, Malek AM, Halbach VV, Phatouros CC, Meyers PM, Dowd CF, Higashida RT: Endovascular treatment of ruptured posterior circulation cerebral aneurysms. Clinical and angiographic outcomes. Stroke 2000;31:100–110.

41 Levy DI, Ku A: Balloon-assisted coil placement in wide necked aneurysms. J Neurosurg 1997; 86:724–727.

42 Levy DI: Embolization of wide-necked anterior communicating artery aneurysms: Technical note. Neurosurgery 1997;41:979–982.

43 Lot G, Houdart E, Cophignon J, Casasco A, George B: Combined management of intracranial aneurysms by surgical and endovascular treatment. Modalities and results from a series of 395 cases. Acta Neurochir 1999;141:557–562.

44 Luessenhop AJ, Velasquez AC: Observations on the tolerance of intracranial arteries to catheterization. J Neurosurg 1964;21:85–91.

45 Macdonald RL, Wallace C, Kestle JRW: Role of angiography following aneurysm surgery. J Neurosurg 1993;79:826–832.

46 Malisch TW, Guglielmi G, Vinuela F, Duckwiler G, Gobin P, Martin NA, Frazee JG: Intracranial aneurysms treated with the Guglielmi detachable coil: Midterm clinical results in a consecutive series of 100 patients. J Neurosurg 1997;87:176–183.

47 McDougall CG, Halbach VV, Dowd CR, Higashida RT, Larsen DW, Hieshima GB: Endovascular treatment of basilar tip aneurysms using electrolytically detachable coils. J Neurosurg 1996;84: 393–399.

48 Mericle RA, Wakhloo AK, Rodriguez R, Guterman LR, Hopkins LN: Temporary balloon protection as an adjunct to endovascular coiling of wide-necked cerebral aneurysms: Technical note. Neurosurgery 1997;41:975–978.

49 Moret J, Boulin A, Mawad M, Castaings L: Endovascular treatment of berry aneurysms by endosaccular balloon occlusion. Neuroradiology 1991;33(suppl):135–136.

50 Moret J, Cognard C, Weill A, Castaings L, Rey A: The 'remodelling technique' in the treatment of wide neck intracranial aneurysms. Angiographic results and clinical follow-up in 56 cases. Intervent Neuroradiol 1997;3:21–35.

51 Mullan S, Beckman F, Vailati G: An experimental approach to the problem of cerebral aneurysms. J Neurosurg 1964;21:838–845.

52 Mullan S, Raimondi AJ, Dobben G, Vailati G, Hekmatpanah J: Electrically induced thrombosis in intracranial aneurysms. J Neurosurg 1965;22:539–547.

53 Mullan S: Experiences with surgical thrombosis of intracranial berry aneurysms and carotid cavernous fistulas. J Neurosurg 1974;41:657–670.

54 Murayama Y, Vinuela F, Duckwiler GR, Gobin YP, Guglielmi G: Embolization of incidental cerebral aneurysms using the Guglielmi detachable coil system. J Neurosurg 1999;90:207–214.

55 Murayama Y, Vinuela F, Tateshima S, Song JK, Nestor GR, Wallace MP: Bioabsorbable polymeric material for embolization of intracranial aneurysms: A preliminary experimental study. J Neurosurg 2001;94:454–463.

56 Murayama Y, Vinuela F, Suzuki Y, Akiba Y, Ulihoa A, Duckwiler GR, Gobin YP, Vinters HV, Iwaki M, Abe T: Development of the biologically active Guglielmi detachable coil for the treatment of cerebral aneurysms. II. An experimental study in a swine aneurysm model. AJNR Am J Neuroradiol 1999;20:1992–1999.

57 Nichols DA, Brown RD, Thielen KR, Meyer FB, Atkinson JLD, Piepgras DG: Endovascular treatment of ruptured posterior circulation aneurysms using electrolytically detachable coils. J Neurosurg 1997;87:374–380.

58 Payner TD, Horner TG, Leipzig TJ, Scott JA, Gilmor RL, DeNardo AJ: Role of intraoperative angiography in the surgical treatment of cerebral aneurysms. J Neurosurg 1998;88:441–448.

59 Pierot L, Boulin A, Castaings L, Rey A, Moret J: Selective occlusion of basilar artery aneurysms using controlled detachable coils: Report of 35 cases. Neurosurgery 1996;38:948–954.

60 Pride GL Jr, Horowitz MB, Purdy PD: Endovascular problem solving with intravascular stents. AJNR Am J Neuroradiol 2000;21:532–540.

61 Raymond J, Roy D, Bojanowski M, Moumdjian R, L'Esperance: Endovascular treatment of acutely ruptured and unruptured aneurysms of the basilar bifurcation. J Neurosurg 1997;86: 211–219.

62 Raymond J, Roy D: Safety and efficacy of endovascular treatment of acutely ruptured aneurysms. Neurosurgery 1997;41:1235–1246.

63 Regli L, Uske A, de Tribolet N: Endovascular coil placement compared with surgical clipping for the treatment of unruptured middle cerebral artery aneurysms: A consecutive series. J Neurosurg 1999;90:1025–1030.

64 Richling B, Gruber A, Bavinzski G, Killer M: GDC-system embolization for brain aneurysms-location and follow-up. Acta Neurochir (Wien) 1995;134:177–183.

65 Roy D, Raymond J, Bouthillier A, Bojarowski MW, Moumdjian R, L'Esperance G: Endovascular treatment of ophthalmic segment aneurysms with Guglielmi detachable coils. AJNR Am J Neuroradiol 1997;18:1207–1215.

66 Sanders WP, Burke TH, Mehta BA: Embolization of intracranial aneurysms with Guglielmi detachable coils augmented by microballoons. AJNR Am J Neuroradiol 1998;19:917–920.

67 Sekhon LHS, Morgan MK, Sorby W, Grinnell V: Combined endovascular stent implantation and endosaccular coil placement for treatment of a wide-necked vertebral artery aneurysm: Technical case report. Neurosurgery 1998;43:380–384.

68 Serbinenko FA: Balloon catheterization and occlusion of major cerebral vessels. J Neurosurg 1974;41:125–145.

69 Sheptak PE, Zanetti PH, Susen AF: The treatment of intracranial aneurysms by injection with a tissue adhesive. Neurosurgery 1977;1:25–29.

69a Siddique K, Alvernia J, Fraser K, Lanzino G: Treatment of aneurysms with wires and electricity: A historical review. J Neurosurg 2003;99:1102–1107.

70 Solander S, Ulhoa A, Vinuela F, Duckwiler GR, Gobin P, Martin NA, Frazee JG, Guglielmi G: Endovascular treatment of multiple intracranial aneurysms by using Guglielmi detachable coils. J Neurosurg 1999;90:857–864.

71 Steiger HJ, Medele R, Bruckmann H, Schroth G, Reulen HJ: Interdisciplinary management results in 100 patients with ruptured and unruptured posterior circulation aneurysms. Acta Neurochir 1999;141:359–366.

72 Turjman F, Massoud TF, Sayre J, Vinuela F: Predictors of aneurysmal occlusion in the period immediately after endovascular treatment with detachable coils: A multivariate analysis. AJNR Am J Neuroradiol 1998;19:1645–1651.

73 Vanninen R, Koivisto T, Sari T, Hernesniemi J, Vapalahti M: Ruptured intracranial aneurysms: Acute endovascular treatment with electrolytically detachable coils – A prospective randomized study. Radiology 1999;211:325–336.

74 Vinuela F, Duckwiler G, Mawad M: Guglielmi detachable coil embolization of acute intracranial aneurysms: Perioperative anatomical and clinical outcome in 403 patients. J Neurosurg 1997;86: 475–482.

74a Wanke I, Doerfler A, Schoch B, Stolke D, Forsting M: Treatment of wide necked intracranial aneurysms with a self expanding stent system: Intial clinical experience. AJNR Am J Neuroradiol 2003;24:1192–1199.

75 Wilms G, van Calenbergh F, Stockx L, Demaerel P, van Loon J, Goffin J: Endovascular treatment of a ruptured paraclinoid aneurysm of the carotid syphon achieved using endovascular stent and endosaccular coil placement. AJNR Am J Neuroradiol 2000;21:753–756.

76 Yamaura I, Tani E, Yokota M, Nakano A, Fukami M, Kaba K, Matsumoto T: Endovascular treatment of ruptured dissecting aneurysms aimed at occlusion of the dissected site by using Guglielmi detachable coils. J Neurosurg 1999;90:853–856.
77 Zubillaga AF, Guglielmi G, Vinuela F, Duckwiler GR: Endovascular occlusion of intracranial aneurysms with electrically detachable coils: Correlation of aneurysm neck size and treatment results. AJNR Am J Neuroradiol 1994;15:815–820.

Dr. Michael B. Horowitz
Department of Neurosurgery
Director, Neuroendovascular Surgery
UPMC Presbyterian
Suite B-400, 200 Lothrop Street, Pittsburgh, 15213-2582, USA
Tel. +1 412 647 3685, Fax +1 412 647 7000, E-Mail horowitzmb@upmc.edu

Horowitz MB, Levy EI (eds): Neuroendovascular Surgery.
Prog Neurol Surg. Basel, Karger, 2005, vol 17, pp 122–134

Endovascular Management of Wide-Necked Aneurysms

Michael B. Horowitz[a], *Elad I. Levy*[b]

[a] Center for Cranial Nerve Disorders, UPMC Presbyterian, Pittsburgh, Pa., USA
[b] Millard Filmore Hospital, Dept. of Neurosurgery, Buffalo, N.Y., USA

Endovascular management of intracranial aneurysms using detachable platinum coils (Guglielmi detachable coils) was initially developed in 1990 by Guido Guglielmi, an Italian neurosurgeon. Working in collaboration with Fernando Vinuela, MD and others at the University of California at Los Angeles along with Target Therapeutics (Fremont, Calif., USA) the advent of endovascular obliteration of aneurysms became a commonplace practice. Many studies have shown equivalent or improved short- and medium-term outcomes when comparing matched groups of patients undergoing surgical and endovascular therapy. Despite advances, however, the treatment of wide-necked aneurysms (aneurysms with a fundus to neck ratio less than 2) remains problematic. Reasons for incomplete treatment include low volumetirc filling (20–30% of the sac filled with coils), coil compaction, and recanalization. Additionally, the lack of neointimal proliferation across these wide necks leads to a higher rate of recurrence. Results from early studies using single dimensional coils alone demonstrated 72–80% complete occlusion when the ratio was greater than 2 and 53% when it was lower. Inability to keep coils within these lesions, the posttreatment presence of aneurysm residual, and the occurrence of delayed aneurysm recanalization lead investigators to seek new ways to safely and effectively embolize these lesions. Techniques and devices aimed at treating wide-necked aneurysms will be focused upon in this review.

Definition of Wide-Necked Aneurysm

The term wide-necked aneurysm is a relative one. Rather than thinking of a wide neck as having to exceed a particular size, one should think of a wide neck as the neck's size as compared to the maximal fundal width. One characteristic of an aneurysm that is ideal for endovascular therapy is a fundus to neck ratio greater than 2. The greater this ratio the greater the disparity between the orifice and the body, thus making coil deposition easier and coil stability within the lesion higher. As the ratio falls, it is more difficult to prevent coils from herniating out of the fundus, through the neck, and into the parent vessel. In some cases wide-necked can be considered a neck that exceeds the diameter of the widest diameter coil. This diameter will depend upon the system used for embolization.

Techniques or Devices for Repairing Wide-Necked Aneurysms

A number of techniques and devices can be used when treating wide-necked aneurysms. These include balloon remodeling, use of three-dimensional coils (3DC), combined use of stents and coils, use of devices that span the neck, simultaneous deposition of more than one coil in an aneurysm, intentional partial aneurysm embolization, and combined exo- and endovascular treatment.

Balloon Remodeling

The balloon remodeling technique was initially promoted by Moret et al. [1997] in France who achieved total and near total occlusion of wide-necked lesions in 94% of cases. This maneuver involves simultaneous catheterization using both a microcatheter and nondetachable silicon balloon. The interventionalist may opt to pass both catheter and balloon through a single large guiding catheter (8 or 9 french) or work through two smaller guiding catheters (6 french) placed in each femoral artery with a balloon in one catheter and a microcatheter in another. Whichever technique is utilized is based upon the surgeon's comfort as well as the size of the proximal vessels. Advantages of the single guiding catheter technique are that only one femoral artery is punctured, a single guide catheter is placed in a feeding artery, that the surgeon can work from one side of the patient without having to reach across the patient's body, and that fewer catheters are utilized thus making catheter maintenance during the procedure simpler which in turn reduces the risk to the patient. Disadvantages involve the increased size of the guiding catheter which may increase the risk for vessel injury or occlusion. Advantages of the double guide catheter system reside in the smaller individual catheter size. When working in the internal carotid artery (ICA), for instance, one 6-french catheter can be placed in the ICA while the other remains in the common carotid artery. When working in the vertebral artery (VA) one catheter can be placed in the VA while the other is positioned in the

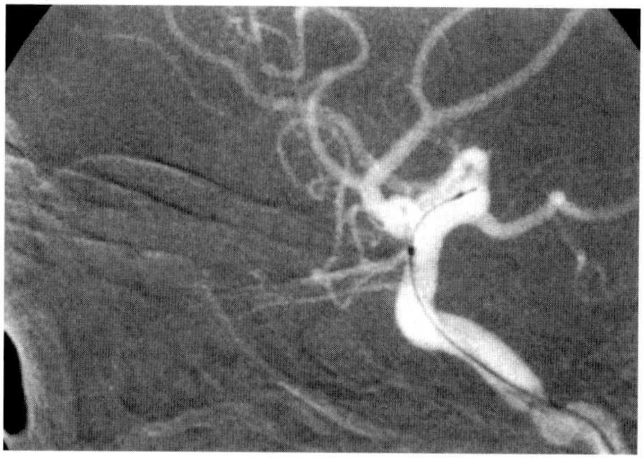

Fig. 1. Deflated angioplasty balloon positioned across the aneurysm neck.

subclavian artery or one catheter can be placed in each VA. In many cases, the ICA or VA diameter will be too small to accommodate a single 8- or 9-french or two 6-french catheters.

Once a stable guiding catheter platform is established, a nondetachable silicon microballoon, an intracranial angioplasty balloon, or a coronary angioplasty balloon is advanced to the level of the aneurysm neck. The microcatheter is then advanced into the aneurysm. Variable sized coils are placed into the aneurysm. If the coils have a tendency to herniate out of the aneurysm the balloon is gently inflated across the aneurysm neck while the coil is introduced. This keeps the coil in the fundus and out of the parent vessel and serves to shape the coil so that it assumes a convex configuration along the balloon interface. Once the coil is completely introduced the balloon is deflated. The coil is observed for a period to determine that it is stable and it is then detached. Sequential coils are introduced into the aneurysm using the same technique until the lesion is maximally filled (fig. 1–5).

Using balloon remodeling it is now possible to occlude many wide-necked aneurysms that were formerly not amenable to endovascular therapy. Nevertheless, this technique is not without its risks and drawbacks. While the procedure can be carried out by a single operator, it is easier to work with two endovascular surgeons one of whom maneuvers the balloon while the other introduces the coils. This requires manpower that is not always readily available. Inflation of the balloon across an unsecured aneurysm can lead to neck deformation and aneurysm rupture. Inflation of a balloon in a 5-mm or smaller vessel, if not performed carefully, can lead to vessel rupture or thrombosis. Use of a large guiding catheter or two smaller guiding catheters can increase the risk

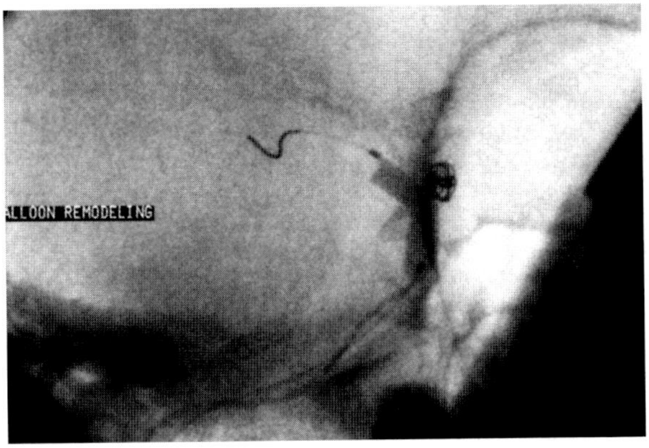

Fig. 2. Angioplasty balloon inflated across the aneurysm neck with coil deposited in the aneurysm.

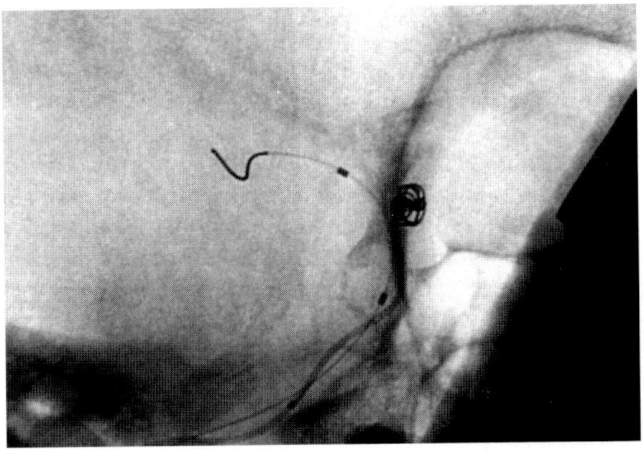

Fig. 3. Deflated angioplasty balloon across the aneurysm neck with coil in the aneurysm.

of vessel injury. Finally, the procedure requires experience that is only achieved through exposure to a busy endovascular practice. Many enodvascular surgeons may not have the opportunity to practice the technique often enough so as to develop the necessary skills. In the series of Moret et al. technique-related morbidity and mortality was 2 and 0%, respectively.

Three-Dimensional Coils

3DC are coils that assume a complex 3-dimensional configuration once exiting the catheter and entering the aneurysm fundus. Those manufactured by

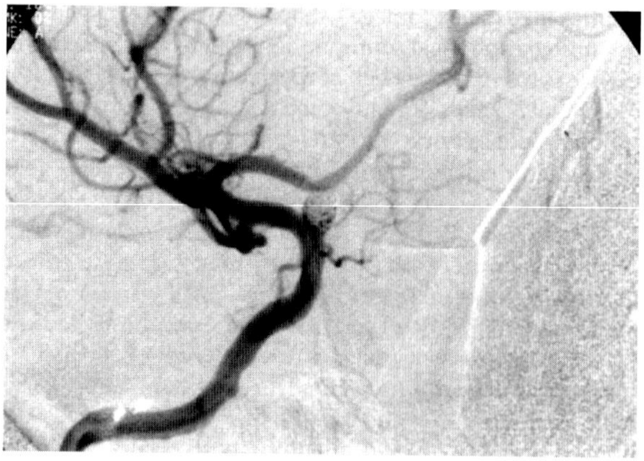

Fig. 4. Coiled wide-neck aneurysm following balloon remodeling procedure.

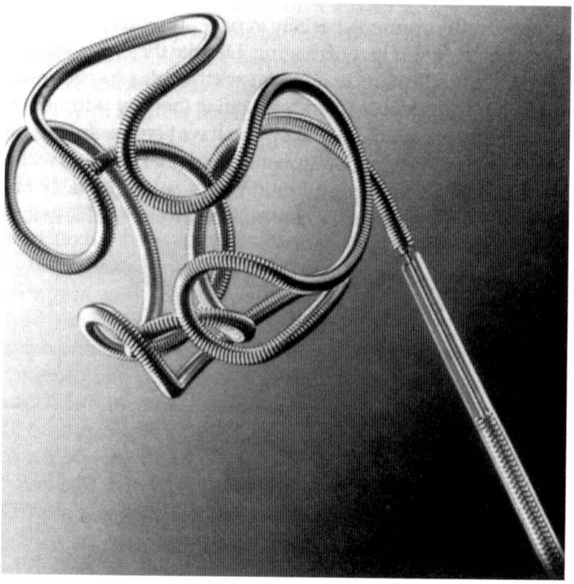

Fig. 5. Target 3-dimensional coil.

Target Therapeutics take on an omega shape at each turn eventually taking the configuration of a sphere (fig. 6). The goal of this device is to cover the aneurysm's neck making it less likely that subsequently introduced 3DC or regular coils will herniate out into the parent vessel.

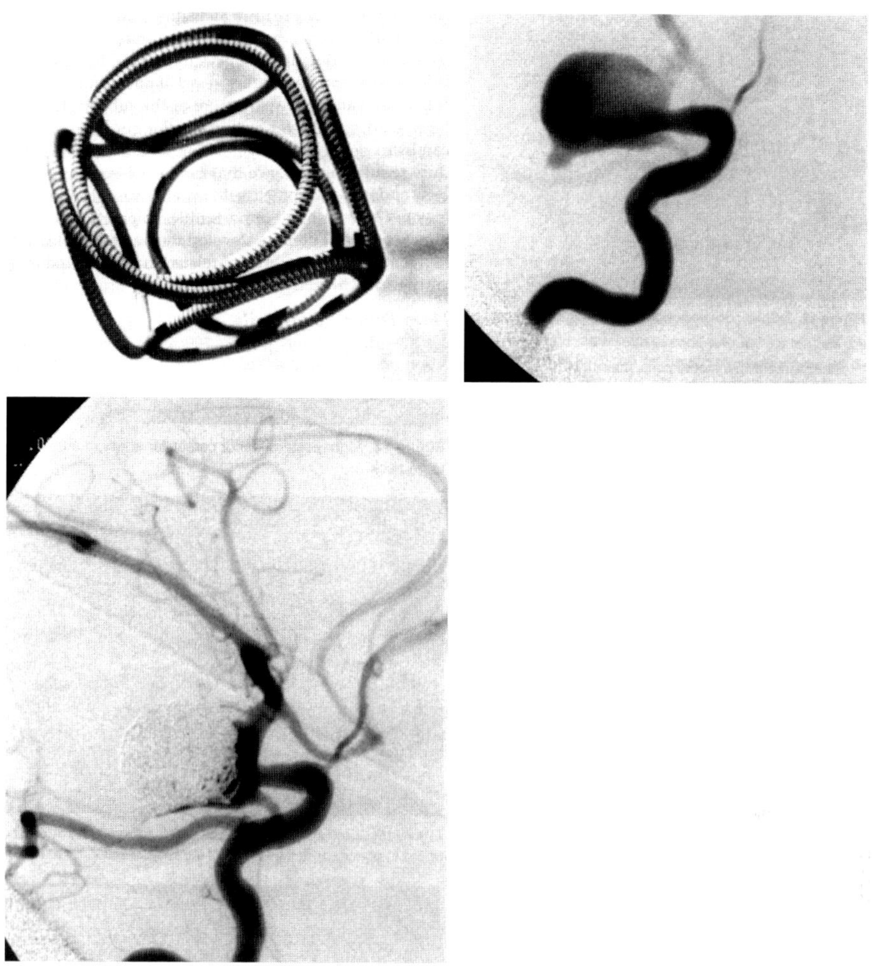

a b c

Fig. 6. ***a*** Micrus 3-dimensional coil. ***b*** Large wide-necked posterior carotid wall aneurysm. ***c*** Coiled posterior carotid wall aneurysm using 3DC.

3DC have proven very useful in the management of wide-necked aneurysms, obviating the need for balloon remodeling in many cases. Often either an initial framing coil is inserted into the aneurysm followed by helical coils which remain in the aneurysm due to the framing coil that covers the aneurysm neck. An alternative is to place framing coils of progressively smaller diameters into the aneurysm (analogous to Russian dolls) until the entire lesion is filled. These coils, however, are not a panacea and may make successful aneurysm obliteration at times difficult. These difficulties arise from the stiffer, less compliant quality

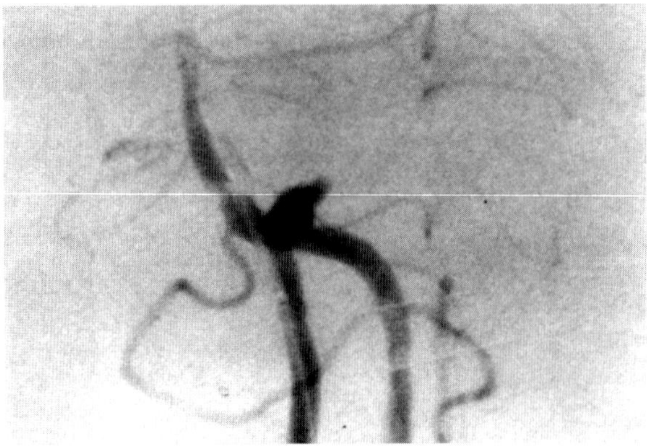

Fig. 7. Wide-necked vertebral confluence aneurysm.

of the coil. At times once the 3DC is deposited compartments can develop in the aneurysm that are difficult to later fill with regular coils. This is often not a long-term problem because the aneurysm's neck is ultimately well covered and thrombosis within the small fundal compartments occurs once the heparin wears off or is reversed. 3DC also have a tendency to place increased forces on the aneurysm wall due to the rigidity of the omega turns. This rigidity can increase the risk of aneurysm rupture especially in patients with recent subarachnoid hemorrhage. Despite these qualities, 3DC have made many aneurysms with fundus to neck ratios less than two amenable to endovascular therapy without the use of balloon remodeling. They have also been useful in cases where balloon remodeling alone could not keep coils within the fundus. Used in combination with an angioplasty balloon, 3DC can occlude many previously untreatable lesions.

Other 3DC manufactured by Micrus (Micrus, Mountain View, Calif., USA, Cordis-Johnson & Johnson, Miami Lakes, Fla., USA) also form a scaffolding within the aneurysm thus allowing for further deposition of coils without occluding the parent vessel (fig. 7). These devices are mechanically rather than electrolytically detached. Experience is limited and further work needs to be done to determine the long-term efficacy of this technology.

Stents and Coils

In certain situations an aneurysm neck is so wide relative to its fundus that it is impossible to keep coils within the lesion. In these situations it is often possible to cover the aneurysm neck with a coronary stent and then use the stent to hold the coils within the fundus (fig. 8–11). The patient is prepared with one

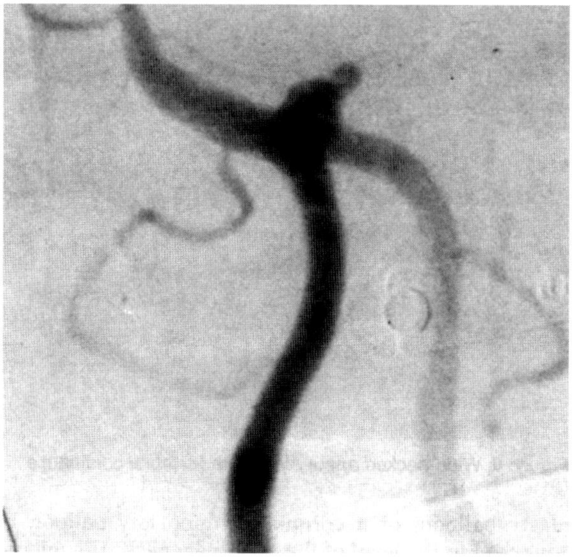

Fig. 8. Stent across aneurysm neck.

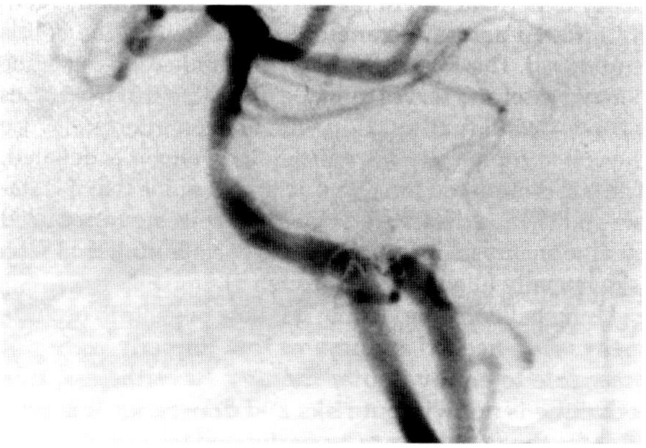

Fig. 9. Vertebral confluence aneurysm coiled with stent across neck.

or two guiding catheters as described in the section for balloon remodeling. A coronary stent is then advanced across the aneurysm neck and deposited. A 300-cm 0.014-inch guidewire is left across the stent until the end of the entire procedure in case access to the stent lumen is required. Once the stent is in position a microcatheter is advanced over a wire through a stent cell and into the aneurysm fundus. The aneurysm is then embolized with coils until it is

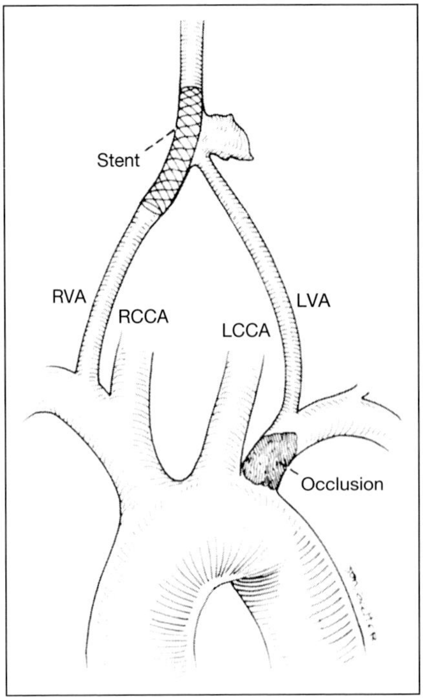

Fig. 10. Diagram of a stent across the vertebral confluence aneurysm neck. LCCA = Left common carotid artery; RCCA = right common carotid artery; LVA = left vertebral artery; RVA = right vertebral artery.

completely filled. The stent wall acts as a scaffolding holding the coils in the aneurysm and out of the parent vessel.

The combined use of stents and coils is not free of difficulties and risks. In some situations stents cannot expand to the degree needed. The largest coronary stent is manufactured at a diameter of 4.5 mm and will only open to a diameter of 4.7 mm (when overinflated). When the parent vessel is greater than 4.7 mm it may be impossible to open the stent and have it appose the vessel walls. If apposition fails to occur the stent will move and become either a source of emboli or an embolus itself. In other situations, despite the flexibility of newer coronary devices, the stent cannot be advanced through the numerous turns inherent in the intracranial vasculature. This makes it impossible to advance the stent to the required location. Attempts to place it through these turns can lead to vessel injury, dissection, occlusion, and subsequent stroke. Finally, the long-term sequelae of placing stents into small intracranial vessels are unknown. Intimal hyperplasia, the bane of interventional cardiologists, can lead to vessel stenosis over time thus predisposing patients to delayed cerebral ischemic symptoms.

The Neuroform stent (Target Therapeutics, Boston Scientific, Boston, Mass., USA) is the first stent manufactured specifically for intracranial aneurysm treatment. This device consists of a catheter-loaded stent that is unsheathed and

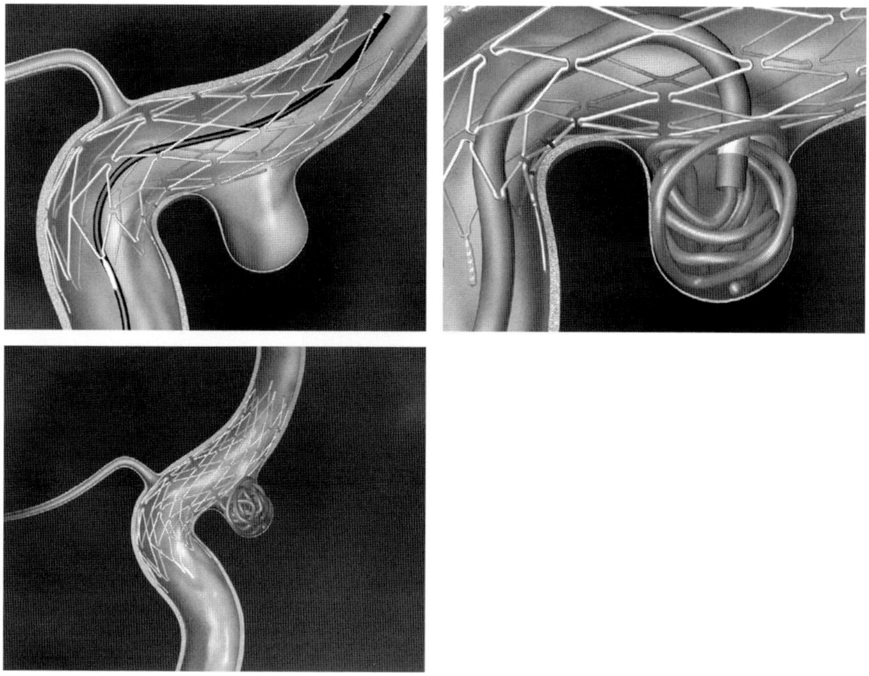

a b c

Fig.11. ***a*** Diagram of Neuroform stent across the aneurysm neck. ***b*** Catheter and coil in aneurysm and through stent. ***c*** Final coiling result of Neuroform stent and coil.

released from the catheter across the aneurysm neck. The stent self-expands to a predetermined diameter. Once the aneurysm neck is covered a microcatheter (0.014 inch or smaller) is advanced through the stent's cells and into the aneurysm. Coils are then deployed with the stent preventing the coils from entering the parent vessel's lumen. An alternative technique is to first catheterize the aneurysm and then place the stent across the aneurysm neck. Once coils are deposited and the aneurysm is treated the catheter is withdrawn from the aneurysm with the stent remaining in place across the neck.

Simultaneous Coil Deposition

Another technique that can be used to occlude wide-necked aneurysms is to deploy two coils simultaneously in the hope that a complex shape will form that covers the neck while the intertwining of the two coils restrains each from herniating out into the parent vessel. This maneuver requires one large or two smaller guiding catheters with the drawbacks of each technique that are mentioned above. It also necessitates placing two catheters into the aneurysm which may not be possible or safe in a smaller, wide-necked lesion. Finally, the deposition of simultaneous coils requires two interventionalists, a commodity which may not be available at all institutions.

Liquid Embolic Agents

Liquid embolic agents such as Onyx (ethylene-vinyl alcohol copolymer; MTI, Irvine, Calif., USA) are currently under clinical investigation for obliteration of wide-necked aneurysms. This alcohol copolymer is delivered via microcatheter into an aneurysm whose neck is temporarily covered by a balloon to reduce the risk of polymer leakage into the parent vessel. Upon contact with blood there is immediate solidification of the liquid agent within the aneurysm fundus. The theoretical advantages of this device are that the aneurysm can be completely filled with polymer thus eliminating the incidence of aneurysm recurrence through compaction or recanalization as is seen with coils. In addition, residual neck posttreatment can be obviated by introducing polymer until it is flush with the intra-arterial balloon-aneurysm interface.

Intentional Incomplete Embolization

While the issue of incomplete coiling is a sensitive one, especially when competing procedures like exo- and endovascular therapy are being considered, it is important to realize that the goal of aneurysm therapy is to reduce or eliminate the incidence of hemorrhage while at the same time preserving patient function. It is not clear whether or not incomplete coiling of an aneurysm reduces the incidence of delayed hemorrhage. This information will only be available with increased patient follow-up. However, as with aneurysm clipping, there are some instances where an aneurysm cannot be completely obliterated due to afferent and efferent vessel relationships to the fundus and neck. This is especially true for large aneurysms with large necks and aneurysms of the middle cerebral artery M1 bifurcation. In such instances, it may be desirable to plan on managing the wide-necked lesion by intentionally placing coils in the fundus and not trying to place material flush with the neck. This might strengthen the weaker fundus wall and reduce the incidence of future bleeding.

Combined Therapies

It may often be necessary to treat a wide-necked aneurysm in two stages. If the above techniques fail and clipping of the entire lesion is judged too risky, the surgeon may opt to partially clip the aneurysm neck thus turning a wide-necked lesion into a small-necked lesion. The aneurysm can then be endovascularly treated with a reduced risk for coil herniation into the parent vessel. This technique should be reserved for those rare lesions which cannot be remedied using exo- or endovascular therapy alone. If it is performed, both procedures should be carried out on the same day to minimize the risk of aneurysm rupture following partial clipping. Surgical hemostasis needs to be impeccable as the patient will be heparinized during the endovascular stage and may need to remain anticoagulated following the coiling.

Conclusion

Wide-necked aneurysms remain difficult lesions to treat and occlude permanently. A variety of techniques and devices are currently available or in development to improve upon the interventionalist's ability to embolize these lesions. Only time and well-organized studies will reveal whether or not endovascular approaches to these entities are safe and effective.

References

Aletich VA, Debrun GM, Misra M, Charbel F, Ausman JI: The remodeling technique of balloon-assisted Guglielmi detachable coil placement in wide-necked aneurysms: Experience at the University of Illinois at Chicago. J Neurosurg 2000;93:388–396.

Baxter BW, Rosso D, Lownie SP: Double microcatheter technique for detachable coil treatment of large, wide-necked intracranial aneurysms. AJNR Am J Neuroradiol 1998;19: 1176–1178.

Cloft HJ, Joseph GJ, Tong FC, Goldstein JH, Dion JE: Use of three-dimensional Guglielmi detachable coils in the treatment of wide-necked cerebral aneurysms. AJNR Am J Neuroradiol 2000; 21:1312–1314.

Cockroft KM, Marks MP, Steinberg GK: Planned direct dual-modality treatment of complex broad-necked intracranial aneurysms: Four technical case reports. Neurosurgery 2000;46: 226–231.

Debrun GM, Aletich VA, Kehrli P, Misra M, Ausman JI, Charbel F: Selection of cerebral aneurysms for treatment using Guglielmi detachable coils: The preliminary University of Illinois at Chicago experience. Neurosurgery 1998;43:1281–1297.

Debrun GM, Aletich VA, Kehrli P, Misra M, Ausman JI, Charbel F, Shownkeen H: Aneurysm geometry: An important criterion in selecting patients for Guglielmi detachable coiling. Neurol Med Chir Suppl (Tokyo) 1998;38:1–20.

Fessler RD, Ringer AJ, Qureshi AI, Guterman LR, Hopkins LN: Intracranial stent placement to trap an extruded coil during endovascular aneurysm treatment: Technical note. Neurosurgery 2000;46:248–253.

Gruber A, Killer M, Bavinski G, Richling B: Clinical and angiographic results of endosaccular coiling treatment of giant and very large intracranial aneurysms: A 7-year, single center experience. Neurosurgery 1999;45:793–804.

Gruber DP, Zimmerman GA, Tomsick TA, Van Loveren HR, Link MJ, Tew JM: A comparison between endovascular and surgical management of basilar artery apex aneurysms. J Neurosurg 1999; 90:868–874.

Guglielmi G, Vinuela F, Dion J, Duckwiler G: Electrothrombosis of saccular aneurysms via endovascular approach. Part 1. J Neurosurg 1991;75:8–14.

Guglielmi G, Vinuela F, Sepetka I, Macellari V: Electrothrombosis of saccular aneurysms via endovascular approach. Part 1. J Neurosurg 1991;75:1–7.

Hacein-Bey L, Connolly S, Mayer SA, Young WL, Pile-Spellman J, Solomon RA: Complex intracranial aneuryms: Combined operative and endovascular approaches. Neurosurgery 1998;43: 1304–1313.

Higashida RT, Smith W, Gress D, Urwin R, Dowd CF, Balousek PA, Halbach VV: Intravascular stent and endovascular coil placement for a ruptured fusiform aneurysm of the basilar artery. Case report and review of the literature. J Neurosurg 1997;87:944–949.

Hope Ayton JK, Byrne JV, Molyneaux J: Factors influencing successful angiographic occlusion of aneurysms treated by coil embolization. AJNR Am J Neuroradiol 1999;20:391–399.

Johnston SC, Dudley A, Gress DR, Ono L: Surgical and endovascular treatment of unruptured cerebral aneurysms at university hospitals. Neurology 1999;52:1799–1805.

Lanzino G, Wakhloo AK, Fessler RD, Hartney ML, Guterman LR, Hopkins LN: Efficacy and current limitations of intravascular stents for intracranial internal carotid, vertebral, and basilar artery aneurysms. J Neurosurg 1999;91:538–546.

Lavine SD, Larsen DW, Giannotta SL, Teitelbaum GP: Parent vessel Guglielmi detachable coil herniation during wide-necked aneurysm embolization: Treatment with intracranial stent placement: Two technical case reports. Neurosurgery 2000;46:1013–1017.

Lefkowitz MA, Gobin YR, Akiba Y, Duckwiler GR, Murayama Y, Guglielmi G, Martin N, Vinuela F: Balloon-assisted Guglielmi detachable coiling of wide necked aneurysms. II. Clinical results. Neurosurgery 1999;45:531–538.

Levy DI, Ku A: Balloon-assisted coil placement in wide-necked aneurysms. J Neurosurg 1997; 86:724–727.

Levy DI: Embolization of wide-necked anterior communicating artery aneurysm: Technical note. Neurosurgery 1997;41:979–982.

Lownie SP, Pelz DM, Fox AJ: Endovascular therapy of a large vertebral artery aneurysm using stent and coils. Can J Neurol Sci 2000;27:162–165.

Malek AM, Higashida RT, Phatouros CC, Dowd CF, Halbach VV: Treatment of an intracranial aneurysm using a new three dimensional shape Guglielmi detachable coil: Technical case report. Neurosurgery 1999;44:1142–1145.

Marks MP, Steinberg GK, Lane B: Combined use of endovascular coils and surgical clipping for intracranial aneurysms. AJNR Am J Neuroradiol 1995;16:15–18.

Mericle RA, Lanzino, G, Wakhloo AK, Guterman LR, Hopkins LN: Stenting and secondary coiling of intracranial internal carotid artery aneurysm: Technical case report. Neurosurgery 1998;43: 1229–1234.

Mizoi K, Takahashi A, Yoshimoto T, Fujiwara S, Koshu K: Combined endovascular and neurosurgical approach for paraclinoid internal carotid aneurysms. Neurosurgery 1993;33:986–992.

Moret J, Cognard C, Castaings WL, Rey A: The 'remodelling technique' in the treatment of wide neck intracranial aneurysms. Intervent Neuroradiol 1997;3:21–35.

Richling B, Bavinski G, Gross C, Gruber A, Killer M: Early clinical outcome of patients with ruptured cerebral aneurysms treated by endovascular (GDC) or microsurgical techniques. Intervent Neuroradiol 1995;1:19–27.

Sanders WP, Burke TH, Mehta BA: Embolization of intracranial aneurysms with Guglielmi detachable coils augmented by microballoons. AJNR Am J Neuroradiol 1998;19:917–920.

Sekhon LH, Morgan MK, Sorby W, Grinnell V: Combined endovascular stent implantation and endosaccular coil placement for the treatment of a wide-necked vertebral artery aneurysm: Technical case report. Neurosurgery 1998;43:380–383.

Wakhloo AK, Lanzino G, Lieber BB, Hopkins LN: Stents for intracranial aneurysms: The beginning of a new endovascular era? Neurosurgery 1998;43:377–379.

Zubillaga AF, Guglielmi G, Vinuela F, Duckwiler GR: Endovascular occlusion of intracranial aneurysms with electrically detachable coils: Correlation of aneurysm neck size and treatment results. AJNR Am J Neuroradiol 1994;15:815–820.

Dr. Michael B. Horowitz
Department of Neurosurgery
Director, Neuroendovascular Surgery
UPMC Presbyterian
Suite B-400, 200 Lothrop Street, Pittsburgh, 15213-2582, USA
Tel. +1 412 647 3685, Fax +1 412 647 7000, E-Mail horowitzmb@upmc.edu

Horowitz MB, Levy EI (eds): Neuroendovascular Surgery.
Prog Neurol Surg. Basel, Karger, 2005, vol 17, pp 135–147

Liquid Embolic Agents in the Treatment of Intracranial Arteriovenous Malformations

Jay U. Howington[a], *Charles W. Kerber*[b], *Lee R. Guterman*[a], *L. Nelson Hopkins*[a]

[a]Department of Neurosurgery and Toshiba Stroke Research Center, School of Medicine and Biomedical Sciences, University at Buffalo, State University of New York, Buffalo, N.Y., and [b]Departments of Radiology and Neurosurgery, University of California, San Diego, Calif., USA

Historical Background

The morbidity associated with the surgical treatment of intracranial arteriovenous malformations (AVMs) has decreased over the past two decades owing mainly to advances in endovascular therapy. Several studies have demonstrated the direct relationship between AVM size and both surgical difficulty and operative morbidity [1–5]. The aim of endovascular therapy is to obliterate the AVM or to reduce its size and enhance the patient's outcome through either surgery or radiosurgery. Luessenhop and Spence [6] performed the first embolization of an AVM in 1960 by injecting silastic spheres through a surgical exposure of the cervical carotid artery. Although this method was technically simple to perform, it was nonselective and often resulted in inadvertent occlusion of normal vessels and neurological injury [7, 8]. In 1973, Djindjian et al. [9] developed a technique of selective catheterization involving the external carotid artery, but it was Serbinenko [10] in 1974 who succeeded in accessing the cerebral arteries using a detachable balloon mounted on a floating catheter. Unfortunately, this technique was limited to single-vessel therapy as the balloons could not penetrate the nidus of the malformation.

Several studies reported the first use of polyvinyl alcohol (PVA) particles for embolization, but this agent was problematic in the treatment of AVMs for several reasons [11–13]. First, the particles need to be large enough to effectively embolize the lesion but small enough to be injected through the catheter without blocking the lumen. This problem was solved by later catheter innovations but other problems remaining are that occlusion caused by the particles is temporary and leads to reperfusion of the lesion, and the particles are not radiopaque.

Zanetti et al. [14] described the use of the monomer isobutyl-2-cyanoacrylate for endovascular embolizations in canine renal arteries in 1972, but it was not until 1976 that Kerber [15] reported the use of a calibrated-leak balloon mounted on a microcatheter to successfully navigate the intracranial circulation and deliver the adhesive agent to the small feeding vessels of an AVM. This technique required the repeated inflation and deflation of the balloon to advance the microcatheter, which was associated with a number of complications and was technically difficult [16–19]. Moreover, although the initial acrylates were excellent embolic agents, they were associated with toxic reactions and reported to have carcinogenic properties [20, 21]. Structural modifications of the basic cyanoacrylate monomer were made and resulted in N-butyl cyanoacrylate (NBCA), which has become the standard liquid acrylic adhesive agent in endovascular neurosurgery. Another adhesive monomer, 2-hexyl-cyanoacrylate (neuracryl M; Provasis Therapeutics, El Cajon, Calif., USA), is currently being evaluated for embolization of AVMs as well. Most recently, a nonadhesive liquid embolic agent known as Onyx (Micro Therapeutics, Irvine, Calif., USA) has undergone evaluation for embolization in several centers [22]. These three agents have in common the ability to be injected in liquid form through a microcatheter, although they differ significantly in their various properties and chemical composition. These agents and the techniques used for intracranial AVM embolization with each are the focus of this report.

Provocative Testing

Extremely helpful for endovascular treatment of an intracranial AVM is provocative testing with either amobarbital or methohexital. (Lidocaine is added to the testing process if the AVM is dural-based, intimately involved with the cranial nerves, or has supply from the external circulation.) It is for this reason that we feel provocative testing deserves mentioning in any discussion of AVM embolization. Although a negative provocative test predicts the safety of permanent vessel occlusion, it does not eliminate the risk of neurological injury. Any transient neurological deficit produced by pharmacologic testing, however, should be expected to produce a permanent deficit with arterial embolization [23, 24]. The authors prefer to treat the patient without general anesthesia in an effort to better evaluate the territory supplied by the particular vessel or vessels selected for embolization.

N-Butyl Cyanoacrylate

Prior to the advances in microcatheter technology, particulate agents such as PVA were the mainstay of preoperative embolic therapy for AVMs. One of the major drawbacks with this type of treatment is that the occlusion is the result of thrombosis. The thrombus can be broken down over time so that there is a relatively high recanalization rate when using PVA [25]. Histopathological studies of NBCA demonstrate that the glue provokes a more intense inflammatory reaction than that caused by PVA and involves both the wall of the vessel and the adjacent interstitial areas [26–30]. The inflammatory reaction provoked by NBCA ultimately leads to vessel necrosis, fibrous ingrowth, and a fairly permanent occlusion [28, 31]. NBCA was recently approved by the US Food and Drug Administration (FDA) for endovascular treatment of AVMs; the results of the NBCA Trial, which demonstrated that NBCA was equivalent to PVA as a preoperative embolic agent for the treatment of cerebral AVMs, have been published [11].

Liquid monomeric NBCA is converted to a solid long chain polymer by anionic initiators (nucleophiles), which are found in excess in blood and on endothelium. Once the polymerization reaction begins, it proceeds rapidly and generates heat. The reaction proceeds so rapidly that the NBCA will solidify in a catheter without the addition of another medium that permits adjustments in polymerization time. Cromwell and Kerber [16] published their experience with iophendylate oil as an additive, and other investigators later found the optimal ratio of cyanoacrylate to oil to be from 1:5 to 2:5 [32, 33]. At those ratios, the polymerization time could be extended to allow for adequate penetration of the nidus. Iophendylate oil has been replaced by other oil-based mediums such as ethiodized oil and lipiodol. Unfortunately, diluting the glue with oil changes the character of the adhesive so that it comes out of the tip of the catheter in droplets, which can then pass uncontrolled through the AVM and to the lung. Powdered tantalum is also added to the adhesive to increase radiopacity during the procedure, and glacial acetic acid is sometimes used to prolong the polymerization times in AVMs with low-flow hemodynamics.

Proponents of embolization with cyanoacrylate glue argue that it causes permanent occlusion and can even cure small AVMs if adequate nidal penetration is accomplished [19, 31, 34–37]. Figure 1 demonstrates the treatment of such a lesion. Larger AVMs usually cannot be cured with this technique because the multiplicity of arterial feeders precludes complete occlusion of the nidus. The patent areas of the nidus retain flow, recruit secondary feeders, and require further treatment in the form of either surgery or radiosurgery to affect a cure [38, 39]. Advocates of NBCA embolization claim that the portion of the nidus that has been well cast is permanently occluded and effectively transforms an

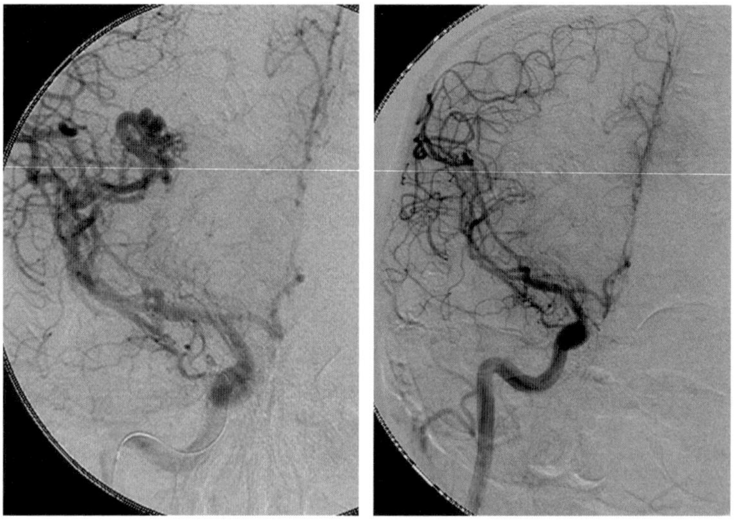

a b

Fig. 1. ***a*** Anteroposterior intracranial angiogram of the right internal carotid artery in a 26-year-old woman obtained 2 months after she presented with an intracerebral hemorrhage. This small AVM is supplied by only one feeder. ***b*** Right common carotid artery angiogram obtained after embolization with NBCA (Trufill, Cordis Neurovascular, Miami Lakes, Fla., USA) demonstrating complete obliteration of the malformation.

inoperable AVM into an operable one by reducing its size as well as the number of its arterial feeders [31, 34, 40–46]. The permanence of the occlusion appeals to the radiosurgeon because it reduces the risk of hemorrhage during the time it takes the radiation to treat the AVM. For the neurosurgeon, NBCA embolization has the advantage of making the vessels soft and retractable and decreasing the amount of blood loss and serves to establish a boundary zone between the AVM vessels and those of normal brain. Embolization with NBCA is also used in the palliative treatment of large and giant AVMs that possess complex angioarchitecture in an effort to decrease the shunt volume and achieve seizure control or reduce focal hypoxia.

The following is a general description of the technique used at the authors' institution for NBCA embolization. After superselectively guiding the microcatheter to a wedge position at the nidus of the AVM, appropriate provocative testing is performed. While this is being done, a second physician mixes the NBCA on a table uncontaminated by any ionizing material, adding as clinically appropriate ethiodized oil, tantalum, and possibly glacial acetic acid. It is critical that the preparation takes place in an ion-free environment to prevent premature polymerization. Each physician changes both gown and gloves before handling the adhesive. The adhesive monomer is added to the mixture of ethiodized oil and tantalum and then collected in a 3-ml syringe. Depending on the hemodynamics of the AVM determined during the angiographic portion of the procedure, the concentration of the adhesive is adjusted so as to provide adequate penetration of the nidus without occlusion of the venous drainage system. The authors prefer to use a standard concentration of 30% (0.9 ml NBCA and 2.1 ml oil mixed with the standard vial of tantalum supplied by the manufacturer) and dilute this concentration further if necessary with glacial acetic acid. After the provocative testing is done and before the embolization is performed, the microcatheter is flushed continuously with nonionic 5% dextrose in water (D5W). In a rapid exchange, the D5W syringe is removed, allowing no air entry, and replaced with the syringe containing the adhesive. With steady force, the NBCA is pushed through the catheter until the first drops appear at the tip of the catheter. The rate of injection is then modified to establish a good nidal cast by keeping the drops from coming out too fast or too slow. Care is taken to avoid reflux, and when the embolization is complete, negative pressure is applied to the syringe containing the adhesive, and the microcatheter is quickly withdrawn. This final maneuver takes the cooperation of two physicians. Whether more pedicles are to be embolized is a decision made by the endovascular surgeon based on the amount of nidus occluded. As a general rule, no more than 50% of the nidus should be embolized in the first attempt. The authors give credence to the theory of normal perfusion pressure breakthrough and feel that a greater percentage of occlusion without complete nidal obliteration increases the risk of postprocedural hemorrhage [47]. Smaller AVMs with only one feeder can often be cured during a single embolization procedure, whereas larger, more complex lesions usually require multiple sessions spaced over several months.

A long-known risk of using cyanoacrylates to embolize AVMs is that of gluing the catheter in place as the result of early polymerization of the agent [11, 48]. Early polymerization can also lead to glue blocking the catheter or feeding vessel, without penetrating the nidus. If the polymerization time is too long, the cyanoacrylate can pass into the venous circulation and into the lung. With a thorough understanding of the flow dynamics of the AVM, along with the ability to titrate the polymerization time with additive mediums, these risks can be largely minimized.

Onyx

Taki et al. [49] first described the use of ethylene-vinyl alcohol copolymer (EVOH) mixed with dimethyl sulfoxide (DMSO) in the embolization of cerebral AVMs in 1990. They used a mixture of 5 g of the solid copolymer and

35 g of metrizamide powder (for opacification) dissolved in 60 g of DMSO. The DMSO is an organic solvent and when the mixture comes in contact with an aqueous medium, such as blood, the DMSO diffuses away, and the EVOH precipitates and solidifies. The resultant embolic material does not adhere to the wall of the vessel or the catheter. Subsequent studies led to a premixed solution of EVOH, tantalum, and DMSO known as Onyx, which comes in three different concentrations of EVOH (6.0, 6.5 and 8.0%) [22, 50, 51]. The higher the concentration of EVOH, the more viscous the solution will be and the sooner it will precipitate in the AVM.

DMSO was chosen as the solvent because it readily diffuses in water, and its physiologic properties in humans have been well studied [49, 52]. This compound is extremely angiotoxic, and its adverse effects range from vasospasm to angionecrosis and arterial rupture. The damage to the vessel can be so great that an occlusion occurs, which alters the flow dynamics of the malformation to the point that premature reflux of the Onyx takes place. This reflux can lead to either inadequate nidal penetration or inadvertent parent artery embolization. Murayama et al. [50] demonstrated that the volume of DMSO used along with the amount of time it was in contact with the arterial wall were the two most important determinants of the compound's angiotoxicity. DMSO is such a powerful solvent that it has also been shown to damage some of the catheters used for its delivery [22, 50, 53]. Therefore, specially designed, DMSO-compatible catheters must be used. The only catheters currently available that meet these criteria are the Radifocus GT III catheter (Terumo, Tokyo, Japan) and the Flow Rider Plus and Rebar catheters (Micro Therapeutics). Another potential drawback to the use of Onyx as an adjunctive modality for the treatment of cerebral AVMs is the discomfort that many awake patients report with its injection. This discomfort can be so great as to obviate the ability to perform embolization without general anesthesia. Institutions that routinely use provocative testing as part of their embolization protocol may have difficulty using Onyx. Finally, the ready-made vials of the EVOH-DMSO-tantalum (Onyx) mixture must be constantly shaken right up to the point of injection. Jahan et al. [22] advocate the use of the Vortex-Genie shaker (Micro Therapeutics) for keeping the tantalum evenly dispersed to maximize radiopacity.

Because Onyx is a nonadhesive liquid embolic agent, it has several advantages over NBCA. Gluing the catheter to the arterial pedicle is not a concern. The nonadhesive nature of Onyx allows for a slower, more controlled injection during which serial angiograms can be used to evaluate the progress of the embolization. After one pedicle is embolized, the same catheter can be repositioned in another pedicle for another embolization. Figure 2 demonstrates an AVM with multiple feeding vessels that was treated with Onyx during one setting. The repeated use of a microcatheter is not possible with NBCA.

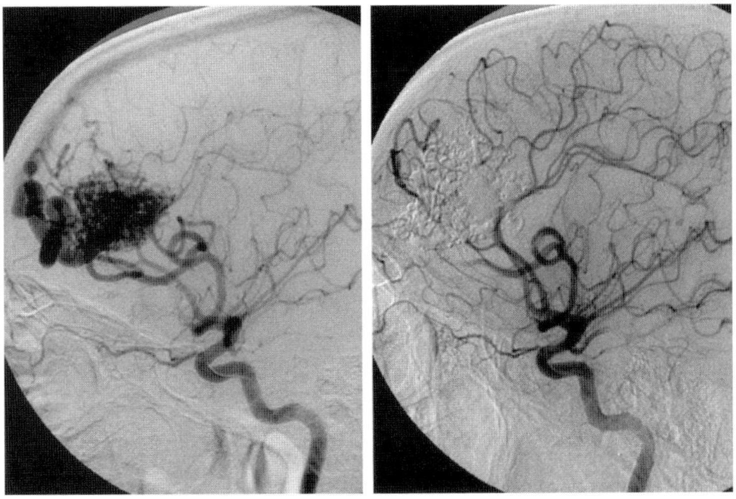

a b

Fig. 2. ***a*** Lateral intracranial angiogram of the right internal carotid artery in a 37-year-old woman who presented with refractory epilepsy. The malformation is fed by branches from both the anterior and middle cerebral arteries. ***b*** Lateral intracranial angiogram obtained after embolization with Onyx (Micro Therapeutics) demonstrating no residual malformation.

Like NBCA, Onyx acts as an aid to surgical resection by delineating AVM vessels from normal ones. At the time of operation, the Onyx-filled nidus is reported to be spongy and easily retractable, which also benefits surgical resection [22, 49, 54].

The basic technique of embolization with Onyx is similar to that of NBCA. No preparation of the embolic material in an ion-free environment is necessary, but the catheter must be primed with normal saline and then with 0.27 ml of DMSO to fill the dead space of the catheter and prevent premature solidification of the Onyx. The particular concentration of EVOH is chosen based on the flow dynamics of the AVM. Using a 1-ml syringe, the 0.27 ml of DMSO is slowly (over the course of 40 s) replaced by the Onyx. Slow injection of the Onyx is performed under fluoroscopy until adequate nidal penetration is achieved or reflux is noted. The catheter is then either removed or reprimed with DMSO if further embolization is warranted.

Histopathologically, vessels embolized with EVOH show mild inflammatory changes in the acute setting and chronic inflammatory changes after only several days [22, 49–51, 53, 54]. These changes are usually found within the lumen of the vessel with only focal areas of elastica disruption and without histological evidence of vessel wall angionecrosis. The lack of necrosis and continued viability of the vessel makes future recanalization a possibility. Angionecrosis can occur, but this is felt to be due to the improper injection of DMSO. Examination of resected AVMs treated with Onyx has revealed complete filling of some vessels and others only partially filled with the embolic material. The remainder of the vessel lumen was filled with thrombus, which can undergo recanalization over time. To date, there have been no long-term angiographic follow-up analyses of patients treated with Onyx. Late recanalization of AVMs treated with Onyx is possible given the histopathologic findings published thus far and needs to be further evaluated.

Neuracryl M

In an effort to avoid the inconsistent polymerization rates, premature beading, and inadvertent gluing of the catheter to the vessel wall associated with NBCA and the lack of angionecrosis and associated recanalization potential seen with Onyx, Kerber, Knox, and Krall began work on neuracryl M [Kerber et al., pers. commun.]. They sought to develop a radiopaque, injectable embolic agent composed primarily of the basic cyanoacrylate monomer that would stay together as much as possible when exposed to rapidly flowing blood and cause the inflammatory reaction necessary to result in permanent occlusion. The new agent, once polymerized, also had to have a soft consistency so that surgeons could easily manipulate embolized vessels. After working with many different mixtures, they produced a cyanoacrylate-based polymer named neuracryl M.

Initial studies comparing the behavioral characteristics of neuracryl M and NBCA were done using porcine blood in four different settings [55]. Drops of the two substances were placed on and beneath the surface of stagnant blood, and they were also injected into a linear flow model as well as a standardized AVM model. In the stagnant models, NBCA and neuracryl M had equivalent polymerization times; however, when placed beneath the surface of the blood, the neuracryl formed a rubbery mass, which remained at the tip of the needle, while the NBCA dropped to the bottom of the beaker, forming a friable mass. When injected in the flow models, the neuracryl remained as a cohesive mass that filled the entire linear flow model and yielded better penetration of the AVM model than did the NBCA. In the linear flow model, the NBCA formed small droplets that embolized downstream in the tubing. Unfortunately, neuracryl M is a cyanoacrylate derivative and as such still has the potential to glue the catheter to the vessel wall. As with NBCA, a significant learning curve accompanies the use of neuracryl M. Once one has mastered the technique of using cyanoacrylates in the treatment of AVMs and takes the proper precautions, inadvertent adherence to the vessel wall can be largely avoided.

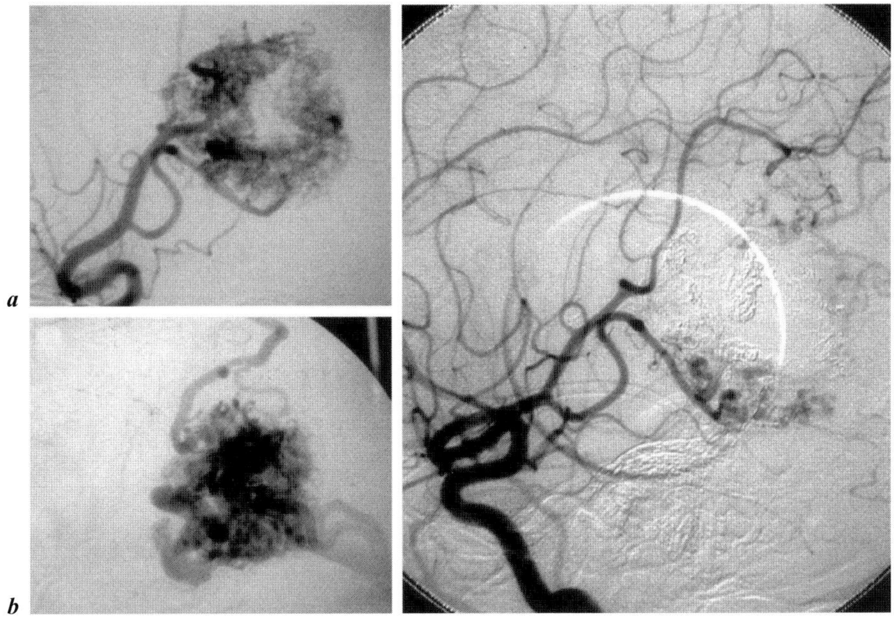

Fig. 3. ***a*** Lateral intracranial left internal carotid artery angiogram taken in a 40-year-old man who presented with an intracerebral hemorrhage. This image was obtained 0.5 s after injection of contrast agent. The lack of filling in the center of the nidus is caused by the hemorrhage. ***b*** Pretreatment image taken 1 s after injection of contrast agent demonstrating early venous drainage through multiple veins. The malformation was then embolized with neuracryl M (Provasis Therapeutics). ***c*** Posttreatment image taken 1 s after injection of contrast agent. There is a small amount of nidus remaining, but the early draining veins are no longer visualized.

A randomized clinical trial comparing neuracryl M to PVA for the treatment of AVMs was then conducted [56]. Complete embolization of the AVM was achieved in 5 of 10 patients who received neuracryl M. Among the remaining 5 patients, the nidus size was reduced by 50–99% in 2 AVMs, by less than 50% in 2 others, and felt to have increased slightly in 1. It was felt that in this latter case the nidus was inadequately penetrated and enlarged by recruiting other feeding vessels. Figure 3 shows a recently ruptured AVM that was partially treated with neuracryl M. The trial was an angiographic study only and did not focus on the histopathologic changes induced by the neuracryl M. Chopko et al. [57] reported the first human histopathologic results in a 34-year-old man who was treated with neuracryl M 4 days before surgical resection. Histopathologic analysis revealed scattered foci of neuracryl M that filled the lumen and did not breach the vessel wall (fig. 4). A profound acute inflammatory response

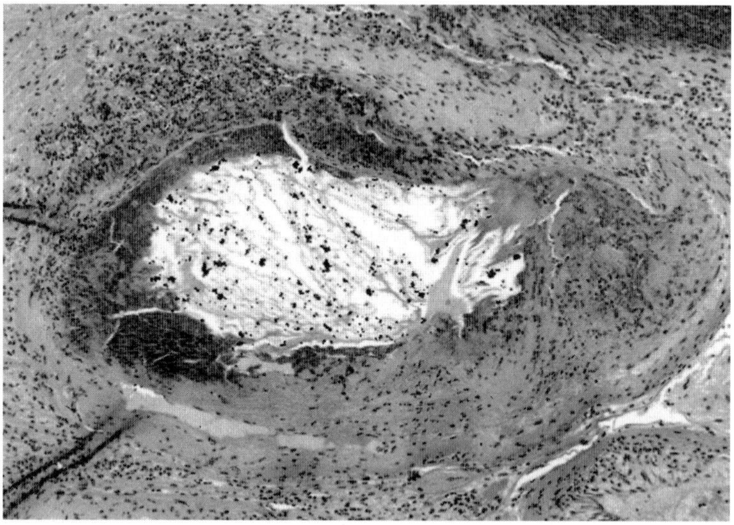

Fig. 4. Hematoxylin and eosin-stained section of a human brain AVM embolized with neuracryl M. Note the acute inflammatory response. The black specks within the vessel are gold, which is part of the polymer. The majority of the cyanoacrylate is dissolved during the fixation process. The transverse diameter of the vessel lumen is approximately 90 μm.

surrounding many of the AVM vessels along with a giant cell foreign body reaction and angionecrosis were also noted.

The results of long-term follow-up of patients treated with neuracryl M are not yet available but such an analysis is planned. At present, NBCA is the only cyanoacrylate approved by the FDA for use in the endovascular treatment of AVMs. Given the early success with neuracryl M, it is likely that the FDA will soon approve of its use in this arena.

Conclusions

The endovascular treatment of cerebral AVMs has advanced greatly in the four decades since Luessenhop and Spence [6] first used silastic spheres to embolize an AVM. Innovations with regard to the embolic materials used as well as the catheters used for access to these lesions have radically altered the methods for the treatment of intracranial AVMs. Endovascular therapies have helped to decrease operative morbidity by making it easier for the surgeon to resect the AVM or by eliminating the need for surgery altogether. The reduction in size of the AVM caused by embolization also improves the efficacy of radiosurgery. With continued advances, the surgical morbidity should drop even lower.

References

1 Heros RC, Tu YK: Unruptured arteriovenous malformations: A dilemma in surgical decision making. Clin Neurosurg 1986;33:187–236.
2 Luessenhop AJ, Gennarelli TA: Anatomical grading of supratentorial arteriovenous malformations for determining operability. Neurosurgery 1977;1:30–35.
3 Pasqualin A, Barone G, Cioffi F, Rosta L, Scienza R, Da Pian R: The relevance of anatomic and hemodynamic factors to a classification of cerebral arteriovenous malformations. Neurosurgery 1991;28:370–379.
4 Spetzler RF, Martin NA: A proposed grading system for arteriovenous malformations. J Neurosurg 1986;65:476–483.
5 Tamaki N, Ehara K, Lin TK, et al: Cerebral arteriovenous malformations: Factors influencing the surgical difficulty and outcome. Neurosurgery 1991;29:856–863.
6 Luessenhop AJ, Spence WT: Artificial embolization of cerebral arteries: Report of use in a case of arteriovenous malformation. JAMA 1960;172:1153–1155.
7 Wolpert SM: Silastic sphere embolization of intracranial arteriovenous malformations; in Wilson CB, Stein BM (eds): Intracranial Arteriovenous Malformations. Baltimore, Williams & Wilkins, 1988, pp 274–294.
8 Wolpert SM, Stein BM: Catheter embolization of intracranial arteriovenous malformations as an aid to surgical excision. Neuroradiology 1975;10:73–85.
9 Djindjian R, Cophignon J, Rey Theron J, Merland JJ, Houdart R: Superselective arteriographic embolization by the femoral route in neuroradiology. Study of 50 cases. 3. Embolization in craniocerebral pathology. Neuroradiology 1973;6:143–152.
10 Serbinenko FA: Balloon catheterization and occlusion of major cerebral vessels. J Neurosurg 1974;41:125–145.
11 The n-BCA Trial Investigators: N-Butyl cyanoacrylate embolization of cerebral arteriovenous malformations: Results of a prospective, randomized, multi-center trial. AJNR Am J Neuroradiol 2002;23:748–755.
12 Porstmann W, Wierny L, Warnke H, Gerstberger G, Romaniuk PA: Catheter closure of patent ductus arteriosus. 62 cases treated without thoracotomy. Radiol Clin North Am 1971;9:203–218.
13 Sorimachi T, Koike T, Takeuchi S, et al: Embolization of cerebral arteriovenous malformations achieved with polyvinyl alcohol particles: Angiographic reappearance and complications. AJNR Am J Neuroradiol 1999;20:1323–1328.
14 Zanetti PH, Sherman FE: Experimental evaluation of a tissue adhesive as an agent for the treatment of aneurysms and arteriovenous anomalies. J Neurosurg 1972;36:72–79.
15 Kerber C: Balloon catheter with a calibrated leak. A new system for superselective angiography and occlusive catheter therapy. Radiology 1976;120:547–550.
16 Cromwell LD, Kerber CW: Modification of cyanoacrylate for therapeutic embolization: Preliminary experience. AJR Am J Roentgenol 1979;132:799–801.
17 Merland JJ, Rufenacht D, Laurent A, Guimaraens L: Endovascular treatment with isobutyl cyano acrylate in patients with arteriovenous malformation of the brain. Indications, results and complications. Acta Radiol Suppl 1986;369:621–622.
18 Vinuela F, Fox AJ, Pelz D, Debrun G: Angiographic follow-up of large cerebral AVMs incompletely embolized with isobutyl-2-cyanoacrylate. AJNR Am J Neuroradiol 1986;7:919–925.
19 Vinuela F, Duckwiler G, Guglielmi G: Intravascular embolization of brain arteriovenous malformations; in Maciunas RJ (ed): Endovascular Neurological Intervention. Park Ridge, American Association of Neurological Surgeons, 1995, pp 189–199.
20 Samson D, Marshall D: Carcinogenic potential of isobutyl-2-cyanoacrylate. J Neurosurg 1986;65: 571–572.
21 Vinters HV, Galil KA, Lundie MJ, Kaufmann JC: The histotoxicity of cyanoacrylates. A selective review. Neuroradiology 1985;27:279–291.
22 Jahan R, Murayama Y, Gobin YP, Duckwiler GR, Vinters HV, Vinuela F: Embolization of arteriovenous malformations with Onyx: Clinicopathological experience in 23 patients. Neurosurgery 2001;48:984–997.

23 Mathis JM, Barr JD: Pharmacologic testing as an adjunct to neuroendovascular procedures. Neurosurg Clin N Am 2000;11:21–26, vii.

24 Peters KR, Quisling RG, Gilmore R, Mickle P, Kuperus JH: Intraarterial use of sodium methohexital for provocative testing during brain embolotherapy. AJNR Am J Neuroradiol 1993;14: 171–174.

25 Standard SC, Guterman LR, Chavis TD, Hopkins LN: Delayed recanalization of a cerebral arteriovenous malformation following angiographic obliteration with polyvinyl alcohol embolization. Surg Neurol 1995;44:109–113.

26 Brothers MF, Kaufmann JC, Fox AJ, Deveikis JP: n-Butyl 2-cyanoacrylate – Substitute for IBCA in interventional neuroradiology: Histopathologic and polymerization time studies. AJNR Am J Neuroradiol 1989;10:777–786.

27 Duffner F, Ritz R, Bornemann A, Freudenstein D, Wiendl H, Siekmann R: Combined therapy of cerebral arteriovenous malformations: Histological differences between a non-adhesive liquid embolic agent and n-butyl 2-cyanoacrylate (NBCA). Clin Neuropathol 2002;21:13–17.

28 Kerber CW, Wong W: Liquid acrylic adhesive agents in interventional neuroradiology. Neurosurg Clin N Am 2000;11:85–99, viii–ix.

29 Kish KK, Rapp SM, Wilner HI, Wolfe D, Thomas LM, Barr J: Histopathologic effects of transarterial bucrylate occlusion of intracerebral arteries in mongrel dogs. AJNR Am J Neuroradiol 1983; 4:385–387.

30 Standard SC, Hopkins LN: Principles of neuroendovascular intervention; in Maciunas RJ (ed): Endovascular Neurological Intervention. Park Ridge, American Association of Neurological Surgeons, 1995, pp 1–34.

31 Wikholm G: Occlusion of cerebral arteriovenous malformations with N-butyl cyano-acrylate is permanent. AJNR Am J Neuroradiol 1995;16:479–482.

32 Stoesslein F, Muenster W: A new technique for safe embolization using cyanoacrylate/contrast medium mixtures. Ann Radiol (Paris) 1984;27:296–298.

33 Stoesslein F, Ditscherlein G, Romaniuk PA: Experimental studies on new liquid embolization mixtures (histoacryl-lipiodol, histoacryl-panthopaque). Cardiovasc Intervent Radiol 1982;5:264–267.

34 Fournier D, TerBrugge KG, Willinsky R, Lasjaunias P, Montanera W: Endovascular treatment of intracerebral arteriovenous malformations: Experience in 49 cases. J Neurosurg 1991;75:228–233.

35 Hurst RW, Berenstein A, Kupersmith MJ, Madrid M, Flamm ES: Deep central arteriovenous malformations of the brain: The role of endovascular treatment. J Neurosurg 1995;82:190–195.

36 Mansmann U, Lasjaunias P, Meisel HJ: Treatment of patients with cerebral arteriovenous malformations. Radiology 2002;223:879–881.

37 Wikholm G, Lundqvist C, Svendsen P: Embolization of cerebral arteriovenous malformations. I. Technique, morphology, and complications. Neurosurgery 1996;39:448–459.

38 Fournier D, Terbrugge K, Rodesch G, Lasjaunias P: Revascularization of brain arteriovenous malformations after embolization with bucrylate. Neuroradiology 1990;32:497–501.

39 Gobin YP, Laurent A, Merienne L, et al: Treatment of brain arteriovenous malformations by embolization and radiosurgery. J Neurosurg 1996;85:19–28.

40 Debrun GM, Aletich V, Ausman JI, Charbel F, Dujovny M: Embolization of the nidus of brain arteriovenous malformations with n-butyl cyanoacrylate. Neurosurgery 1997;40:112–121.

41 DeMeritt JS, Pile-Spellman J, Mast H, et al: Outcome analysis of preoperative embolization with N-butyl cyanoacrylate in cerebral arteriovenous malformations. AJNR Am J Neuroradiol 1995;16:1801–1807.

42 Frizzel RT, Fisher WS III: Cure, morbidity, and mortality associated with embolization of brain arteriovenous malformations: A review of 1246 patients in 32 series over a 35-year period. Neurosurgery 1995;37:1031–1040.

43 Jafar JJ, Davis AJ, Berenstein A, Choi IS, Kupersmith MJ: The effect of embolization with N-butyl cyanoacrylate prior to surgical resection of cerebral arteriovenous malformations. J Neurosurg 1993;78:60–69.

44 Pasqualin A, Scienza R, Cioffi F, et al: Treatment of cerebral arteriovenous malformations with a combination of preoperative embolization and surgery. Neurosurgery 1991;29:358–368.

45 Richling B, Killer M: Endovascular management of patients with cerebral arteriovenous malformations. Neurosurg Clin N Am 2000;11:123–145, ix.

46 Vinuela F, Dion JE, Duckwiler G, et al: Combined endovascular embolization and surgery in the management of cerebral arteriovenous malformations: Experience with 101 cases. J Neurosurg 1991;75:856–864.

47 Spetzler RF, Wilson CB, Weinstein P, Mehdorn M, Townsend J, Telles D: Normal perfusion pressure breakthrough theory. Clin Neurosurg 1978;25:651–672.

48 Bank WO, Kerber CW, Cromwell LD: Treatment of intracerebral arteriovenous malformations with isobutyl 2-cyanoacrylate: Initial clinical experience. Radiology 1981;139:609–616.

49 Taki W, Yonekawa Y, Iwata H, Uno A, Yamashita K, Amemiya H: A new liquid material for embolization of arteriovenous malformations. AJNR Am J Neuroradiol 1990;11:163–168.

50 Murayama Y, Vinuela F, Ulhoa A, et al: Nonadhesive liquid embolic agent for cerebral arteriovenous malformations: Preliminary histopathological studies in swine rete mirabile. Neurosurgery 1998;43:1164–1175.

51 Yamashita K, Taki W, Iwata H, et al: Characteristics of ethylene vinyl alcohol copolymer (EVAL) mixtures. AJNR Am J Neuroradiol 1994;15:1103–1105.

52 Marshall LF, Camp PE, Bowers SA: Dimethyl sulfoxide for the treatment of intracranial hypertension: A preliminary trial. Neurosurgery 1984;14:659–663.

53 Chaloupka JC, Vinuela F, Vinters HV, Robert J: Technical feasibility and histopathologic studies of ethylene vinyl copolymer (EVAL) using a swine endovascular embolization model. AJNR Am J Neuroradiol 1994;15:1107–1115.

54 Terada T, Nakamura Y, Nakai K, et al: Embolization of arteriovenous malformations with peripheral aneurysms using ethylene vinyl alcohol copolymer. Report of three cases. J Neurosurg 1991; 75:655–660.

55 Kerber C, Connors J III, Knox K: The behavior of a new liquid embolic agent, Neuracryl M, in blood. AANS/CNS Section on Cerebrovascular Surgery and American Society of Interventional and Therapeutic Neuroradiology Meeting, Nashville, 1999.

56 Kerber CW, Wong W, Knox K, et al: Neuracryl M, a new liquid embolic agent: Initial clinical results (abstract). J Neurosurg 2000;92:196.

57 Chopko BW, Kerber C, Wong W, Knox K, Krall R: Initial neuropathologic observations after treatment of a human arteriovenous malformation with a novel liquid embolic agent, Neuracryl-M. American Association of Neurological Surgery/Congress of Neurological Surgeons Section on Cerebrovascular Surgery and American Society of Interventional and Therapeutic Neuroradiology Meeting, New Orleans, 2000.

L. Nelson Hopkins, MD
University at Buffalo Neurosurgery, Kaleida Gates Hospital
3 Gates Circle, Buffalo NY 14209 (USA)
Tel. +1 716 887 5200, Fax +1 716 887 4378, E-Mail dzbuffns@aol.com

Horowitz MB, Levy EI (eds): Neuroendovascular Surgery.
Prog Neurol Surg. Basel, Karger, 2005, vol 17, pp 148–159

Management of Arteriovenous Malformations Using Liquid Agents

Burak M. Ozgur[a], *David I. Levy*[b]

[a]Division of Neurosurgery, University of California, San Diego and
[b]Department of Neurosurgery, Kaiser-Permanente Medical Center,
San Diego, Calif., USA

Background

Endovascular techniques have been in development for treating intracranial pathology for the past 40 years. Embolization has been a common objective in reducing the blood supply to tumors, initiating thrombosis of aneurysms, and now in attacking the nidus of arteriovenous malformations (AVMs). These goals contribute to management not only as an adjunctive preoperative or prestereotactic radiosurgery treatment, but they are proving, in some cases, to be a complete minimally invasive treatment.

In 1960, Luessenhop [1] demonstrated that they could affect an AVM by sailing plastic beads up from the cervical internal carotid artery and vertebral artery. In 1974, Serbinenko [2] demonstrated more selective catheterization using microballoons to close specific intracranial vessels. The use of microcatheters and calibrated-leak balloons for delivery of cyanoacrylate-based liquid embolic agents was published by Kerber [3] in 1976 and Pevsner and Doppman [4] in 1980. Since then, the many technological advances in microcatheter design have made AVM embolization safer and more reliable.

There has been a wide variety of substances used as embolic agents throughout the years. In 1990, Purdy et al. [5] published an article detailing their experience with polyvinyl alcohol particles. Schumacher and Horton [6] in 1991 described their experience not only with polyvinyl alcohol, but also with silk, coils, gelfoam, and detachable balloons. In 1993, Schweitzer et al. [7] published their microscopic and immunohistochemical analysis from surgically resected AVMs that had been preoperatively embolized with various embolic agents. They explain that Avitene® (microfibrillar collagen) had the mildest tissue reaction, but its use resulted in early recanalization. Cyanoacrylate derivatives were associated with more acute and chronic inflammatory changes, and the effects lasted longer. Additionally, they showed that polyvinyl alcohol foam/ethanol mixtures fell into the intermediate category as regards inflammation and recanalization.

The use of isobutyl-2-cyanoacrylate (IBCA) was reported by Vinuela et al. [9], Fournier et al. [10], and Debrun et al. [11]. In 1993, Jafar et al. [12] published their use of N-butyl cyanoacrylate (NBCA) commenting that NBCA as opposed to IBCA is more amenable to surgical resection postembolization. They argued that preoperative AVM embolization with NBCA enables safer resection of larger and higher grade AVMs with statistically insignificant differences in complications and long-term outcome of smaller and lower grade AVMs. Ethanol endovascular embolization, resulting in progressive AVM thrombosis without recanalization or neovascular recruitment, was reported by Yakes et al. [8].

In 1990, Taki et al. [13] published their experience with a nonadhesive particulate plastic dissolved in dimethyl sulfoxide (DMSO). Subsequently, in 1991, Jahan et al. [14] reported the use of Onyx®, an ethylene vinyl alcohol copolymer, in AVM embolization. However, recently Lagares et al. [15] published their experience using Onyx noting concern for recanalization.

Another factor that has proven significant is the embolization strategy and target. The need for a clear and consistent plan was emphasized by Vinuela et al. [16] 1986 and supported by Fournier et al. [10] in 1991. Some important principles set forth by Debrun et al. [17] include specifically targeting the nidus of the AVM, using dilute cyanoacrylate mixtures, and employing longer injection times in order to penetrate the nidus. Cases of AVM revascularization have been described when AVM arterial feeders have been embolized without including the nidus. If the nidus has not been adequately penetrated, then the AVM characteristically reconstitutes via leptomeningeal, deep medullary, and dural collaterals. Finally, staging of embolic sessions may be indicated in cases of larger AVMs where gradual embolization will allow time for the intracranial circulation to adapt to the increased local pressures as the AVM shunt flow decreases.

Technical Methodology

AVM Embolization Techniques

The goal of AVM embolization with liquids is to reduce the size of the AVM by filling as much of the nidus with the polymer as possible. By comparing the cast of polymer following the embolization to the preembolization angiogram the therapist may objectively evaluate the penetration of the device (see fig. 1–10). If the nidus is not well filled with polymer, recanalization of

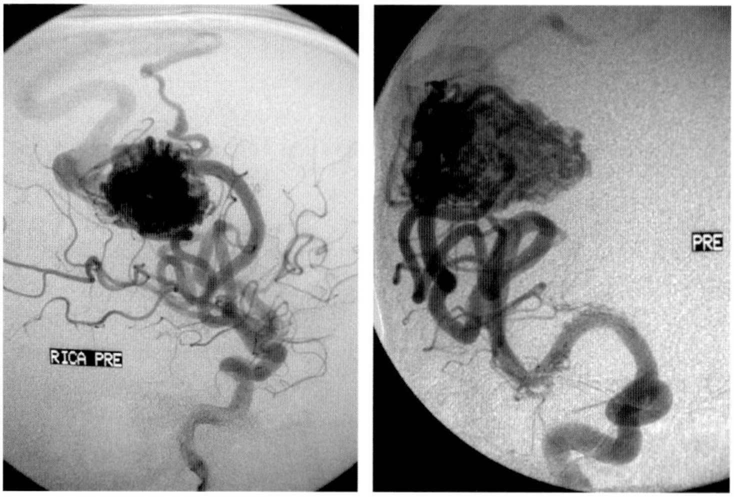

a b

Fig. 1. Case 1: Preembolization lateral (*a*) and AP (*b*) MCA injection.

the AVM is likely. Though recanalization is usually not dangerous because of the slow flow through the pial collaterals, the AVM will persist and present treatment difficulties in the future. While curing an AVM with NBCA is accomplished only in a reported 15% of cases, in a majority of cases, enough of the AVM nidus can be reduced in size and flow so that surgery or radiosurgery become safer options.

Flow-Controlled Injection

The use of flow-controlled injection techniques was pioneered by Kerber. With the invention of the calibrated-leak balloon, cyanoacrylate embolization became widely used in the treatment of AVMs [18]. The design incorporated a silicone or latex balloon that was secured to a catheter and then punctured to create a small hole at the tip allowing a guidewire to pass if needed. The system was then maneuvered to a distal intracranial location by using balloon inflation or the wire to help navigate the system. After removal of the wire, the IBCA or NBCA was injected with a syringe. As the liquid embolic flowed into the balloon, it inflated which slowed or halted blood flow into the feeding pedicle. Through the pinhole, the liquid was expelled toward the AVM allowing polymerization in a flow-controlled environment. Although there were many advantages to the technique, some difficulty was encountered in positioning the pinhole in the system so that the liquid embolic would exit into the center of the artery and was not injected against the arterial wall.

As other flow-directed catheters were developed and introduced, more distal positioning in the intracranial circulation was possible. It became possible to wedge a catheter in a small AVM vessel and establish flow-controlled injections without using a balloon. The advantages of flow-controlled injections are several. They allow a slower and more controlled injection using dilute cyanoacrylate mixtures. Because dilute agent is used, longer injection times are possible and the risk of gluing the catheter to the vessel is significantly reduced. The situations allowing utilization of wedged positions or flow-controlled injections are less than 50% of cases in our experience. This inability to achieve perfect positioning is the main limitation of this technique. It takes more time to safely wedge catheters in small, diseased vessels. However, once a wedged-position is obtained, the injection of glue is often rewarding with extensive filling of the nidus.

Another technique that creates a flow-controlled situation involves letting the liquid reflux around the catheter and begin to harden around the catheter tip thus creating a seal between the external surface of the catheter and the internal surface of the artery. Once hardened, this initial material blocks the forward flow of blood and prevents reflux of the embolic agent. The liquid can then be pushed forward by the operator who can expect better penetration of the liquid into multiple compartments. This technique has been recommended for Onyx injection, but also has been used successfully with dilute NBCA. Because of the long injection times, combined with the polymerization around the catheter, removing of the catheter can be difficult. Braided catheters are recommended to reduce the incidence of catheter fracture or retention in tortuous vascular anatomy.

As therapists have been using hydrophilic catheters and more dilute glue mixtures, fewer retained catheters are reported. If a catheter tip is in distal vasculature and does not come easily when traction is applied, it is not recommended to use great force to remove it. Few complications have been reported from retained catheters. Simply cutting them off at the groin puncture site and burying them beneath the skin has been used as an effective solution since the 1970s when liquid embolics were first used. If appropriate, a platelet inhibitor such as aspirin for 6 weeks may prevent emboli on the retained foreign body.

Flow-guided systems are generally flexible, have low inertia, and small diameter systems that use the high flow nature of AVMs to assist in their placement. A flexible wire may be used to assist in movement through more distal tortuous branches, are well tolerated by awake patients, and have been the mainstay of AVM embolization work for the last decade. Stretching and fracture of these catheters have been reported; however, this complication has been significantly less frequent in the last few years. Micro-guidewires compatible

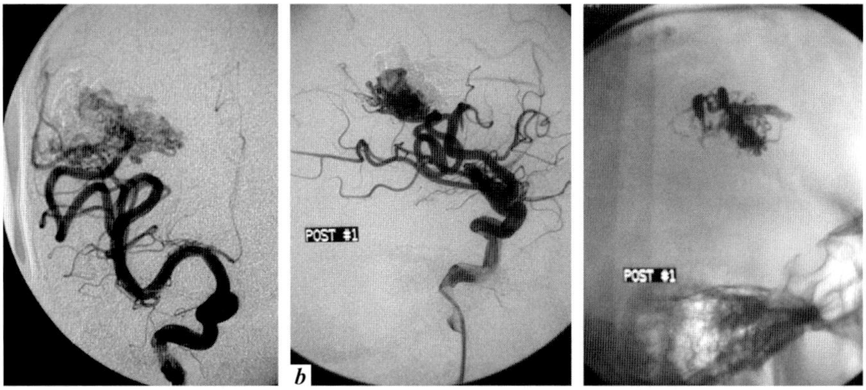

a *b* *c*

Fig. 2. Case 1: Immediate postembolization No. 1 (single injection using 0.021-inch catheter). ***a*** AP. ***b*** Lateral. ***c*** Cast.

with the 0.010-inch diameter flow-directed catheters were recently developed, thus allowing more frequent wedged positions, and so better nidus penetration.

Over-the-Wire Systems

Wire-guided or over-the-wire systems have gained in popularity with the advent of braided, flexible, soft hydrophilic catheters and steerable hydrophilic guidewires. The speed of distal catheterization often rivals the flow-guided systems, and the ability to control and direct these systems around sharper bends is greater than the flow-guided systems. Since the flow to an AVM decreases rapidly after the highest flow compartments of the nidus are occluded, flow-guided systems generally have progressive difficulty in accessing the distal vessels as the treatment becomes successful and the high flow decreases. Wire-guided systems, however, can generally be advanced effectively and equally in low or high flow situations. The ability to deliver larger quantities of liquid quickly is an advantage of the 0.021-inch diameter hydrophilic, braided catheters that are available. Flow control can be accomplished with the larger diameter catheters, but can be dangerous in smaller vessels as significant force can be generated in these braided catheters. Our preference has been not to maneuver in the diseased vessels to extremely distal positions unless absolutely necessary. A wire perforation while attempting to maneuver in these delicate vessels can cause local hemorrhage and often requires stopping the procedure for the day. When a safety zone is determined, we like to position the 0.021-inch catheters in the larger feeding vessels and attempt to close two or more branch vessels in a single injection (fig. 2 illustrates a single injection using a 0.021-inch catheter). If large fistulae within the nidus are encountered, several options are available.

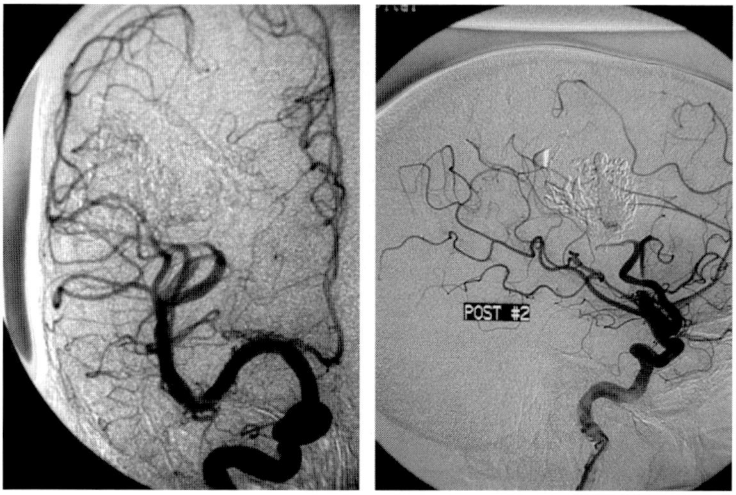

Fig. 3. Case 1: Immediate postembolization stage 2 (using 0.021-inch catheter).

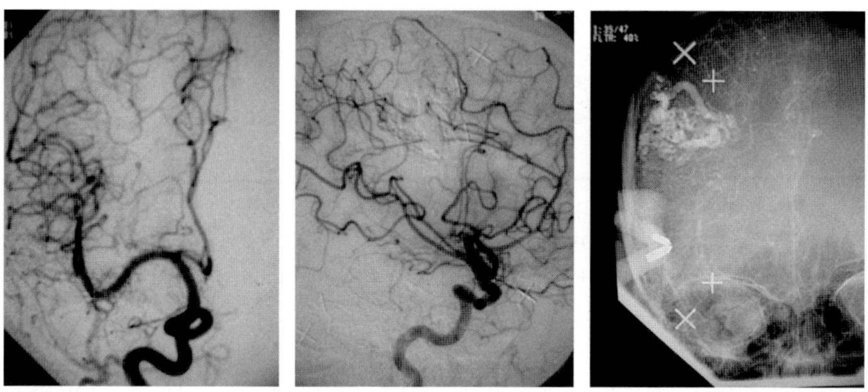

Fig. 4. Case 1: 8-month follow-up. (Note, radiosurgery frame was placed, but patient was not treated because no AVM was identified.)

Pure or concentrated (>75%) NBCA can be injected using 'Bullet' or 'Sandwich' techniques to slow the flow and then subsequently to allow a 'continuous column' of the liquid embolic to be used. These techniques are described in the manuscript by Dion and Mathis [19]. The Bullet or Sandwich technique injects a small amount (0.05–0.1 ml) into the AVM with the intention of closing the largest shunts as well as preserving the catheter position so that further injections can be made without making the journey to the distal vessels

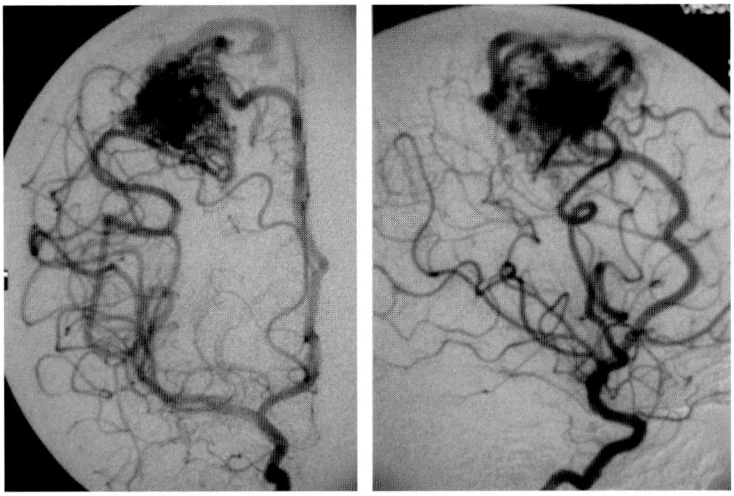

Fig. 5. Case 2: Preembolization. (Note, AVM supplied by both anterior and middle cerebral vessels; treated with five injections during a single session.)

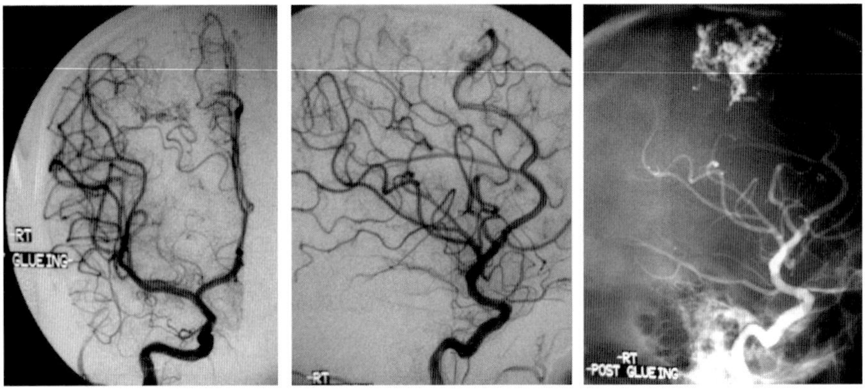

Fig. 6. Case 2: Immediate postembolization (small amount of nidus and shunt present).

with a new catheter. In a 1-ml syringe, 0.9 ml of 5% dextrose in water (D5W) is aspirated, followed by 0.05–0.1 ml of NBCA. Another syringe is used to flush the catheter and hub with D5W. When the syringe with the Bullet of NBCA is secured to the hub there is D5W in front and behind the NBCA creating the Sandwich. The entire syringe is injected using the D5W to push the Bullet into the largest of the AVM shunts. Several of these Bullets can be injected until the

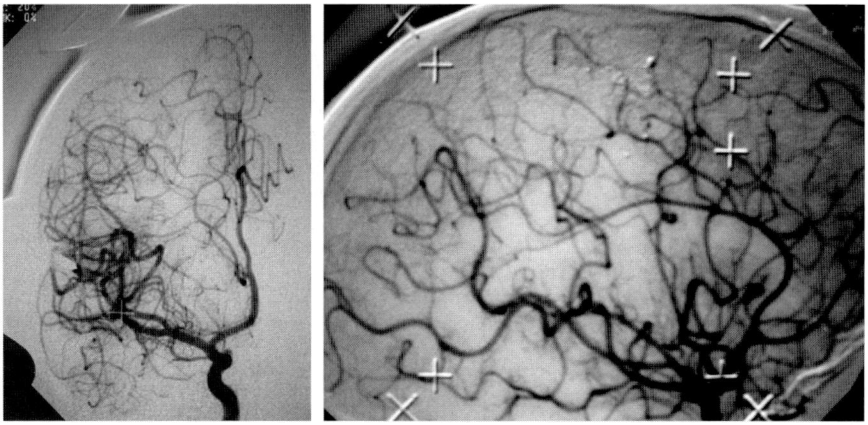

Fig. 7. Case 2: Late postembolization follow-up (patient lost to follow-up, returned 4 years later; patient was set up for adjuvant radiosurgery, but no residual AVM remained).

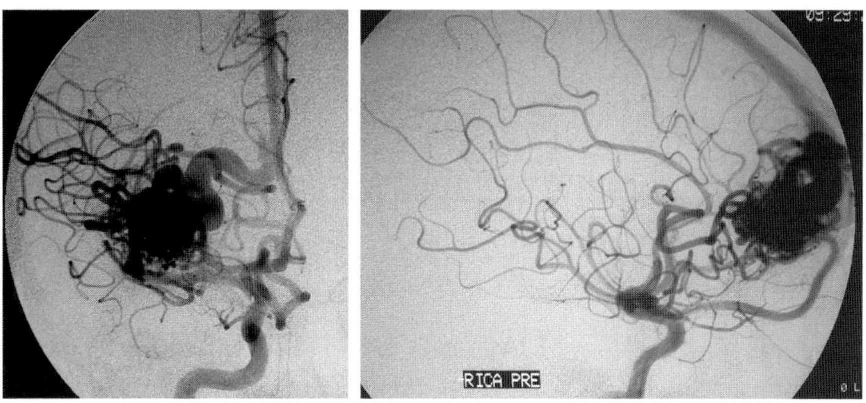

Fig. 8. Case 3: Preembolization.

flow is slowed enough to allow a continuous column of NBCA to be used. Detachable or nondetachable coils can also be used to slow these large shunts. If the largest shunts are not closed before a continuous column is used, the liquid embolic will go into the venous system before the arterial side is closed causing a potentially dangerous situation. Once the highest-flow shunts in a compartment are closed, a continuous column of glue can be used. The entire syringe is filled with the NBCA mixture and injected until it is seen refluxing back to the tip of the catheter.

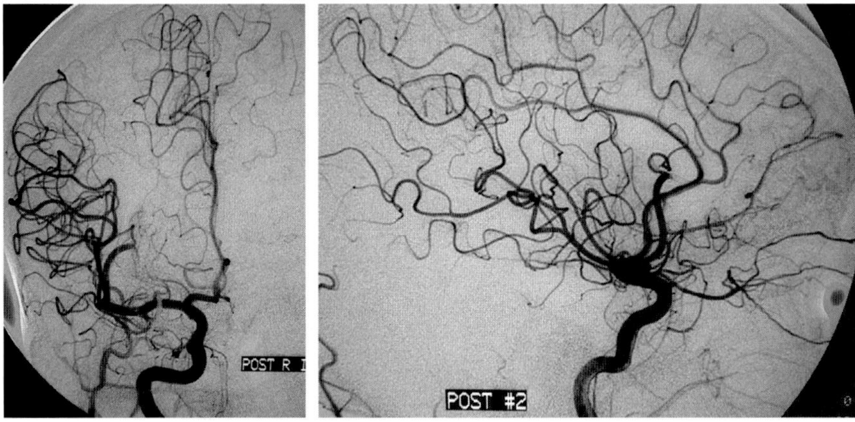

Fig. 9. Case 3: Immediate postembolization (following second staged session).

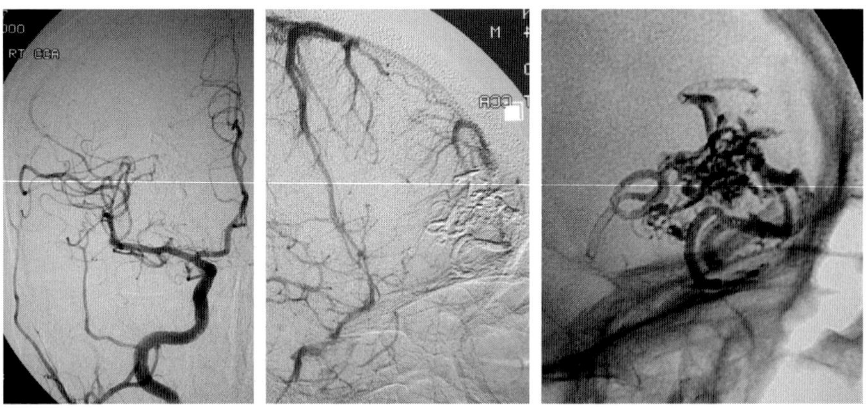

Fig. 10. Case 3: 6 months postembolization follow-up (no AVM remains; glue cast resembles AVM).

Staged Embolization

In our practice, AVM embolizations are usually accomplished in several sessions if the AVM is larger than 3 cm in diameter, or if several high-flow shunts are seen. The problems experienced with an overaggressive embolization are many and are primarily a result of creating significant cerebral edema by closing high-flow/low-resistance shunts that have been present for years with the accompanying venous dilatation. We typically close one or two high-flow shunts or 3 or 4 low-flow shunts during the first session. The patients typically stay overnight in the hospital, being watched for signs of cerebral swelling, then are discharged the following morning. They return in 4–12 weeks for another session of the treatment.

Embolic Materials

Embolic agents may be divided into four classes: first, particles that block flow mechanically then elicit some degree of tissue reaction. Polyvinyl alcohol or silk suture are the commonest. Sclerosing agents such as ethyl alcohol have also been used in the treatment of AVMs. Alcohol acts by destroying the vessel endothelium. Particulate agents such as Onyx rely on the solvent DMSO to remain in liquid form during introduction. As the solvent dissipates, the precipitate comes out of solution and remains in the AVM. Finally, polymers based upon the cyanoacrylate molecule rely on a polymerization reaction initiated by a substance with basic properties such as blood. Polymers such as NBCA can be diluted and made radiographically visible by adding ethiodized oil or microparticulate heavy metals such as tantalum powder. Diluting the NBCA allows longer polymerization times. For example, we have used up to 90% ethiodized oil and 10% NBCA for AVMs with slow artery-to-vein shunting. As more oil is added, the viscosity of the glue is increased so penetration of the embolic device into small vessels and fine nidal networks is prevented. In cases of small nidal networks such as those found in some dural AVMs, we have found glacial acetic acid to be of great benefit. Acetic acid delays the polymerization time of NBCA by adding H^+ to the glue mixture. It is important not to use tantalum and only as much ethiodized oil as is needed to see the mixture in these cases. We typically use a 50% mixture of NBCA and ethiodized oil when using acetic acid. This mixture allows a low viscosity while the acetic acid delays the polymerization time. We titrate the dose (1–5 ml) of acetic acid to delay the polymerization time and allow glue penetration as needed.

Discussion

Embolic agents and devices used for treating AVMs have evolved and improved over the past 40 years. We continue to see new products tested and introduced. The goal remains filling the nidus rather than solely occluding the feeding vessels. Depending on the size and flow of the lesion, some malformations must be staged; most require adjuvant therapies including radiosurgery and microsurgical resection. As devices evolve and improve, and as operator experience is gained, more angiographic cures may be expected.

Today, the embolization techniques and choice of agent depend largely on the technical skill and experience of the operator. Control of the physical behavior of the device is available when using an agent such as NBCA. Currently, we believe flexibility and control to be a significant advantage in customizing each injection for each particular target.

Each year, new products emerge that reshape our understanding and treatments of AVMs. (For example, Hamada et al. [20] published in 2002 their experience using an ethylene vinyl alcohol copolymer/ethanol mixture). In all, the future looks bright for this treatment paradigm. Though the numbers of AVM patients are small, the disease is worthy of our respect, perhaps even a little fear, and our full attention.

References

1 Luessenhop A: Artificial embolization of cerebral arteries. JAMA 1960;172/11:119–121.
2 Serbinenko FA: Balloon catheterization and occlusion of major cerebral vessels. J Neurosurg 1974; 41:125–145.
3 Kerber CW: Balloon catheter with a calibrated leak. Radiology 1976;120:547–550.
4 Pevsner PH, Doppman JL: Therapeutic embolization with a microballoon catheter. AJR Am J Roentgenol 1980;134:949–958.
5 Purdy P, Samson D, Batjer H, Risser R: Preoperative embolization of cerebral arteriovenous malformations with polyvinyl alcohol particles: Experience in 51 adults. AJNR Am J Neuroradiol 1990;11:501–510.
6 Schumacher M, Horton J: Treatment of cerebral arteriovenous malformations with PVA. Neuroradiology 1991;33:101–105.
7 Schweitzer J, Chang B, Madsen P, Vinuela F, Martin N, Marroquin C, Vinters H: The pathology of arteriovenous malformations of the brain treated by embolotherapy: Results of embolization with multiple agents. Neuroradiology 1993;35:468–474.
8 Yakes WF, Krauth L, Ecklund J, Swengle R, Dreisbach JN, Seibert CE, Baker R, Miller M, VanderArk G, Fullager T, Prenger E: Ethanol endovascular management of brain arteriovenous malformations: Initial results. Neurosurgery 1997;40:1145–1152.
9 Vinuela F, Fox A, Debrun G, Drake C, Peerless S, Girvin J: Progressive thrombosis of brain arteriovenous malformations after embolization with isobutyl-2-cyanoacrylate. AJNR Am J Neuroradiol 1983;4:1233–1238.
10 Fournier D, TerBrugge K, Willinsky R, Lasjaunias P, Montanera W: Endovascular treatment in intracerebral arteriovenous malformations: Experience in 49 cases. J Neurosurg 1991;75:228–233.
11 Debrun G, Vinuela F, Fox A, Drake C: Embolization of cerebral arteriovenous malformations with bucrylate. J Neurosurg 1982;56:615–627.
12 Jafar J, Davis A, Berenstein A, Berenstein A, Choi I, Kupersmith M: The effect of embolization with N-butyl cyanoacrylate prior to surgical resection of cerebral arteriovenous malformations. J Neurosurg 1993;78:60–69.
13 Taki T, Yonekawa Y, Iwata H, Uno A, Yamashita K, Amemiya H: A new liquid material for embolization of arteriovenous malformations. AJNR Am J Neuroradiol 1990;11:163–168.
14 Jahan R, Murayama Y, Gobin YP, Duckwiler GR, Vinters HV, Vinuela F: Embolization of arteriovenous malformations with Onyx®: Clinicopathological experience in 23 patients. Neurosurgery 2001;48:984–995.
15 Lagares A, Lobato R, Ricoy JR, Campollo J: Embolization of arteriovenous malformations with Onyx®: Clinicopathological experience in 23 patients. Neurosurgery 2002;51:1525–1526.
16 Vinuela F, Fox A, Pelz D, Debrun G: Angiographic follow-up of large cerebral AVMs incompletely embolized with isobutyl-2-cyanoacrylate. AJNR Am J Neuroradiol 1986;7:919–925.
17 Debrun GM, Aletich V, Ausman JI, Charbel F, Dujovny M: Embolization of the nidus of brain arteriovenous malformations with n-butyl cyanoacrylate. Neurosurgery 1997;40/1:112–120.

18 Kerber CW, Bank WO, Cromwell LD: Calibrated leak balloon catheter – A devise for arterial exploration and occlusive therapy. AJR Am J Roentgenol 1979;132:207–212.
19 Dion J, Mathis J: Cranial arteriovenous malformations. The role of embolization and stereotactic surgery. Neurosurg Clin N Am 1994;5:459–474.
20 Hamada J, Kai Y, Morioka M, Kazekawa K, Ishimaru Y, Iwata H, Ushiro Y: A mixture of ethylene vinyl alcohol copolymer and ethanol yielding a nonadhesive liquid embolic agent to treat cerebral arteriovenous malformations: Initial clinical experience. J Neurosurg 2002;97:881–888.

David I. Levy, MD
Department of Neurosurgery, San Diego Medical Center
4647 Zion Ave, San Diego, CA 92120 (USA)
Tel. +1 619 528 5478, E-Mail bozgur@ucsd.edu, David.I.Levy@KP.org

Horowitz MB, Levy EI (eds): Neuroendovascular Surgery.
Prog Neurol Surg. Basel, Karger, 2005, vol 17, pp 160–179

Treatment of Dural Arteriovenous Fistulas

Lei Feng, Philip M. Meyers, Randall T. Higashida

Departments of Radiology and Neurological Surgery, New York Presbyterian Hospitals, Columbia University, New York, N.Y., USA

Dural arteriovenous fistulas (DAVFs), or dural arteriovenous malformations, are acquired artery-to-vein shunts within dural mater, often without a distinctive vascular nidus. They constitute 10–15% of all intracranial arteriovenous malformations [1]. Symptoms depend upon the location of the fistula and range from pulse-synchronous tinnitus and exophthalmos to cranial nerve deficits, dementia, venous infarct, intracranial hemorrhage and even death.

Etiology

Although the pathogenesis remains elusive, DAVFs are likely to be acquired lesions with genetic predisposition in a proportion of cases. Many reports have suggested that DAVFs develop following trauma, infection, or surgery [2–9]. Disruption of adjacent arteries and veins can result in arteriographic shunt in the healing process. However, only a very small number of patients develop DAVFs following skull fracture or sinus surgery, implicating other pathogenic factors.

The association of sinus thrombosis and DAVFs has long been recognized [10–15]. Cases with hypercoagulable states, such as protein S deficiency [16, 17], prothrombin mutation [18] and factor V Leiden [19], have been reported. However, it is not clear whether sinus thrombosis is the cause or consequence of DAVFs. The high flow rate through the dural sinuses can result in disruption of normal laminar flow potentially denuding the endothelium thus predisposing the sinuses to thrombosis.

Because some DAVFs of the cavernous sinus occur in puerperal and postmenopausal women, the association of low estradiol level and development of

DAVFs have been proposed [20, 21]. However, there have been no further data to substantiate this hypothesis [22].

Recent evidence points to a role for potent angiogenic factors. Angiogenesis is stimulated by ischemia secondary to sinus thrombosis or cytokines produced by inflammatory cells in organizing thrombus. Elevated levels of basic fibroblast growth factor and vascular endothelial growth factor have been found in the sinus wall and perivascular connective tissues of DAVFs [23–26]. These chemical mediators induce neovascularity in the organizing thrombus, which may contain small shunts between the terminal arteries and veins previously demonstrated in tumor vessels [27]. As the thrombus resolves, these small shunts may then communicate with the dural sinus. Alternatively venous hypertension and ischemia due to primary sinus thrombosis may cause enlargement of normally present, but quiescent, microscopic arteriovenous shunts to facilitate development of collateral blood flow [28]. Such 'microshunts' may continue to grow in the patients with genetic predisposition or under the influence of other unknown factors and eventually develop into DAVFs.

Classification

Numerous classification systems have been proposed to categorize DAVFs. Several of the primary grading systems are summarized in table 1. However, the venous drainage pattern determines their clinical behavior and is the most clinically important feature for classification [29–33]. Pathophysiologically, elevated venous pressure and turbulent flow can lead to intimal proliferation and venous stenosis [34]. Venous outflow obstruction in turn aggravates venous hypertension. As the venous pressure rises, cerebral perfusion pressure decreases, resulting in interstitial exudates, brain edema, venous infarct, and hemorrhage [35, 36].

To guide treatment decisions, Djindjian and Merland [37] classified DAVFs into four types based on the venous drainage pattern: type I with immediate drainage into a dural sinus or meningeal vein, type II with initial drainage into the sinus and retrograde flow into other sinuses or cortical veins, type III with initial drainage into a cortical vein, and type IV with initial drainage into a cortical vein with venous ectasia. The type I DAVFs are considered relatively benign. With types II–IV, there are increased risks of neurological symptoms and hemorrhage.

To emphasize the importance of venous hypertension as the cause of clinical symptoms, two modifications of this classification have been proposed based on the causes and consequences of venous hypertension, respectively.

Table 1. Three major classification guides for assessment of venous drainage patterns in DAVFs

Venous drainage pattern	Djindjian and Merland [37]	Cognard et al. [32]	Lalwani et al. [38]
Antegrade flow into dural sinus	I	I	1
Retrograde flow in dural sinus only	**II**	IIa	2
Retrograde flow into cortical vein only	**II**	**IIb**	**3**
Retrograde flow into dural sinus and cortical vein	**II**	**IIa + b**	**3**
Retrograde venous drainage, no antegrade drainage	**III**	**III**	**3**
Cortical venous ectasia >5 mm or 3× larger than normal draining vein	**IV**	**IV**	**4**
Perimedullary venous drainage		**V**	

Bold Roman and Arabic numbers represent higher-risk lesions for complications including stroke and hemorrhage.

Lalwani et al. [38] proposed a grading system incorporating features of venous restrictive diseases. Grade 1 DAVFs are characterized by normal antegrade venous drainage without venous restriction or cortical venous drainage. Grade 2 patients have antegrade venous drainage in the ipsilateral transverse/sigmoid sinuses but have developed retrograde venous flow through the transverse sinus to the torcular herophili with or without cortical venous drainage. Grade 3 patients have retrograde and cortical venous drainage without antegrade flow through the sigmoid sinus. In grade 4 disease, there is severe antegrade and retrograde venous obstruction in the transverse and sigmoid sinuses such that the dural AVF is drained exclusively through cortical veins. Grade 1 and 2 diseases have a benign clinical presentation, such as tinnitus and headache. Grade 3 and grade 4 patients have much higher risks of intracranial hemorrhage and visual symptoms and should be treated aggressively.

Cognard et al. [32] realized retrograde sinus flow differed significantly from cortical venous drainage in that it did not necessarily increase the hemorrhagic risk. They thus expanded type II of Djindjian's classification into three subtypes: type IIa, which has retrograde venous drainage into a sinus only, type IIb, which has retrograde venous drainage into a cortical vein only, and type IIa + b, which has retrograde venous drainage into both sinus and cortical veins. Venous ectasia, distinguishing type IV from type III, was defined as veins larger than 5 mm in diameter and 3 times larger than the diameter of the draining vein. Type V was added to describe those intracranial DAVFs that drain into perimedullary veins. Mechanistically, Cognard et al. suggested that sinus stenosis/occlusion and very high rates of arteriovenous shunting can result in venous insufficiency with elevated hemorrhagic risk. In their case series of 205 patients, only 1 of 84 patients with type I DAVFs had severe neurological symptoms. Among the AVFs with cortical venous drainage, less than 25% of patients with type IIb and IIa + b had hemorrhage, whereas 40% of patients with type III DAVFs had hemorrhage and the presence of venous ectasia increased this risk to 65% in the type IV patients.

It is especially important to be aware that the venous drainage patterns of DAVFs are dynamic and frequently progress to higher grades over time. Thus, a type IIa lesion can progress to type IIa + b, and then to type III following sinus occlusion. Should a patient's symptoms change, even subjectively resolve, reevaluation and follow-up imaging are warranted.

Fistulas involving the cavernous sinus have been traditionally divided into four types by their arterial supply [39]. Type B are DAVFs involving meningeal branches of the internal carotid artery; type C are DAVFs involving the meningeal branches of the external carotid artery; type D are DAVFs fed by both internal and external carotid branches. Type A, also called 'direct' carotid-cavernous fistulas, due to a recently ruptured aneurysm of the internal carotid artery, was more common than types B–D (indirect carotid-cavernous fistulas), but is not dural fistula. Since the introduction of automobile airbags, these type A fistulas are much less common.

Clinical Presentation and Diagnostic WorkUp

The clinical presentation of DAVFs is variable, depending on the location, venous drainage patterns, and duration of the disease. The symptoms change as the disease progresses. DAVFs may be completely asymptomatic and incidentally identified during evaluation for other disease entities. Most patients present with symptomatic DAVFs in the 5th to 6th decades of life, although DAVF has been reported in neonates and octogenarians [32, 40]. DAVF is more common in women (M:F = 1.3–1.5:1) [28, 32], particularly those types involving the cavernous and transverse sinuses [41–43]. However, male patients may present with more severe symptoms, as they tend to develop DAVFs in locations where these lesions remain indolent until venous hypertension or hemorrhage occurs [32].

Pulse-synchronous tinnitus is the most common symptom of DAVF due to the confluence of venous drainage near the auditory apparatus; other symptoms are predominantly related to venous hypertension. Therefore, DAVFs of the transverse/sigmoid and cavernous sinuses frequently present with tinnitus.

The physician may appreciate a bruit in the retroauricular or the periorbital region on physical exam. These patients should be referred for complete diagnostic cerebral arteriography to stratify the risk profile of the DAVF.

Cavernous sinus fistula classically presents with a constellation of three findings: proptosis, chemosis, and ophthalmoparesis. In a series of 135 patients evaluated for DAVF of the cavernous sinus, we found that arterialization of the conjunctival veins is the most common finding (93%), followed by conjunctival swelling or chemosis (87%), and ophthalmoparesis (81%) [40]. The symptoms are more prominent when there is venous outflow restriction resulting in pressurization of the orbital veins. Findings that warrant emergency treatment include uncontrollable open angle glaucoma, subretinal effusion, and retinal detachment resulting in visual deterioration. Ophthalmoparesis likely results from venous hypertension with ischemia of the vasa nervosum of cranial nerves within the cavernous sinus. Atypical facial pain may result from involvement of the gasserian ganglion. The patients should undergo angiography to confirm the diagnosis and risk stratification. Duplex ultrasound of the superior ophthalmic vein has been used to assess flow direction in the superior ophthalmic vein and look for evidence of cortical venous drainage [44], but transorbital ultrasound cannot be used reliably to exclude cortical venous drainage or flow direction in the ophthalmic veins especially if the veins within the orbital apex have become stenotic.

The symptoms and signs of intracranial venous hypertension can be quite subtle, possibly delaying diagnosis of high-risk DAVFs. Headaches are usual complaints. Dizziness, ataxia, memory loss, dementia, and seizures can all result from chronic venous hypertension and venous ischemia [45–47]. Communicating hydrocephalus can also develop as a result of impaired CSF reabsorption. Such patients may present with papilledema, nausea, and vomiting. When a patient presents with a bizarre constellation of neurological symptoms, DAVF should be included in the differential diagnosis even if unapparent on noninvasive imaging.

Intracranial DAVFs that drain into perimedullary veins of the spinal cord can cause myelopathy [48–52]. Spinal DAVF is a separate topic not covered in this article. Cerebral arteriography must be considered in the workup of myelopathy if the more common causes have been excluded. In pediatric patients with high-flow fistulas cardiac failure and respiratory distress may ensue.

Although cross-sectional imaging modalities are neither sensitive nor specific for all DAVFs and may not permit adequate risk stratification, noninvasive imaging is the initial study of choice, and pertinent findings must be recognized in order to reach the correct diagnosis. Proptosis, increased attenuation of the intraorbital fat, extraocular muscle enlargement, superior ophthalmic vein enlargement and enlargement of the cavernous sinus can be seen on noncontrast head CT in patients with cavernous sinus fistulas. Noncontrast head CT can also demonstrate brain edema secondary to venous hypertension and hemorrhagic complications. In contrast, dilated cortical veins, venous varices and sinus thrombosis may also be revealed. Dynamic contrast CT with three-dimensional reconstruction using modern multidetector CT may improve detection. On MRI, dilated flow voids, occluded dural sinuses or abnormal curvilinear or serpiginous enhancement of dilated cortical veins may be found. MRA can also be used to detect DAVFs. Phase-contrast MRA eliminates some artifacts found with time-of-flight technique and can be used to assess the direction of flow within the dural sinuses and other draining veins.

Angiography remains the gold standard for diagnosis, risk stratification, and treatment planning for DAVFs. Complete arteriographic evaluation including selective injections of bilateral internal carotid, external carotid, and vertebral arteries, possibly involving superselective injections must be performed. Injections of the thyrocervical and costocervical trunks should also be obtained to exclude feeder arteries coming off the ascending and deep cervical arteries when the suspected lesion is at the craniocervical junction. Magnified and oblique views should be obtained with a rapid filming sequence to document the exact anatomy of each fistula. The vast majority of DAVFs are fed by meningeal arteries, while only 5% are supplied by both meningeal and cortical arteries. The presence of cortical arterial involvement may not be associated with severe neurological symptoms [32] but may have significant bearings on treatment planning. Assessment of arteriovenous transit through the normal brain structures may require prolonged filming during the venous phase and a large contrast bolus. Venous access to the fistula site is particularly important in cases with high-risk angiographic features in which endovascular treatment is contemplated.

Transverse and sigmoid sinuses are the most common sites of DAVFs, followed by cavernous sinus, tentorial incisura and superior sagittal sinuses [32]. The arterial supply to transverse or sigmoid sinus DAVFs is typically from transmastoid perforators of the occipital artery, branches off the middle meningeal artery (fig. 1), posterior auricular artery, neuromeningeal division of the ascending pharyngeal artery, posterior meningeal branches of the ipsilateral vertebral artery (fig. 1) and marginal tentorial branches of the meningohypophyseal trunk (fig. 2) [33]. Venous stenosis can occur, often at the junction of the draining vein and the draining dural sinus. Occasionally, the transverse sinus can be occluded on both ends, resulting in a trapped sinus with exclusive cortical venous drainage (fig. 1). Cortical venous drainage with distal venous stenosis is highly predictive of repeated hemorrhage and severe neurological symptoms.

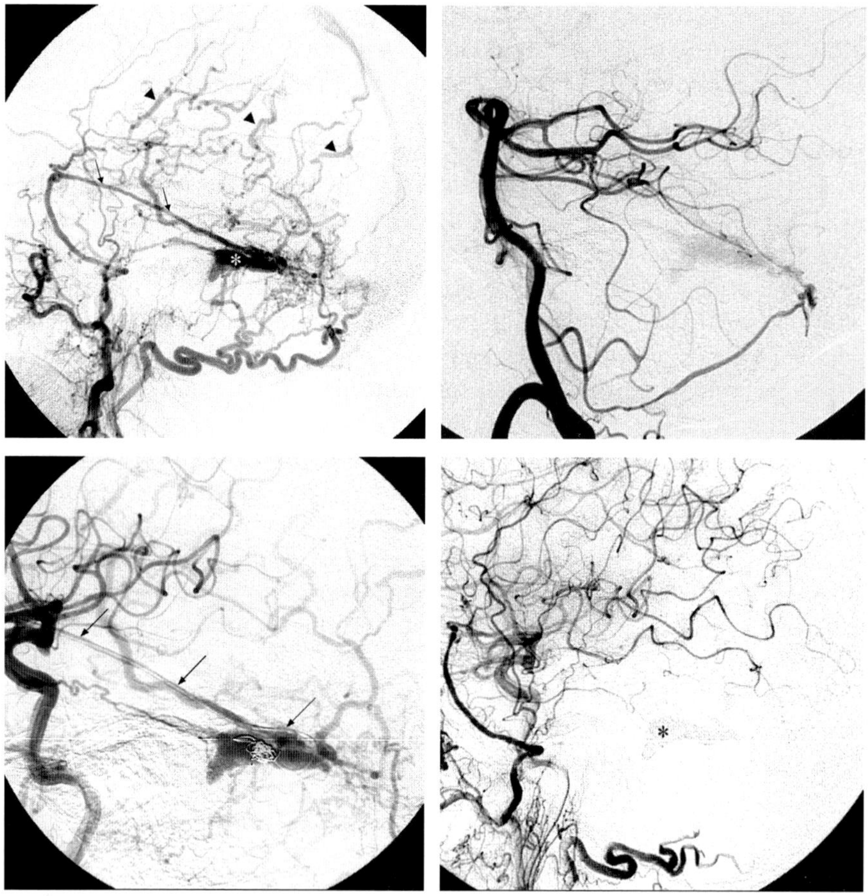

Fig. 1. Trapped transverse sinus DAVF. A 64-year-old woman presented with a 2-year history of headaches. ***a*** Lateral view of left external carotid artery injection demonstrates a transverse sinus DAVF with dominant supplies from middle meningeal artery (short arrows) and mastoid perforators of the occipital artery. The transverse sinus is occluded at both ends (*). The venous drainage is exclusively through cortical veins (arrowheads). ***b*** Lateral view of left vertebral artery injection also shows contribution from the posterior meningeal branch of the vertebral artery. ***c*** A microcatheter is placed into the trapped transverse sinus through the middle meningeal feeder artery and an electrolytically detachable coil is deployed in the sinus. ***d*** After complete packing of the trapped transverse sinus with fibered coils, arterio-venous shunting is no longer seen.

The anatomy and venous drainage of the cavernous sinus are rather complex. The meningeal branches of both internal and external carotid arteries and the internal carotid artery itself are in or around the cavernous sinus and can contribute to carotid-cavernous fistulas. The cavernous sinus normally receives

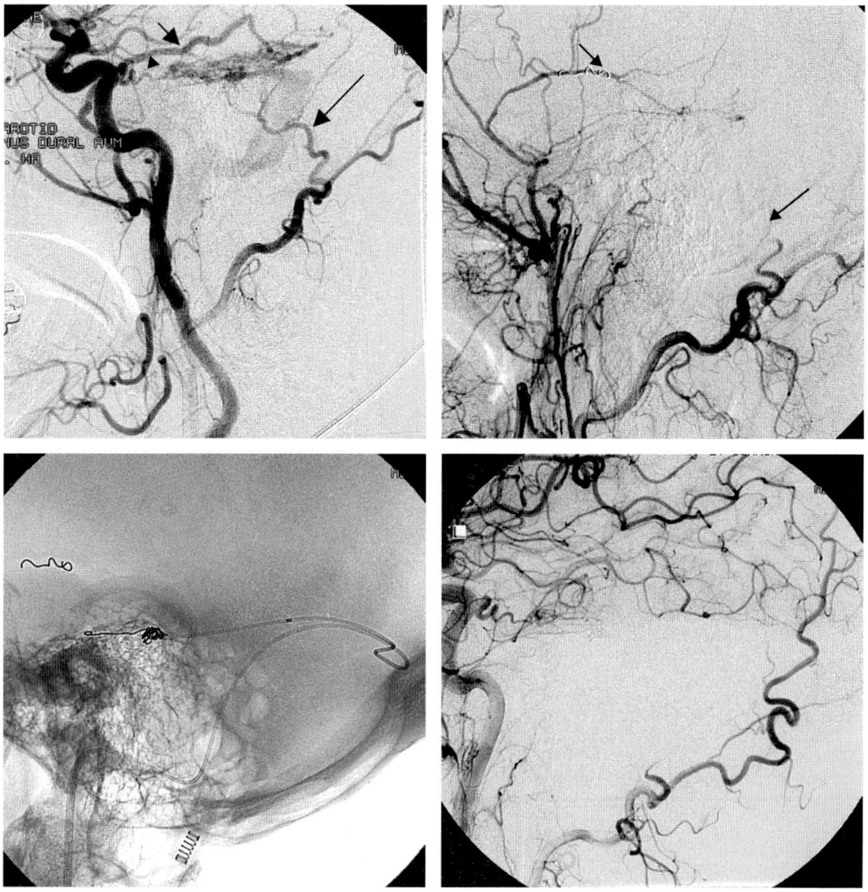

a *b* *c* *d*

Fig. 2. Superior petrosal sinus DAVF. A 52-year-old woman presented with relentless left periauricular headache and unbearable tinnitus. ***a*** Lateral view of left common carotid injection reveals a superior petrosal sinus DAVF, supplied by middle meningeal artery (long arrow), mastoid perforator of occipital artery (short arrow) and a corkscrew marginal tentorial branch of the internal carotid artery (arrowhead). ***b*** The middle meningeal feeder has been occluded with a coil and the occipital supply is embolized with absolute alcohol. ***c*** The reduced flow allows successful catheterization of the superior petrosal sinus. Electrolytically detachable coils are deployed to occlude the superior petrosal sinus. ***d*** Postembolization angiogram of the left common carotid artery demonstrates complete obliteration of the DAVF.

venous inflow from the superior and inferior ophthalmic veins and superficial middle cerebral veins via the sphenoparietal sinuses. Its outflow tract is through the superior and inferior petrosal sinuses, basilar plexus and anteroinferior emissary veins that drain into the pterygoid plexus (fig. 3). The cavernous sinus DAVFs frequently receive blood supply from the meningohypophyseal trunk,

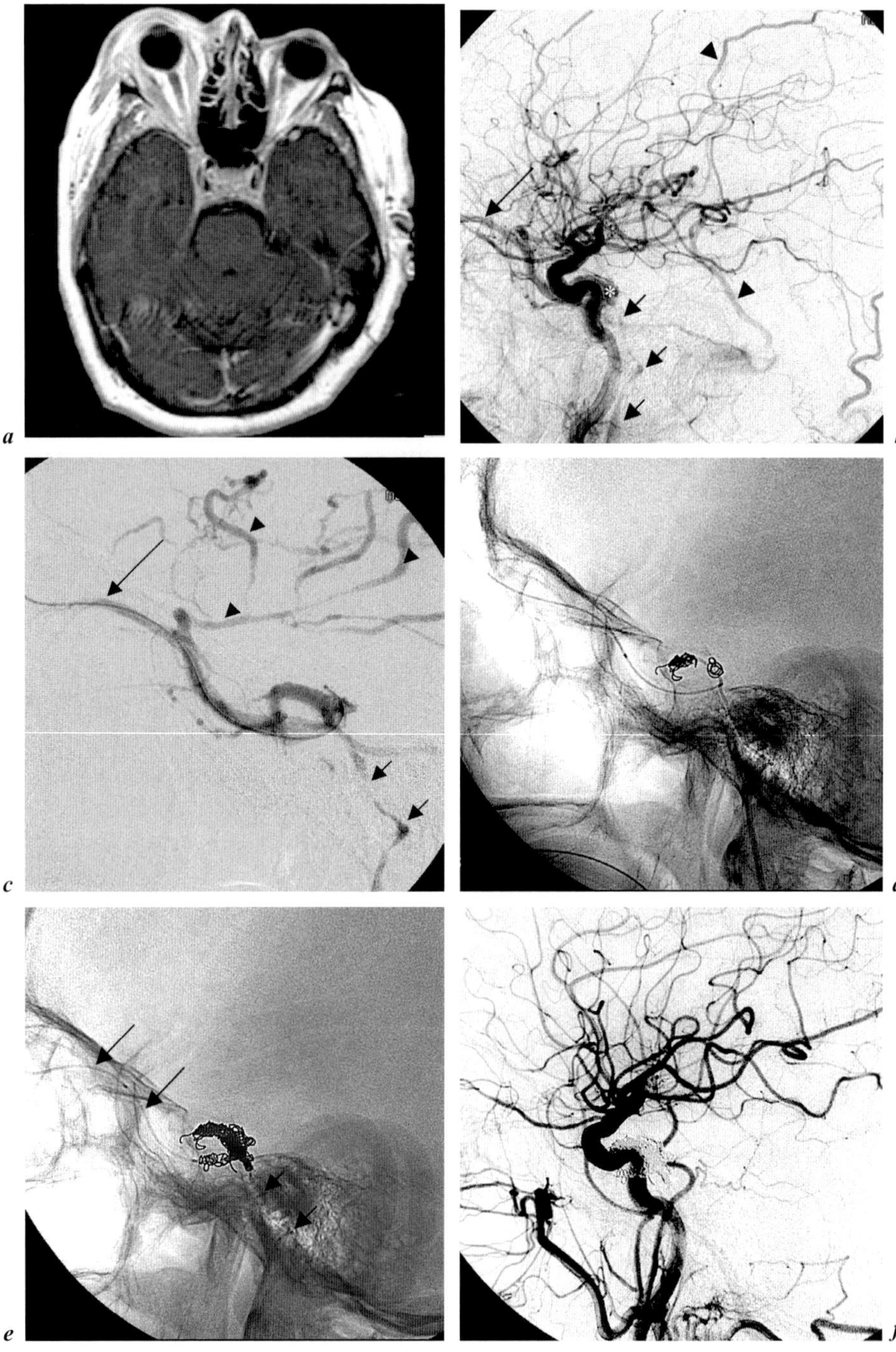
a
b
c
d
e
f

the inferolateral trunk, McConnell's capsular arteries and ophthalmic branches of the internal carotid artery and external carotid branches including the jugal and hypoglossal divisions of the ascending pharyngeal artery, the middle and accessory meningeal arteries, and arteries of foramen rotundum and pterygoid canal that come off the internal maxillary artery [53]. Supply from the contralateral internal and external carotid arteries can also occur. The venous drainage of cavernous sinus DAVFs are highly variable, depending on the preexisting venous anatomy, fistula flow rate and duration of disease. Retrograde drainage through the ophthalmic veins is the cause of visual symptoms, which frequently bring the patients to medical attention. On the other hand, cortical venous drainage with stenosis of the proximal superior ophthalmic vein can be indolent until hemorrhage occurs.

Superior sagittal sinus DAVFs usually involve the mid to posterior third of the superior sagittal sinus [54]. The arterial supply is mostly from the middle meningeal arteries, symmetrically on both sides. Small contributions from the falcine branch of the ophthalmic artery and the posterior meningeal branch of the vertebral artery may also be seen (fig. 4).

DAVFs of the anterior cranial fossa are uncommon. They are usually supplied by bilateral anterior and posterior ethmoidal branches of the ophthalmic artery, and drain cortically or infrequently through the cavernous sinus [55]. DAVFs involving the anterior cranial fossa, tentorium and superior sagittal sinus are more likely to develop the advanced types of venous drainage, and are thus at higher risk of hemorrhage [32].

DAVFs can also occur in the deep venous system [56]. The arterial feeders usually come from bilateral middle meningeal artery, marginal tentorial branches of internal carotid artery, occipital artery and possibly anterior cerebral and superficial temporal arteries. The vein of Galen is often involved and associated with hydrocephalus.

Fig. 3. Cavernous sinus DAVF. A 76-year-old woman presented with 6 months of right proptosis and tinnitus. ***a*** T1-weighted axial MRI through the orbit demonstrates periorbital edema, swelling of the extraocular muscles and enlarged superior ophthalmic vein. ***b*** Lateral view of right common carotid artery injection demonstrates a cavernous sinus DAVF with venous drainage through an enlarged superior ophthalmic vein (long arrow), stenotic inferior petrosal sinus (short arrows) and several cortical veins (arrowheads). ***c*** Cavernous sinus venogram confirms the above venous anatomy and drainage pattern. Stenosis of the superficial middle cerebral veins is also seen. ***d*** Electrolytically detachable coils are deployed in the cavernous sinus through two microcatheters placed into the cavernous sinus via superior ophthalmic vein and inferior petrosal sinus, respectively. ***e*** Complete packing of the cavernous sinus is achieved with additional fibered coils. ***f*** Postembolization angiogram of the right common carotid artery shows obliteration of arteriovenous shunting.

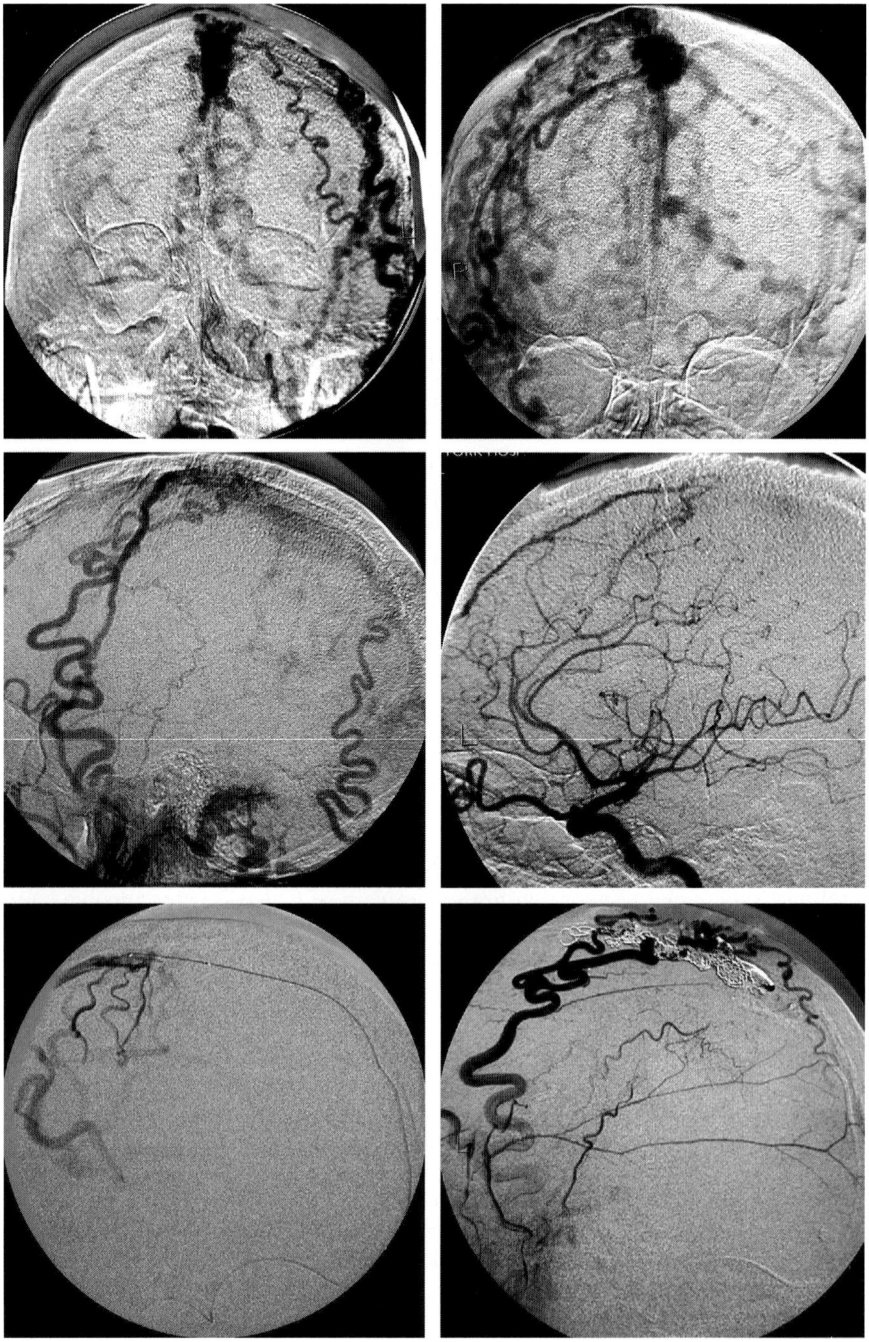

a b c d e f

Treatment

The decision to treat a patient with DAVF depends on the signs, symptoms and the angiographic risk strata of the lesion. Patients with decreasing visual acuity, visual loss, ophthalmoplegia, intracranial hemorrhage or infarct require emergent treatment. The presence of cortical venous drainage and venous varix represents a risk factor that should prompt treatment in a timely fashion. On the other hand, DAVFs that demonstrate slow arteriovenous shunting may spontaneously resolve, presumably from rethrombosis of the involved dural sinus. A 10–20% rate of spontaneous resolution has been reported in several case series [30, 43, 57], but the exact rate is unknown because some patients are managed expectantly by their primary physicians. Early reports of fistula resolution following arteriography alone were likely due to the caustic nature of the early hypertonic contrast agents. Modern nonionic contrast agents are not likely to induce thrombosis. Over time, some patients with pulsatile tinnitus improve without treatment [30]. Some DAVFs remain stable for long periods of time. DAVFs without venous restrictive disease are more likely to improve and remain stable. Detailed discussion will help patients develop an understanding of the benefits and risks of treatment.

Patients with mild symptoms such as tinnitus and absence of cortical venous drainage at arteriography can be managed expectantly. These patients should avoid the use of antiplatelet therapy, such as nonsteroid anti-inflammatory drugs, to best promote spontaneous thrombosis of the fistulas. Repeat arteriography should be considered whenever signs or symptoms change to monitor for escalation in risk factors. Despite low-risk angiographic features, some patients will describe severe pulsatile tinnitus that impairs their activities of daily living. In these cases, palliative transarterial embolization may be performed, although great care must be taken to avoid complications in excess of the natural history of the disease.

Compression therapy has been used to treat DAVF and may still be useful in selected patients with low-risk fistulas [58]. These patients should be

Fig. 4. Superior sagittal sinus DAVF. A 58-year-old man with anticardiolipin antibodies developed headaches and progressive memory loss. ***a*** Anterior projection of left external carotid angiogram demonstrates a superior sagittal sinus DAVF supplied by several middle meningeal feeders. The posterior sagittal sinus is thrombosed. Extensive cortical venous drainage is seen bilaterally. ***b*** Symmetrical arterial supply also comes from the right side. ***c*** Lateral view of the left external carotid artery injection reveals a second DAVF of the transverse sinus. ***d*** Pial supply of the DAVF is also seen and drains anteriorly. ***e*** A microcatheter is placed into the anterior superior sagittal sinus by a transjugular approach. ***f*** Postembolization angiogram of the left external carotid artery shows that the mid superior sagittal sinus has been packed with coils, obliterating the DAVF.

self-motivated and free of atherosclerotic disease in the cervical carotid arteries. For patients with slow-flow cavernous DAVFs, manual compression of the ipsilateral carotid-jugular sheath with the contralateral hand stands the best chance for affecting a cure. We did not experience as high a success rate for compression therapy in our larger series [40]. For patients with transverse/sigmoid sinus AVFs that are predominantly supplied by the occipital artery, compression of the pulsatile occipital artery over the mastoid bone with the ipsilateral hand may be effective. As many as 27% of these patients have been reported to benefit from this simple treatment [53, 58].

For lesions that warrant treatment, craniotomy and endovascular therapy are the primary treatment modalities. Although surgical resection or skeletonization of the involved segment of the sinus is effective, bleeding complications are not infrequent given the highly vascular nature of DAVFs [59]. Recent reports have also shown that disconnection of cortical draining veins near the fistulas is safe and effective [60–62]. Detailed arteriography will help direct the surgeon to the appropriate site for ligation. To reduce the surgical morbidity, preoperative embolization is often warranted. However, in some cases, preoperative embolization may add an unnecessary risk. For example, DAVFs of the anterior cranial fossa are better suited for surgery because these fistulas are supplied by the anterior and posterior ethmoidal branches of the ophthalmic artery. Embolization of these vessels in proximity to the retinal artery risks blindness, whereas a subfrontal craniotomy can give easy access to these feeder arteries and the draining vein [63].

Stereotactic radiosurgery has been used to treat patients with DAVFs. In general, radiation has not been effective against high-flow DAVFs. Treatment success of 75% has been reported for low-flow cavernous sinus DAVFs but only 20% success was found with high-flow DAVFs [64]. Improved success rates for radiosurgery have been reported when patients undergo transarterial embolization prior to radiotherapy [65].

Endovascular treatment strategies can be divided into transarterial and transvenous approaches. Transarterial embolization is more often palliative or preparative treatment before more definitive therapy, either by transvenous embolization or open surgical resection. Under appropriate circumstances, transvenous embolization is highly effective to achieve curative obliteration of high-risk DAVFs. Deposition of embolic materials within the recipient venous pouch of the fistula functions in a manner similar with surgical clipping of the draining cortical veins described previously. Moreover, transvenous embolization when used appropriately is generally safer than transarterial embolization and probably carries a lower risk of stroke [66].

Transarterial embolization reduces arterial inflow hence relieving venous hypertension and its associated symptoms. Platinum coils, particulates, and liquid adhesive and sclerosing agents have been used for transarterial embolization of DAVFs [67–69]. There are benefits to each. Electrolytically detachable coils (GDC) can be passed through smaller caliber microcatheters with precise control but are not thrombogenic and are very expensive. Fibered platinum coils are easy to deposit and are highly thrombogenic but require a larger lumen microcatheter. Proximal deposition of embolic materials of any type is undesirable because collateral circulation to the fistula will soon develop and future access through these primary channels is precluded. Particulate agents usually provide only temporary occlusion and are generally used as temporizing agents. Care must be taken in patients with intrapulmonary or cardiac shunts when using particulate agents to prevent passage of the embolic materials and arterial recirculation. If the use of particulate agents results in slow flow within the fistula, there is a better chance of fistula thrombosis either alone or with compression therapy.

Transarterial injection of liquid adhesive and sclerosing agents are anecdotally more effective at occluding the fistula site, but these agents are more difficult to control and carry a higher risk of neurological injury. If the liquid agent reaches the fistula site within the wall of the dural sinus, then a durable cure can be achieved [68, 70]. N-Butyl cyanoacrylate is the commonly used adhesive agent. Absolute ethanol is a nonviscous liquid that is highly effective in penetrating the fistula resulting in immediate endothelial injury, vasospasm, and thrombosis. However, its use remains controversial because of the potential side effects. Superselective angiograms should be performed and studied carefully before embolization to avoid inadvertent embolization of cranial nerves or extracranial to intracranial collateral arteries. Provocative testing with amytal and xylocaine is used in an effort to reduce the risks of transarterial embolization.

Some DAVFs are difficult to treat using transarterially embolization. These fistulas derive blood supply from small or distal branches of meningeal arteries that are difficult to access, or are supplied by meningeal branches of pial arteries that pose a risk of stroke if occluded, or have innumerable minute branches that are poorly visualized and cannot be individually cannulated.

Transvenous embolization is best suited for high-risk DAVFs with venous outflow restriction. The safety profile of transvenous embolization depends on the presence of anatomic or functional outflow obstruction. Careful examination of the venous drainage pattern before embolization is crucial to determine if the patient will tolerate sinus occlusion. The presence of a cortical vein that uses the involved sinus for drainage should suggest a high risk of venous infarct or worsening of neurological deficit if the sinus is occluded. Occlusion of major cortical veins such as Labbe, Trolard, internal cerebral veins and vein of Galen should also be avoided unless it is clearly demonstrated at arteriography that these veins no longer serve to drain blood from the brain parenchyma. Patients with fast-flow DAVFs have arterialized sinuses with high pressure that is unlikely to receive cortical venous drainage. Patients with chronic venous restrictive diseases are more likely to have developed alternative venous drainage pathways and are more likely to tolerate the occlusion of involved sinuses.

The success of transvenous embolization depends on complete occlusion of the recipient draining vein to achieve thrombosis of the fistula. Failure to completely occlude the sinus or venous drainage pathway may create a trapped sinus with worsening cortical venous hypertension requiring craniotomy to repair. Moreover, additional transvenous embolization is again precluded by the previously placed embolic materials. Therefore, it is very important to clearly identify the fistula site and the sinus segments that need to be occluded before embarking on transvenous embolization.

Venous access can usually be achieved with modern imaging equipment and excellent microcatheter technique. Even occluded sinuses can be recannulated for embolization [71, 72]. If necessary, open surgical exposure [73] and transarterial approach [74] can also help gaining access to the targeted venous segment. Preoperative transarterial embolization may be necessary to reduce the arteriovenous shunt volume and pressure in the involved sinus to facilitate catheterization and stabilization of embolic material. There is usually ample arterial supply to allow road mapping and identification of the fistula site during the transvenous occlusion process.

Both liquid adhesive agent and coils have been successfully used for transvenous embolization [67, 75, 76]. The preferred technique is to initially deploy electrolytically detachable coils to form an anchoring basket to prevent migration of the following coils. Another advantage of the detachable coils is excellent control of coil deposition such that coils can be placed at the precise location in the sinus. Pushable fibered coils, which are more thrombogenic, can be subsequently added to achieve complete occlusion of the venous segment.

Type B and D cavernous sinus DAVFs are ideal for the transvenous approach because the internal carotid feeders are difficult to cannulate and risky to embolize. Even type C cavernous sinus DAVFs are rarely embolized to completion by transarterial embolization alone and transvenous embolization should be favored. The superior ophthalmic vein [77–81], inferior petrosal sinus [72], and superior petrosal sinus [82] can all be used as venous access. The inferior petrosal sinus is probably the easiest transfemoral access as it joins the internal jugular vein at a favorable angle. The superior ophthalmic vein can be surgically exposed if the transfemoral approach turns out to be difficult [83]. The cavernous sinus can be safely occluded without significant risk on normal cortical venous drainage. However, it is important to completely disconnect the cavernous sinus from the superior ophthalmic vein and the superficial middle cerebral vein to resolve visual symptoms and to prevent hemorrhage from cortical draining vein (fig. 3).

Caution should be taken when embolizing lateral sinus DAVFs with the transvenous approach. Acute thrombosis of a normal transverse/sigmoid sinus with antegrade flow is not well tolerated. Djindjian type I and II or Lalwani grade 1 and 2 patients are not candidates for transvenous embolization. For the high-grade patients, particularly, patients with stenosis or occlusion at both ends of the sinus, the so-called 'trapped sinus', transvenous embolization can be safely performed. Microcatheters can be navigated through thrombosed sinus or transarterially into the trapped sinus if the fistula is large enough. Complete packing of the trapped sinus will achieve a durable cure (fig. 1).

Tentorial DAVFs can be treated similarly as cavernous sinus DAVFs. The meningeal feeder arteries are usually tortuous and difficult to cannulate distally for transarterial embolization. Occlusion of the superior and inferior petrosal sinuses is well tolerated (fig. 2).

The sagittal sinus may be difficult to access transfemorally, particularly when it is thrombosed. Direct surgical exposure of the anterior sagittal sinus may be required. The anterior third of the sagittal sinus can be safely occluded. The middle third may be occluded if the patient had long-standing venous hypertension and developed an alternative drainage pathway. The posterior third of the sagittal sinus should be preserved (fig. 4).

Conclusion

Patients with DAVFs present with a wide range of symptoms. Risk stratification by cortical venous drainage is important for the treatment decision. Low-risk patients can be managed expectantly or treated palliatively. Endovascular treatment is the first-line therapy for high-risk patients. Surgical resection or disconnection of the cortical draining vein is preferred for DAVFs of the anterior cranial fossa or those that failed endovascular therapy. Stereotactic radiosurgery has a limited role in the treatment of slow-flow DAVFs, and may be combined with endovascular treatment as an adjunct therapy.

References

1 Newton TH, Cronqvist S: Involvement of dural arteries in intracranial arteriovenous malformations. Radiology 1969;93:1071–1078.

2 Kawaguchi T, et al: Traumatic lesions of the bilateral middle meningeal arteries – Case report. Neurol Med Chir (Tokyo) 2002;42/5:221–223.

3 Field M, et al: Dural arteriovenous fistula after ventriculostomy. Case illustration. J Neurosurg 2002;97/1:227.
4 Komiyama M, et al: Traumatic carotid cavernous sinus fistula: Serial angiographic studies from the day of trauma. AJNR Am J Neuroradiol 1998;19:1641–1644.
5 Sakaki T, et al: Dural arteriovenous fistula of the posterior fossa developing after surgical occlusion of the sigmoid sinus. Report of five cases. J Neurosurg 1996;84/1:113–118.
6 Sasaki T, et al: Postsurgical development of dural arteriovenous malformations after transpetrosal and transtentorial operations: Case report. Neurosurgery 1995;37:820–825.
7 Yoshimura S, et al: Arteriovenous fistula around the ventriculoperitoneal shunt system in a patient with a dural arteriovenous malformation of the posterior fossa. Case report. J Neurosurg 1995; 82/2:288–290.
8 Freckmann N, Sartor K, Herrmann HD: Traumatic arteriovenous fistulae of the middle meningeal artery and neighbouring veins or dural sinuses. Acta Neurochir 1981;55/3–4:273–281.
9 Chaudhary MY, et al: Dural arteriovenous malformation of the major venous sinuses: An acquired lesion. AJNR Am J Neuroradiol 1982;3/1:13–19.
10 Nishio A, et al: Dural arteriovenous fistula involving the superior sagittal sinus following sinus thrombosis – Case report. Neurol Med Chir (Tokyo) 2002;42/5:217–220.
11 Kuncz A, et al: Venous cerebral infarction due to simultaneous occurrence of dural arteriovenous fistula and developmental venous anomaly. Acta Neurochir (Wien) 2001;143:1183–1184.
12 Vilela P, Willinsky R, terBrugge K: Dural arteriovenous fistula associated with neoplastic dural sinus thrombosis: Two cases. Neuroradiology 2001;43:816–820.
13 Phatouros CC, et al: Acquired pial arteriovenous fistula following cerebral vein thrombosis. Stroke 1999;30:2487–2490.
14 Arnautovic KI, et al: Dural arteriovenous malformations of the transverse/sigmoid sinus acquired from dominant sinus occlusion by a tumor: Report of two cases. Neurosurgery 1998;42:383–388.
15 Kollar C, et al: Dural arteriovenous fistula in association with heterotopic brain nodule in the transverse sinus. AJNR Am J Neuroradiol 1998;19:1126–1128.
16 Yassari R, Jahromi B, Macdonald R: Dural arteriovenous fistula after craniotomy for pilocytic astrocytoma in a patient with protein S deficiency. Surg Neurol 2002;58/1:59–64.
17 Witt O, Pereira PL, Tillmann W: Severe cerebral venous sinus thrombosis and dural arteriovenous fistula in an infant with protein S deficiency. Childs Nerv Syst 1999;15/2–3:128–130.
18 Singh V, et al: Dural arteriovenous fistula associated with prothrombin gene mutation. J Neuroimaging 2001;11:319–321.
19 Kraus JA, Stuper BK, Berlit P: Association of resistance to activated protein C and dural arteriovenous fistulas. J Neurol 1998;245:731–733.
20 Kurata A, et al: Spontaneous carotid cavernous fistulas with special reference to the influence of estradiol decrease. Neurol Res 1999;21:631–639.
21 Toya S, et al: Spontaneous carotid-cavernous fistula during pregnancy or in the postpartum stage. Report of two cases. J Neurosurg 1981;54/2:252–256.
22 Terada T, et al: The effect of oestrogen on the development of arteriovenous fistulae induced by venous hypertension in rats. Acta Neurochir 1998;140/1:82–86.
23 Terada T, et al: The role of angiogenic factor bFGF in the development of dural AVFs. Acta Neurochir 1996;138:877–883.
24 Uranishi R, Nakase H, Sakaki T: Expression of angiogenic growth factors in dural arteriovenous fistula. J Neurosurg 1999;91:781–786.
25 Hamada Y, et al: Histopathological aspects of dural arteriovenous fistulas in the transverse-sigmoid sinus region in nine patients. Neurosurgery 1997;40:452–458.
26 Lawton MT, Jacobowitz R, Spetzler RF: Redefined role of angiogenesis in the pathogenesis of dural arteriovenous malformations. J Neurosurg 1997;87/2:267–274.
27 Barth KH, White RI Jr, Marshall FF: Quantification of arteriovenous shunting in renal cell carcinoma. J Urol 1981;125/2:161–163.
28 Malek AM, et al: Treatment of dural arteriovenous malformations and fistulas. Neurosurg Clin N Am 2000;11/1:147–166, ix.
29 Awad IA, et al: Intracranial dural arteriovenous malformations: Factors predisposing to an aggressive neurological course. J Neurosurg 1990;72:839–850.

30 Brown RD Jr, Wiebers DO, Nichols DA: Intracranial dural arteriovenous fistulae: Angiographic predictors of intracranial hemorrhage and clinical outcome in nonsurgical patients. J Neurosurg 1994;81:531–538.

31 Castaigne P, et al: Meningeal arteriovenous fistulas with cortical venous drainage. Rev Neurol (Paris) 1976;132/3:169–181.

32 Cognard C, et al: Cerebral dural arteriovenous fistulas: Clinical and angiographic correlation with a revised classification of venous drainage. Radiology 1995;194:671–680.

33 Halbach VV, et al: Dural fistulas involving the transverse and sigmoid sinuses: Results of treatment in 28 patients. Radiology 1987;163:443–447.

34 Duckwiler GR, et al: Delayed venous occlusion following embolotherapy of vascular malformations in the brain. AJNR Am J Neuroradiol 1992;13:1571–1579.

35 Kurita H, et al: Congestive brain oedema associated with a pial arteriovenous malformation with impaired venous drainage. Acta Neurochir (Wien) 2001;143:339–342.

36 Miyamoto K, Heimann A, Kempski O: Microcirculatory alterations in a Mongolian gerbil sinus-vein thrombosis model. J Clin Neurosci 2001;8(suppl 1):97–105.

37 Djindjian R, Merland JJ: Superselective Arteriography of the External Carotid Artery. New York, Springer, 1978.

38 Lalwani AK, Dowd CF, Halbach VV: Grading venous restrictive disease in patients with dural arteriovenous fistulas of the transverse/sigmoid sinus. J Neurosurg 1993;79/1:11–15.

39 Barrow DL, et al: Classification and treatment of spontaneous carotid-cavernous sinus fistulas. J Neurosurg 1985;62/2:248–256.

40 Meyers PM, et al: Dural carotid cavernous fistula: Definitive endovascular management and long-term follow-up. Am J Ophthalmol 2002;134/1:85–92.

41 Newton TH, Hoyt WF: Dural arteriovenous shunts in the region of the cavernous sinus. Neuroradiology 1970;1:7181.

42 Houser OW, et al: Arteriovenous malformation affecting the transverse dural venous sinus – An acquired lesion. Mayo Clin Proc 1979;54:651–661.

43 Fermand M, et al: Long term follow-up of 43 pure dural arteriovenous fistulae (AVF) of the lateral sinus. Neuroradiology 1987;29:348–353.

44 Kawaguchi S, Sakaki T, Uranishi R: Color Doppler flow imaging of the superior ophthalmic vein in dural arteriovenous fistulas. Stroke 2002;33:2009–2013.

45 Matsuda S, et al: Intracranial dural arteriovenous fistula (DAVF) presenting progressive dementia and parkinsonism. J Neurol Sci 1999;165:43–47.

46 Datta NN, et al: Reversible dementia due to dural arteriovenous fistula: A simple surgical option. Neurosurg Rev 1998;21/2–3:174–176.

47 Hurst RW, et al: Dementia resulting from dural arteriovenous fistulas: The pathologic findings of venous hypertensive encephalopathy. AJNR Am J Neuroradiol 1998;19:1267–1273.

48 Perkash I, et al: Intracranial dural arteriovenous fistula causing a myelopathy. Spinal Cord 2002;40:438–442.

49 Kalamangalam GP, et al: Myelopathy from intracranial dural arteriovenous fistula. J Neurol Neurosurg Psychiatry 2002;72:816–818.

50 Wiesmann M, et al: Intracranial dural arteriovenous fistula with spinal medullary venous drainage. Eur Radiol 2000;10:1606–1609.

51 Ricolfi F, et al: Intracranial dural arteriovenous fistulae with perimedullary venous drainage. Anatomical, clinical and therapeutic considerations. Neuroradiology 1999;41:803–812.

52 Ernst RJ, et al: Cervical myelopathy associated with intracranial dural arteriovenous fistula: MR findings before and after treatment. AJNR Am J Neuroradiol 1997;18:1330–1334.

53 Halbach VV, et al: Dural fistulas involving the cavernous sinus: Results of treatment in 30 patients. Radiology 1987;163:437–442.

54 Halbach VV, et al: Treatment of dural arteriovenous malformations involving the superior sagittal sinus. AJNR Am J Neuroradiol 1988;9:337–343.

55 Halbach VV, et al: Dural arteriovenous fistulas supplied by ethmoidal arteries. Neurosurgery 1990;26:816–823.

56 Halbach VV, et al: Treatment of dural fistulas involving the deep cerebral venous system. AJNR Am J Neuroradiol 1989;10:393–399.

57 Bavinzski G, et al: Evolution of different therapeutic strategies in the treatment of cranial dural arteriovenous fistulas – Report of 30 cases. Acta Neurochir 1996;138:132–138.
58 Higashida RT, et al: Closure of carotid cavernous sinus fistulae by external compression of the carotid artery and jugular vein. Acta Radiol Suppl 1986;369:580–583.
59 Sundt TM Jr, Piepgras DG: The surgical approach to arteriovenous malformations of the lateral and sigmoid dural sinuses. J Neurosurg 1983;59/1:32–39.
60 Thompson BG, Doppman JL, Oldfield EH: Treatment of cranial dural arteriovenous fistulae by interruption of leptomeningeal venous drainage. J Neurosurg 1994;80:617–623.
61 Collice M, et al: Surgical interruption of leptomeningeal drainage as treatment for intracranial dural arteriovenous fistulas without dural sinus drainage. J Neurosurg 1996;84:810–817.
62 Hoh BL, et al: Surgical management of high-grade intracranial dural arteriovenous fistulas: Leptomeningeal venous disruption without nidus excision. Neurosurgery 1998;42:796–805.
63 Lawton MT, et al: Ethmoidal dural arteriovenous fistulae: An assessment of surgical and endovascular management. Neurosurgery 1999;45:805–811.
64 Hirai T, et al: Dural carotid cavernous fistulas: Role of conventional radiation therapy – Long-term results with irradiation, embolization, or both. Radiology 1998;207:423–430.
65 Friedman JA, et al: Results of combined stereotactic radiosurgery and transarterial embolization for dural arteriovenous fistulas of the transverse and sigmoid sinuses. J Neurosurg 2001;94: 886–891.
66 Roy D, Raymond J: The role of transvenous embolization in the treatment of intracranial dural arteriovenous fistulas. Neurosurgery 1997;40:1133–1134.
67 Jansen O, et al: Endovascular therapy of arteriovenous fistulae with electrolytically detachable coils. Neuroradiology 1999;41:951–957.
68 Iizuka Y, et al: Successful transarterial glue embolisation by wedged technique for a tentorial dural arteriovenous fistula presenting with a conjunctival injection. Neuroradiology 2001;43: 677–679.
69 Nakstad PH, Bakke SJ, Hald JK: Embolization of intracranial arteriovenous malformations and fistulas with polyvinyl alcohol particles and platinum fibre coils. Neuroradiology 1992;34: 348–351.
70 Barnwell SL, et al: Dural arteriovenous fistulas involving the inferior petrosal sinus: Angiographic findings in six patients. AJNR Am J Neuroradiol 1990;11:511–516.
71 Gobin YP, et al: Percutaneous transvenous embolization through the thrombosed sinus in transverse sinus dural fistula. AJNR Am J Neuroradiol 1993;14:1102–1105.
72 Benndorf G, et al: Transvenous occlusion of dural cavernous sinus fistulas through the thrombosed inferior petrosal sinus: Report of four cases and review of the literature. Surg Neurol 2000;54/1:42–54.
73 Houdart E, et al: Transcranial approach for venous embolization of dural arteriovenous fistulas. J Neurosurg 2002;97/2:280–286.
74 Fukai J, et al: Transarterial intravenous coil embolization of dural arteriovenous fistula involving the superior sagittal sinus. Surg Neurol 2001;55:353–358.
75 Halbach VV, et al: Transvenous embolization of dural fistulas involving the transverse and sigmoid sinuses. AJNR Am J Neuroradiol 1989;10:385–392.
76 Halbach VV, et al: Transvenous embolization of dural fistulas involving the cavernous sinus. AJNR Am J Neuroradiol 1989;10:377–383.
77 Klink T, Hofmann E, Lieb W: Transvenous embolization of carotid cavernous fistulas via the superior ophthalmic vein. Graefes Arch Clin Exp Ophthalmol 2001;239:583–588.
78 Miller NR, et al: Treatment of carotid-cavernous sinus fistulas using a superior ophthalmic vein approach. J Neurosurg 1995;83:838–842.
79 Monsein LH, et al: Treatment of dural carotid-cavernous fistulas via the superior ophthalmic vein. AJNR Am J Neuroradiol 1991;12:435–439.
80 Quinones D, et al: Embolization of dural cavernous fistulas via superior ophthalmic vein approach. AJNR Am J Neuroradiol 1997;18:921–928.
81 Goldberg RA, et al: Management of cavernous sinus-dural fistulas. Indications and techniques for primary embolization via the superior ophthalmic vein. Arch Ophthalmol 1996;114:707–714.

82 Mounayer C, et al: Superior petrosal sinus catheterization for transvenous embolization of a dural carotid cavernous sinus fistula. AJNR Am J Neuroradiol 2002;23:1153–1155.
83 Benndorf G, et al: Treatment of a cavernous sinus dural arteriovenous fistula by deep orbital puncture of the superior ophthalmic vein. Neuroradiology 2001;43:499–502.

Philip M. Meyers, MD
Neurological Institute of New York
710 West 168th Street, Room 404, New York, NY 10032
Tel. +1 212 305 6384, Fax +1 212 342 1229, E-Mail pmm2002@columbia.edu

Horowitz MB, Levy EI (eds): Neuroendovascular Surgery.
Prog Neurol Surg. Basel, Karger, 2005, vol 17, pp 180–193

Tumor Embolization

Elad I. Levy[a], *Richard Spiro*[b], *Michael B. Horowitz*[b], *Ricardo Hanel*[b]

[a] Millard Filmore Hospital, Dept. of Neurosurgery, Buffalo, N.Y., USA
[b] Center for Cranial Nerve Disorders, UPMC Presbyterian, Pittsburgh, Pa., USA

Patients with facial, cervical, spinal, and intracranial neoplasms are often referred to the endovascular surgeon for preoperative evaluation and embolization. The purpose of these investigations and treatments is to define the relevant arterial and venous anatomy and possibly administer therapy to either aid with subsequent surgical resection or provide primary tumor control thus avoiding an open surgical intervention. Prior to undertaking such a case the interventionalist must be sure he/she understands the purpose of the study along with the patient's disease stage so that appropriate therapy can be applied.

Background and Routine Indications

The earliest reports of tumor embolization surfaced in 1974 when Hekster et al. [1] described the use of preoperative embolization to reduce blood loss during tumor resection. Since that time embolization has developed into a routine procedure for many hypervascular neoplasms including metastatic renal cell carcinomas in the spine, hemangioblastomas, hemangiopericytomas, choroid plexus papillomas, juvenile nasopharyngeal angiofibromas, paragangliomas, and some meningiomas. Indications, however, at times remain variable and at times subjective. With regard to meningiomas, for example, as modern surgical techniques and tools such as microscopy, endoscopy, electrocautery, skull base approaches for tumor and dural exposure, and development of newer hemostatic agents have become available it has been less necessary to devascularize these lesions ahead of time. Bendszus et al. [2, 3] reported on 60 patients, 30 of whom underwent embolization and resection and 30 of whom underwent resection alone. The rates of surgical morbidity with permanent neurological worsening were 16% in the embolization group and 20% in the nonembolization group. If the one patient that suffered a neurological injury as

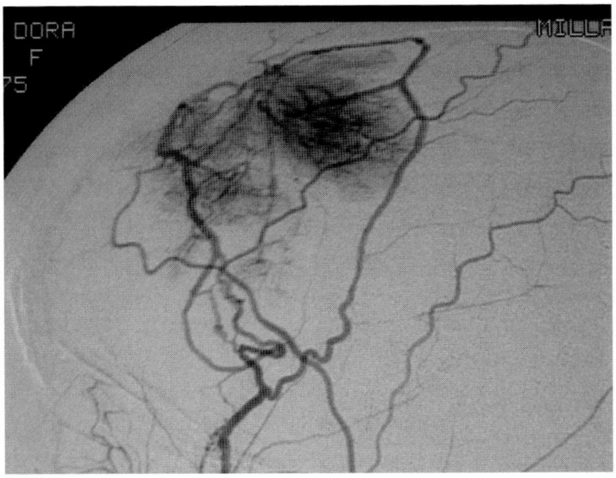

Fig. 1. Lateral ECA angiogram showing supply to meningioma.

a consequence of the embolization is added to the total complication numbers then overall morbidity and mortality were identical for the embolized and non-embolized patients. The only significant difference between the two groups was intraoperative blood loss, which was lower in the embolized cohort.

A variety of lesions are commonly referred for endovascular therapy. These include hemangiopericytomas, meningiomas, hemangioblastomas, paragangliomas of the head and neck, juvenile nasopharyngeal angiofibromas, choriocarcinomas, choroid plexus tumors, malignant head and neck cancers (squamous cell carcinomas), nasal papillomas, metastatic renal cell carcinoma, and aneurysmal bone cysts. For the majority of these lesions the embolization is geared towards reducing tumor blood supply prior to surgical extirpation. Reducing blood supply prospectively provides the surgeon with reduced intraoperative bleeding thus improving intraoperative visualization of vital structures, and reducing the need for transfusions or staged procedures. The later is especially relevant in children with lower overall total blood volume and patients with an aversion to blood transfusions. Embolization may also benefit the surgeon by allowing him/her to attack the tumor directly without first having to access and obliterate the vascular supply. This is especially useful for large tumors that obtain their blood supply from regions deep to the surgical exposure such as some sphenoid wing meningiomas, choroid plexus tumors, and hemangioblastomas. This direct attack permits for tumor debulking as the embolization reduces the bleeding that occurs when a tumor is debulked with its blood supply intact. Bendszus et al. [2, 3] reviewed 60 cases and found that while complete embolization of a tumor's blood supply was beneficial, less than 90% devascularization had no effect on intraoperative blood loss. Oka et al. [4]

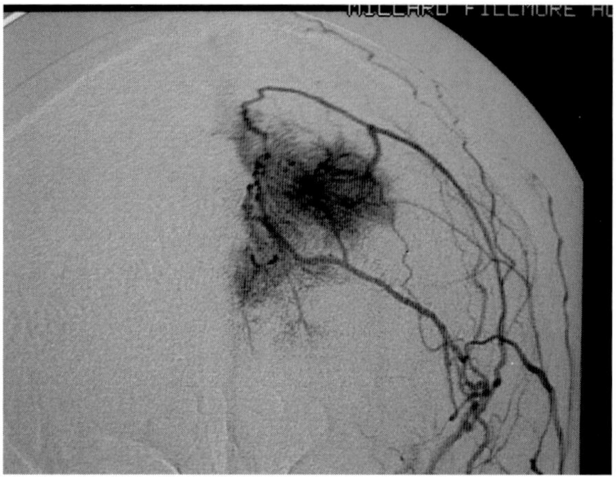

Fig. 2. AP view of external carotid artery angiogram supply to meningioma.

studied 20 embolized skull base meningiomas and found that in lesions smaller than 6 cm in diameter blood loss was significantly less in embolized versus nonembolized lesions. For lesions greater than 6 cm blood loss was no different with or without embolization. This lack of difference might relate to poor infiltration of the tumor bed in these larger lesions or to the overall greater vascularity of these larger lesions. Ng et al. [5] documented a lower need for transfusions, shorter resection times and increased necrosis in tumors treated with superselective catheterization and embolization. Macpherson [6] studied 52 patients, 28 of whom underwent embolization. He noted reduced intraoperative bleeding, decreased surgical complications, and better follow-up result in those who underwent initial endovascular occlusions.

Perhaps the best study to date was carried out by Dean et al. [7]. These authors used matched samples of embolized and nonembolized groups of meningiomas and studied blood loss, number of transfusions, surgical resection time, length of hospitalization, and overall cost effectiveness. Results indicated that for large tumors (mean 5.7 cm) endovascular devascularization translated into decreased blood loss (533 vs. 866 ml), reduced transfusion requirements (0.39 vs. 1.56 units), shorter hospitalization (10.6 vs. 15 days), and overall diminished costs (USD 29.605 vs. USD 38.449). Only blood loss and units transfused were statistically significant .

Embolization for the purpose of changing a tumor's consistency is a newer concept. Embolization performed several days prior to tumor resection may devascularize a tumor to an extent that the tumor begins to necrose and almost liquify making resection easier and faster, as tumor necrosis can change a

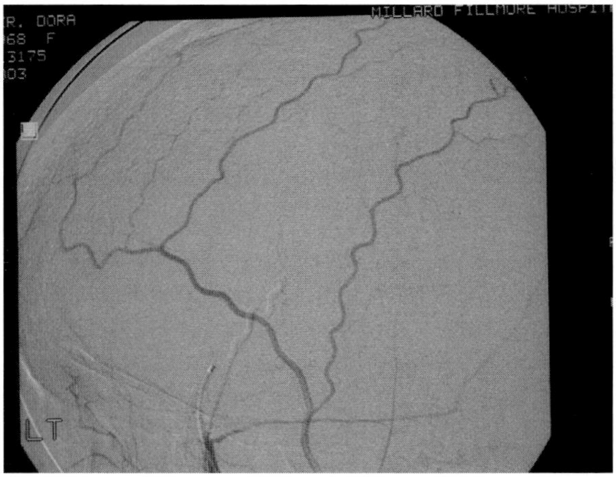

Fig. 3. Lateral view of ECA supply to meningioma after embolization. No tumor slush seen.

fibrous tumor into a soft partially liquified lesion that can be removed at times with vigorous suction alone. The optimal time for resection of meningiomas with at least 50% tumor supply embolization is felt to be 7–9 days, after which there is no additional tissue death [8]. Others have found that tumor necrosis is apparent 4 days after embolization when proton spectroscopy is performed [9, 10].

Despite the fact that most patients are referred for preoperative embolization as an adjunct to surgery, some individuals are referred for endovascular therapy as definitive therapy. These cases include tumor embolizations to induce tumor necrosis and possible shrinkage or growth arrest over time. Other embolization procedures are carried out for the purpose of introducing chemotherapeutic agents into tumors at concentrations that cannot be achieved with systemic administration without unacceptable or intolerable side effects. Schemes for slowing a tumor's growth or actually causing a reduction in tumor volume have been explored. Some elderly patients with large meningiomas have been managed with embolization alone with documented tumor shrinkage over time. This reduction in mass effect can potentially alleviate an individual's symptoms. Intra-arterial therapies for malignant brain neoplasms have also been reported [11–14]. Kerber et al. [15] treated patients with advanced squamous cell carcinoma of the head and neck with intra-arterial cisplatin along with intravenous thiosulfate to counteract systemic toxicity. Tumor control was documented in more than 90% of the patients studied.

Other nontraditional embolization indications are pain control. Patients with metastatic spine lesions such as those from renal cell carcinoma can be embolized to assist with surgical resection. For those patients, however, who have pain and are not candidates for surgery or radiation, embolization of radicular aortic pedicles feeding the tumor can often provide pain relief by reducing the lesions blood supply and the associated periosteal and soft tissue pressure from the normally engorged mass. Such treatment would be indicated in a minimally ambulatory patient whose life expectancy is short in an attempt to improve on quality of life.

General Technique

Regardless of the lesions being treated, the fundamental tenets for tumor embolization remain constant. The goal is to saturate the lesion with material so that the tumor vasculature itself is obliterated. Simply sacrificing large feeding vessels proximally provides no significant benefits and should be avoided in most cases. Superselective catheterization of feeding vessels is accomplished through the use of a variety of guidewires and microcatheters. Particulate or liquid embolic agents are then injected using live road mapping angiography. When the tumor no longer opacifies and reflux is seen the feeding vessel embolization is either stopped or the rate of particulate introduction is slowed so that tumor saturation is achieved. The vessel may or may not be occluded proximally with a platinum-fibered coil. The catheter is then placed into another feeding vessel until all treatable sources are obliterated.

Preembolization Testing

It is often wise to first test a feeding pedicle for concomitant supply to normal neural structures such as cranial nerves. This can be carried out by injecting 3 ml of lidocaine into the artery and then performing a neurological examination on the relevant structures. This test may have to be carried out during the embolization. As the tumor is filled with embolic agent the resistance within the tumor bed rises and previously nonfilling vessels that can potentially go to normal neural structures can begin to fill with embolic agent thus inadvertently embolizing nontarget tissue. If one injects lidocaine and finds a new deficit the embolization within the pedicle should be halted and a new vessel should be selected.

Embolization with Sclerotic Agents

For tumors with very small arterial feeders that cannot accept a catheter it is often necessary to consider using alcohol, D50, sodium morhuate, or another sclerotic agent that permeates the tumor, causes tumor vessel intimal injury, and vessel occlusion. These agents often induce tumor necrosis. When feeding vessels arise from large vessels that supply blood to vital tissue it may be necessary to temporarily occlude the artery distal to the small vessels with a balloon mounted on a catheter. This distal occlusion will make the liquid flow directly into the tumor and at the same time stop it from entering the intracranial circulation. Once the embolization is complete the parent vessel proximal to the balloon is thoroughly irrigated and suctioned out through the guide catheter so that any residual agent or lysed cell products are removed from the lumen before the balloon is deflated and the flow to the brain is restored. Even if some agent remains when the balloon is deflated it is quickly diluted by the incoming blood so that the risk of cerebral injury is minimal. Temporary distal balloon occlusion and liquid embolization is often useful for meningiomas supplied by the cavernous carotid artery branches or carotid body tumors that are supplied by numerous hair-like vessels that arise from the internal (ICA) and external (ECA) carotid artery near the carotid bulb.

Choice of Particles

Several particulate agents are currently used for tumor embolization. These include polyvinyl alcohol (PVA), Gelfoam, coils, and trisacryl gelatin microspheres [16]. PVA, Gelfoam and, trisacryl gelatin microspheres are available in sizes as small as 50 μm in diameter. Ideally one would like to start with the smaller particles to supersaturate the tumor's smaller vessels before graduating to larger particles to fill the larger tumor vessels. In reality, however, arteriovenous shunts can exist within the tumor thus allowing smaller particles to simply wash through the tumor into the venous system. It may be necessary, in some instances, to close off these shunts with larger particles before using smaller particles and then returning to larger particles as the embolization proceeds. As mentioned previously, it is necessary to be vigilant for reflux so that normal parenchymal vessels are not inadvertently embolized.

Complications and Complication Avoidance

The specific risks of tumor embolization include inadvertent embolization of brain or spinal cord parenchyma with subsequent infarction, tumor swelling, tumor hemorrhage, damage to parent vessels, skin necrosis, cranial nerve injury, subarachnoid hemorrhage and epidural or subdural hematoma.

Inadvertent Parenchymal Embolization

Inadvertent embolization of neural parenchyma is generally a consequence of not understanding or visualizing dangerous anastomoses that exist between the radicular vessel and the anterior spinal artery (in the case of a spinal tumor embolization) or between the ECA and the ICA and vertebral arteries (VA; in the case of a meningioma embolization). The most common of these connections include middle meningeal artery (MMA) connections to the ophthalmic artery (OA), MMA connections to the ICA via an intermediate anastomosis with the ICA inferolateral trunk, ascending pharyngeal artery connections to the VA, and occipital artery anastomoses with the VA. It is often best to organize the risks of inadvertent embolization by first considering the tumor's location and then thinking of the potential dangerous anastomoses that exist in these settings.

Parasagittal, convexity and falcine meningiomas are often fed by the MMA. For parasagittal and high convexity meningiomas both the right and the left MMA may supply the lesion. These bilateral connections make possible connections to either the right or left OAs possible. We have had one case of left-sided visual loss from retinal embolization following embolization of a right-sided high convexity lesion. In this instance the right MMA supply was embolized and as soon as tumor saturation was achieved retrograde filling of the contralateral left MMA occurred with subsequent immediate embolization of the left retina through an anomalous left MMA to OA connection. By the time this retrograde filling was recognized the retina had already been devascularized with 50-μm PVA particles (fig. 4, 5). Anterior frontal convexity meningiomas and anterior parasagittal lesions may derive supply from meningeal branches of the anterior ethmoidal arteries which in turn anastomose with the OA. Falcine meningiomas may obtain vascular supply from the callosomarginal, pericallosal, and posterior cerebral arteries. As these lesions have their ECA supply embolized the parenchymal vessels may be inadvertently embolized in a retrograde fashion. Such retrograde embolization is often instantaneous as the tumor bed becomes suddenly saturated with particles. When this occurs there is often no time to halt the injection before particles travel to normal brain tissue (fig. 6).

Olfactory groove meningiomas may obtain supply from the sphenoidal and frontal branches of the MMA. Supply also arises from the anterior and posterior ethmoidal arteries making retrograde filling of these vessels possible following MMA embolization. Connections between the ethmoidal arteries and the OA make blindness a risk during embolization of these lesions.

Greater sphenoid wing meningiomas are often supplied by the sphenoidal branch of the MMA, which can connect to the recurrent MMA, which may anastomose with the OA.

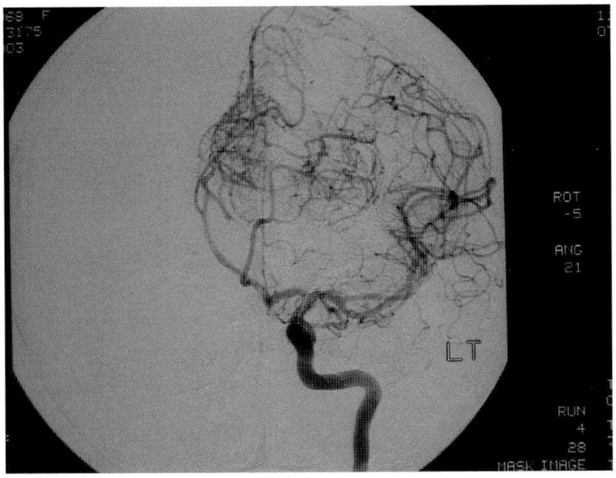

Fig. 4. AP ICA arteriogram showing ACA supply to meningioma.

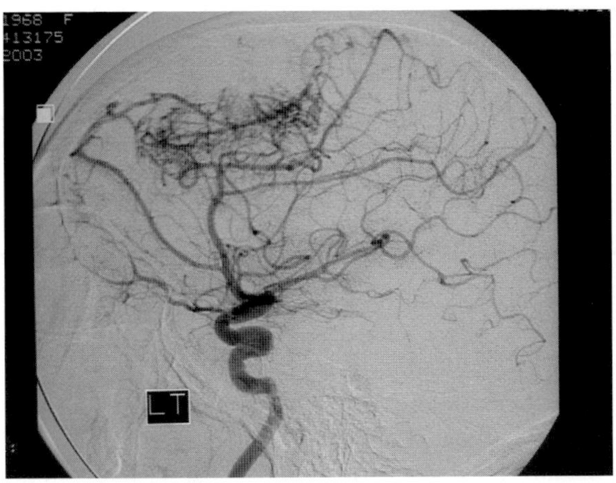

Fig. 5. Lateral ICA angiogram showing ACA supply to meningioma.

Parasellar meningiomas may obtain supply from the meningeal branches of the ICA, MMA along with the accessory MMA, and the internal maxillary artery via the artery of the foramen rotundum. Each of these vessels provides a means for inadvertent embolization of the ICA and OA.

In addition to inadvertent tissue embolization through vascular anastomoses, cerebral stroke can also inadvertently occur in some patients who harbor unrecognized arteriovenous shunts within the lung or heart (patent foramen ovale). Autopsy studies show a patent foramen ovale incidence of

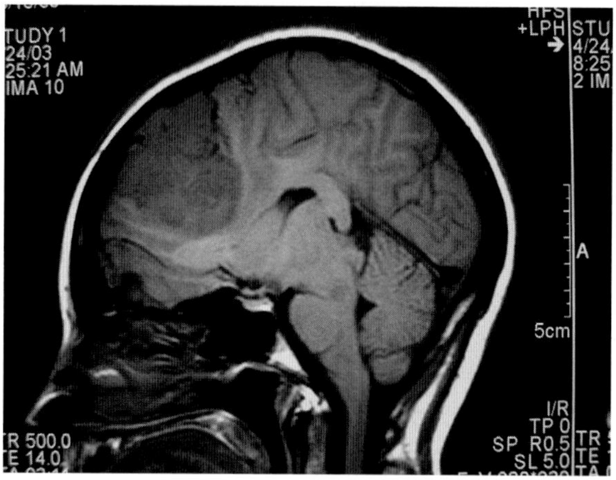

Fig. 6. MRI of meningioma in figure 5.

12–35% with 0.6- to 1.0-cm defects present in 6% of the autopsied population. When particulate emboli are injected into the arterial system to embolize a lesion that contains an arteriovenous shunt such as a tumor, arteriovenous malformation, or arteriovenous fistula the particles can move to the venous circulation, cross a pulmonary or cardiac shunt, and paradoxically embolize the brain. By checking chest radiographs for telltale signs of pulmonary shunts and preembolization bubble study echocardiograms the interventionalist can be aware of these anomalies and adjust the treatment accordingly [17].

It is clear from the above discussion that there are many ways to unexpectedly embolize the retina and cerebral parenchyma while working within the external carotid system. Awareness of the locations of these numerous potential vascular connections is important. Because many do not appear until late in the tumor embolization as hemodynamic balances change extreme vigilance is necessary. Even when extreme care is taken, however, it is often impossible to avoid unwanted consequences.

Cranial Nerve Injury

Branches of the ECA and ICA provide blood supply to the cranial nerves. Embolization of branches that supply both the cranial nerves and tumor tissue risks injury to the nerves secondary to an ischemic insult. Vascular supply of the more commonly embolized vessels is shown in table 1.

Table 1. Vascular supply of the more commonly embolized vessels

Artery	Nerves
MMA	VII, Vm, V3, gasserian ganglion
Accessory meningeal artery	V3, Vm, V2, VII
Inferolateral trunk	III, IV, V1, V2, V3, Vm, gasserian ganglion, VI
Marginal tentorial artery	III, IV
Ascending pharyngeal artery	gasserian ganglion, VI, IX, X, XI, XII, C3 and C4 roots, Jacobson's nerve
Occipital artery	C1 and C2 roots

Vessel Injury

Vascular injury is always a risk whenever a catheter is placed within the internal or external carotid system. Complications, however, that may more commonly arise during tumor embolization include arterial dissection or perforation. These injuries can result in subdural or epidural hematomas, MMA to middle meningeal vein fistulas, or carotid cavernous fistulas.

Tumor Hemorrhage

One of the inherent goals of tumor embolization is tissue necrosis. With necrosis, however, comes the risk for tissue hemorrhage into the necrotic bed. As of 1997 there were seven reported cases although many more certainly exist and have gone unreported in the medical literature [18]. Other etiologies for hemorrhage other than bleeding into necrotic tissue include rupture of feeding artery (MMA) aneurysms and feeding artery rupture as embolization was completed and the resistance within the feeding vessel climbed [19].

Tumor Swelling

As the feeding vessels thrombose and tissue dies tumor tissue can swell just as normal brain parenchyma swells after infarction. This swelling within a body that already may have a significant mass effect can lead to significant increases in intracranial pressure along with distortion of surrounding tissues. Such swelling may be minimized by use of preembolization steroids along with prudent postembolization fluid management. While it is ideal to wait 4–5 days after embolization before performing surgery in order to maximize

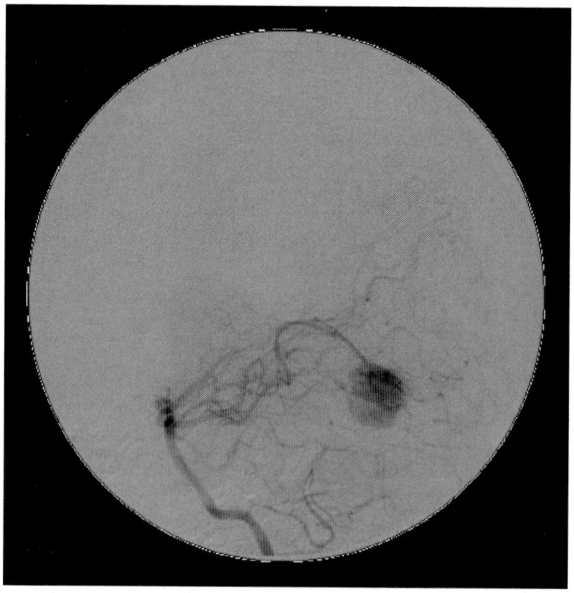

Fig. 7. Lateral VA angiogram showing SCA supply to tumor module.

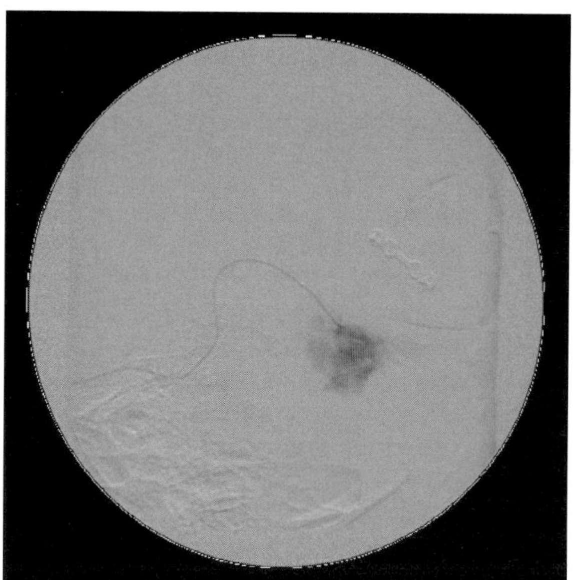

Fig. 8. Superselectives CA arteriogram showing tumor module.

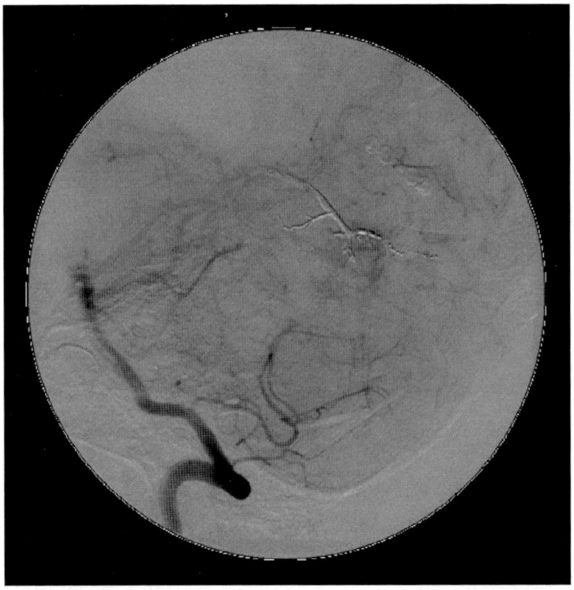

Fig. 9. Lateral VA arteriogram after embolization of set feeder with glue.

necrosis and minimize edema and swelling, early edema may make such plans impossible [20].

Complication Avoidance

Avoidance of complications secondary to tumor embolization can first be realized by choosing cases carefully. Tumors in noneloquent areas that are readily resected with easy access to vascular supply should only be embolized if the surgeon truly feels that endovascular therapy will provide some clear benefit to the patient. For lesions that would benefit from preoperative intervention it is important to carefully study the baseline angiograms so as to be aware of existing and potential dangerous anastomoses. Once this has been done and feeding pedicles are selectively catheterized lidocaine and barbiturate test injections prior to this introduction of embolic material can be carried out to determine ahead of time whether or not vessels that supply the tumor also supply neural structures such as cranial nerves (lidocaine) and/or cerebral parenchyma (barbiturates). Pedicle testing at times must be done at intervals throughout the embolization because as the tumor begins to be saturated with particles hemodynamic shifts may open up previously unopacified shunts and dangerous collaterals. Failure to recognize these hemodynamic changes can result in inadvertent embolization of critical neural structures such as the retina or cranial nerves.

Most cases do not require neurophysiologic monitoring as patients are conscious and can be continually examined throughout the procedure. Neurophysiologic monitoring, however, is useful in those adult patients who are not cooperative and in pediatric patients. These individuals often require a general anesthetic to assure immobility during critical portions of the procedure. General anesthesia may also be necessary when alcohol is being used because of the pain that this agent creates during injection into certain sensitive areas. For ICA branch work we have found EEG, brainstem auditory evoked responses, and somatosensory evoked potentials to be sensitive to inadvertent embolization of cerebral parenchyma. ECA branch work is more difficult to assess. Lower cranial nerve injury from embolic material will not show up as an injury potential when these nerves are being evaluated for ischemic injury. Retinal injury can be evaluated, however, by using visual evoked potentials. We have found this to be useful when working in the presence of dangerous anastomoses between ICA and ECA branches and the OA. Test injections with lidocaine can often reveal transient retinal changes that portend permanent ischemic injury if embolic material is utilized.

Conclusion

Preoperative tumor embolization is useful in carefully selected cases. Knowledge of vascular anatomy and careful intraprocedural testing can reduce the risk of these procedures while at the same time improving outcomes from surgical resection.

References

1 Hekster RE, Matricali B, Luyendijk W: Presurgical transfemoral catheter embolization to reduce operative blood loss. Technical note. J Neurosurg 1974;41:396–398.
2 Bendszus M, Rao G, Burger R, Schaller C, Scheinemann K, Warmuth-Metz M, Hofmann E, Schramm J, Roosen K, Solymosi L: Is there a benefit of preoperative meningioma embolization? Neurosurgery 2000;47:1306–1312.
3 Bendszus M, Klein R, Burger R, Warmuth-Metz M, Hofmann E, Solymosi L: Efficacy of trisacryl gelatin microspheres versus polyvinyl alcohol particles in the preoperative embolization of meningiomas. AJNR Am J Neuroradiol 2000;21:255–261.
4 Okka H, Kurata A, Kawano N, et al: Preoperative embolization of meningiomas. J Neurooncol 1998;40:67.
5 Ng SH, Wan YL, Wong HF, et al: Preoperative embolization of meningiomas: A comparison of selective and subselective techniques. J Formos Med Assoc 1998;97:153.
6 Macpherson P: The value of pre-operative embolization of meningiomas estimated subjectively and objectively. Neuroradiology 1991;33:334.

7 Dean BL, Flom RA, Wallace RC, et al: Efficacy of endovascular treatment of meningiomas: Evaluation with matched samples. AJNR Am J Neuroradiol 1994;15:1675.

8 Kai Y, Hamada J, Morioka M, Yano S, Todaka T, Ushio Y: Appropriate interval between embolization and surgery in patients with meningioma. AJNR Am J Neuroradiol 2002;23:139–142.

9 Kuroiwa T, Tanaka H, Ohta T, Tsutsumi A: Preoperative embolization of highly vascular brain tumors: Clinical and histopathological findings. Noshuyo Byori 1996;13:27–36.

10 Jüngling FD, Wakhloo AK, Hennig J: In vivo proton spectroscopy of meningioma after preoperative embolization. Magn Reson Med 1993;30:155–160.

11 Cloft HJ, Jensen ME, Kallmes DF, Dion JE: Arterial dissections complicating cerebral angiography and cerebrovascular interventions. AJNR Am J Neuroradiol 2000;21:541–545.

12 Herring M: The subclavian steal syndrome: A review. Am Surg 1977;43:220–228.

13 Dorros G, Cohn JM, Palmer LE: Stent deployment resolves a petrous carotid artery angioplasty dissection. AJNR Am J Neuroradiol 1998;19:392–394.

14 Kurata A, Ohmomo T, Miyasaka Y, Fujii K, Kan S, Kitahara T: Coil embolization for the treatment of ruptured dissecting vertebral aneurysms. AJNR Am J Neuroradiol 2001;22:11–18.

15 Kerber CW, Wong WH, Howell SB, Hanchett K, Robbins KT: An organ-preserving selective arterial chemotherapy strategy for head and neck cancer. AJNR Am J Neuroradiol 1998;19:935–941.

16 Bendszus M, Klein R, Burger R, Warmuth-Metz M, Hofmann E, Solymosi L: Efficacy of trisacryl gelatin microspheres versus polyvinyl alcohol particles in the preoperative embolization of meningiomas. AJNR Am J Neuroradiol 2000;21:255–261.

17 Horowitz MB, Carrau R, Crammond D, Kanal E: Risks of tumor embolization in the presence of an unrecognized patent foramen ovale: Case Report. AJNR Am J Neuroradiol 2002;23:982–984.

18 Horowitz MB, Spiro R, Purdy P, Jungreis CC, Levy E, Kassam A: Meningioma embolization. Contemp Neurosurg 2001;23:1–6.

19 Kallmes DE, Evans AJ, Kapstain GJ, et al: Hemorrhagic complications in embolization of a meningioma: Case report and review of the literature. Neuroradiology 1997;39:877.

20 Kai Y, Hamada J, Morioka M, Yano S, Todaka T, Ushio Y: Appropriate interval between embolization and surgery in patients with meningioma. AJNR Am J Neuroradiol 2002;23:139–142.

Dr. Michael B. Horowitz
Department of Neurosurgery
Director, Neuroendovascular Surgery
UPMC Presbyterian
Suite B-400, 200 Lothrop Street, Pittsburgh, 15213-2582, USA
Tel. +1 412 647 3685, Fax +1 412 647 7000, E-Mail horowitzmb@upmc.edu

Horowitz MB, Levy EI (eds): Neuroendovascular Surgery.
Prog Neurol Surg. Basel, Karger, 2005, vol 17, pp 194–215

Acute and Chronic Venous Sinus Thrombosis

Michael B. Horowitz, Ralph G. Greenlee Jr., C.A. Jungreis, Phillip D. Purdy

Center for Cranial Nerve Disorders, UPMC Presbyterian, Pittsburgh, Pa., USA

Historical Perspective

Intracranial dural venous thrombosis is a poorly understood condition, and its etiology, incidence, natural history, treatment, and outcome are debated among clinicians caring for neurological diseases. One fact that is not questioned, however, is that the disease process is unpredictable in terms of course and outcome and has the potential for creating devastating consequences. The advent of magnetic resonance imaging (MRI) and the capacity to selectively deliver thrombolytic agents have opened a new chapter in the diagnosis and treatment of this difficult clinical entity.

Possibly the earliest recorded observations of dural sinus thrombosis were made by Hippocrates who noted apoplexy in association with pregnancy and childbirth [1]. Gowers [2] attributes the first description of dural sinus thrombosis to Ribes, who in 1825 ministered to a 45-year-old man with widespread malignancy, headache, seizures, and delirium. The postmortem examination of this patient revealed superior sagittal sinus (SSS), left transverse sinus (TS), and cortical vein thromboses. In 1888, Gowers [2] himself described aseptic dural sinus thrombosis in a cachectic patient, and in 1915 Holmes and Sargent [3] described posttraumatic thrombosis of the SSS. In 1936, Lhermitte et al. [4] made the association between pediatric congenital heart disease and sinus thrombosis. In the 1940s Martin and Sheehan [5] related thrombosis to the puerperal period. Based on these and other cases, the characterization of cerebral venous thrombosis as a rare, possibly fatal disease characterized by headache, papilledema, seizures, and focal neurological deficits began to evolve. During the period 1942–1990, approximately 203 cases of intracranial venous thrombosis were reported [6].

The finding of hemorrhagic infarction in pathologic material recovered from patients who died secondary to venous sinus thrombosis led to the widely accepted principle that anticoagulants could be dangerous in treating such cases. As will be shown, this view has been modified as our experience has broadened.

Incidence and Demographics

Despite increasing ease of diagnosis, the true incidence of intracerebral venous thrombosis is unknown because many cases continue to go unrecognized. Ehlers and Courville [7] reported 16 cases of SSS thrombosis in 12,500 autopsies. According to Kalbag and Woolf [8], cerebral venous thrombosis was the principle cause of death in only 21.7 persons per year in England and Wales from 1952 to 1961. The female-to-male ratio is 1.29:1. While men of all ages are affected evenly, 61% of cases in women occur between the ages of 20 and 35 years, coinciding with the peak incidence of pregnancy, as well as the use of oral contraceptives [9].

Anatomy and Pathophysiology

The cerebral sinuses are large, valveless, incompletely septated, venous structures, triangular in cross section, with a plexus of adjacent venous channels that act as collateral pathways for drainage in the event of thrombosis. Cerebral veins, as well as calvarial emissary veins, discharge into the sinuses, and the latter may, in pathologic conditions, provide for extracranial drainage. Sinus variations are common. Located over the convexity in the midline, the SSS is the largest of the dural sinuses. The SSS rostral to the coronal suture may be functionally absent in 6% of specimens. In such cases, drainage occurs via cerebral veins. Such a situation should not be confused with pathologic occlusion. The inferior sagittal sinus lies within the inferior margin of the falx cerebri. It joins the vein of Galen to enter the straight sinus (SS). The SS courses to its confluence with SSS to form the torcular herophili, which in turn divides into the TS (lateral) and the less constant occipital sinus (more constant in children). Asymmetry of the TS is common with the right TS draining the SSS and the left TS draining the SS. The right TS provides the dominant drainage in 50–80% of cases. Agenesis or atresia of one of the TSs occurs in up to 5% of the cases and, again, should not be mistaken for dural sinus occlusion [10]. The TS runs inferiorly to join the sigmoid sinus (SgS), which continues into the jugular bulb. The SgS runs within the inner aspect of the mastoid process and is susceptible to thrombosis secondary to infectious processes such as mastoiditis and otitis media, which involve the sinus via emissary veins.

The cavernous sinus (CS) is a mulitseptated, dural-lined collection of venous channels through which the internal carotid artery and the sixth cranial nerve run. Cranial nerves III, IV and V (divisions 1 and 2) are contained within the dural walls. Located on either side of the pituitary fossa, the CS receives drainage from superior and inferior ophthalmic veins, superior petrosal sinus, and the pterygoid plexus (through the foramen of ovale). Each CS communicates with the other across the midline via the circular or intercavernous sinus that surrounds the hypophysis. Communication with the TS/SgS and the juglar bulb occurs via the superior petrosal sinus and inferior petrosal sinus, respectively. Because of its connection with the deep facial veins via the pterygoid plexus and the ophthalmic veins, the CS may become thrombosed as a consequence of sphenoid and ethmoid sinus infections.

Cortical veins can be divided into superficial and deep systems. The largest of the superficial veins are the veins of Trolard and Labbe and the superficial middle cerebral vein (the anastomotic veins). The middle cerebral veins run along the sylvian fissure. Trolard's vein is located over the parietal lobe, while Labbe's vein drains the posterior temporal region. Each vessel's diameter is variable, with the size of one often inversely related to the size of the other.

The organization and presence of veins of the superficial cortex are highly variable, making the angiographic diagnosis of isolated cortical vein thrombosis problematic. In contrast, the deep cerebral venous system that drains the deep white matter, thalamus, brainstem, ventricles, and basal ganglia is more constant. These vessels include the septal, anterior caudate, thalamostriate, internal cerebral, direct lateral, inferior ventricular, and medial atrial veins, the basal vein of Rosenthal, and Galen's vein.

In the case of venous sinus thrombosis, the SSS is the most commonly occluded dural sinus followed by the TS, SgS, and CS [10]. Cortical vein thrombosis is rarely diagnosed in the absence of dural sinus thrombosis (table 1).

Clinical Pathophysiology

Intracranial venous thrombosis is frequently associated with certain predisposing factors and conditions, a partial list of which is outlined in table 1 [1, 6, 9, 11–14]. Such conditions may be divided into infectious and noninfectious categories.

Before the antibiotic era, infection was associated with the vast majority of cases, with frequent spread from the mastoids and other sinuses via the diploic veins. Today, such infectious cases reside primarily within the immunocompromised and diabetic populations.

Table 1. Conditions associated with cerebral venous thrombosis

Infectious conditions
Sinusitis, mastoids, dental infections, facial infections, meningitis, encephalitis
Noninfectious conditions
Pregnancy, puerperium, circulating antiphospholipid antibodies, lupus anticoagulants, oral contraceptives, malignancies, dehydration, jugular vein cannulation, sickle cell disease, surgical trauma, congenital and acquired heart disease
Idiopathic conditions

Noninfectious etiologies now constitute the majority of thrombosis cases. In adults, disorders of coagulation are particularly important. These conditions are especially common during pregnancy and in the 2nd and 3rd weeks after delivery. In the case of the latter, propensity toward thrombosis may be due to elevated plasma fibrinogen as well as factors VII, VIII, IX, and X [15, 16]. Other states that promote thrombosis include antithrombin III, protein C, and protein S deficiencies. Activated protein C inhibits the activity of factors V and VIII, while at the same time stimulating fibrinolysis. Protein S increases the activity of protein C 10,000-fold. Levels of both of these proteins have been found to be deficient in the puerperium but may be congenitally low as well [17–19]. In addition to the above, lupus anticoagulants and antiphospholipid antibodies have been associated with enhanced thrombosis [20] and should be investigated in every patient presenting with thrombosis of unknown etiology.

While cerebral vein thrombosis may present with a wide spectrum of signs and symptoms, headache is the most prominent presenting symptom in almost all series. A common presentation includes headache, focal neurological deficits, seizures, and reduction in the level of consciousness. Many of the abnormalities may be related to increased intracranial pressure due to decreased cerebrospinal fluid absorption secondary to venous hypertension. Others can be attributed to intracranial venous hemorrhage [9, 11, 13]. Ameri and Bousser [9] emphasize that the mode of presentation of symptoms is highly variable. In their series of 110 patients, only 28% presented with acute illnesses, with symptoms developing over 48 h; 42% presented with symptoms between 48 h and 30 days. When the presentation is acute, focal signs are more frequent and the etiologic basis of sinus thrombosis is more often infectious or obstetric, whereas chronic onset was notable for the absence of focal signs and was associated with neoplastic or immune-related illnesses. This slow onset frequently mimics the syndrome of benign intracranial hypertension. Thus, cerebral venous thrombosis must be excluded by either MRI or angiography whenever benign intracranial hypertension is a diagnostic consideration. Finally, an often forgotten complication of sinus thrombosis is pulmonary embolism, 23 cases of which were reported in the literature between 1942 and 1990 [6].

Diagnostic Investigations

When signs and symptoms suggest sinus thrombosis, investigations should be directed first toward confirming the diagnosis and then toward the underlying predisposing factor or factors. Radionuclide studies and electroencephalography are of historical interest and will not be covered. The cornerstones of diagnosis are the findings on computed tomography (CT), cerebral angiography, and MRI. Because CT images of the brain may be normal in 10–20% of cases, MRI and cerebral angiography must be pursued when sinus thrombosis is suspected [9]. While MRI results are fairly diagnostic cerebral angiography remains the gold standard against which all other technologies continue to be compared.

Angiographic findings include partial or complete nonopacification of venous sinuses and veins, dilated cortical collateral veins with a corkscrew appearance, increased cerebral circulation transit time, and reversal of flow away from the obstructed sinus or vein [9, 10]. In the process of interpreting angiographic images, one must be aware of a number of pitfalls. Often the anterior SSS is normally absent, replaced by two superior cerebral veins that join behind the coronal suture. Absent opacification of the anterior SSS alone therefore is insufficient in and of itself to make the diagnosis of sinus thrombosis [9]. The same statement can be made about the TS and SgS, which may normally fail to be visualized during cerebral angiography [21]. Careful attention to technique with visualization of the entire venous phase may help in the delineation of parasagittal sinuses and veins.

Although CT images of the brain may be normal in 10–20% of cases of venous thrombosis, common findings include hemorrhagic venous infarcts, small ventricles, intense contrast enhancement of the falx and tentorium, a cord sign representing fresh thrombus in the posterior SSS, and an empty-delta sign secondary to enhancement of collateral veins in the SSS wall surrounding a nonenhancing thrombus. Ventricles are frequently small and white matter may be edematous.

MRI represents a noninvasive means of assessing the presence of thrombosed sinuses and veins, as well as possibly determining thrombus age by analyzing its T1- and T2-weighted signal intensities [9]. The advantage of MRI is its ability to demonstrate blood flow and parenchymal processes. In acute stages, there is an absence of 'flow void' and the thrombus appears hyperintense on T1-weighted images and hypointense on T2-weighted images. With the appearance of methemoglobin, the absence of flow persists and the thrombus becomes hyperintense on both T1- and T2-weighted images.

Natural History

An important clinical point concerning cerebral venous thrombosis is that the clinical course and prognosis are variable and unpredictable. Some feel that the rate of thrombus formation, presence or absence of coma, focal symptoms, hemorrhagic infarct, and age of presentation (infants and elderly doing worse) are useful prognosticators. While the mortality rate has been reported to approach 70%, more recent reviews estimate the range to be 5–30% [9]. There is little information concerning prognosis for functional recovery after cerebral venous thrombosis. Eighty-eight percent of 35 cases reported in the literature since 1980 survived [22]. Only 15–25% of affiliated patients have any sequelae [9]. Information concerning the outcome in the pediatric population is equally scant. Taha et al. [23] reported a series of 5 patients with traumatic SgS thrombosis, all of whom had normal neurological examinations 6 months after their initial symptoms. Four patients had complete resolution of the sinus obstruction. With SgS thrombosis, however, venous drainage can occur across a patent torcular and into the contralateral sinus system.

Management Strategies

The management of intracerebral venous sinus thrombosis is varied. Controlled, randomized studies are difficult to perform in view of the rarity of symptomatic cases and the multiple etiologies, both of which make adequate randomization nearly impossible. Some physicians espouse a course of watchful waiting in view of the benign nature and uneventful recovery made by the majority of patients. Interventions are reserved for individuals who worsen while being observed [9, 23, 24]. Medical management of these patients includes cerebral dehydrating agents [1, 14]. Steroids [9, 24, 25], acetazolamide, cerebrospinal fluid drainage, barbiturates, decompressive craniectomy [14], sinus thrombectomy [24, 25], heparin/warfarin [1, 25–31], urokinase [11, 25, 32–36], and tissue plasminogen activator [37].

Stansfield [26] was the first to use heparin in a puerperal woman with focal neurological deficits secondary to venous thrombosis. She recovered within 4 days of beginning therapy. Bousser et al. [28] managed 38 patients who were treated with heparin, none of whom died; 19 patients made a complete recovery. While this report answers no questions about heparin therapy versus nonheparin therapy, it does point out the relative safety of using the former in a small group of patients. Einhaupl et al. [31] performed the only randomized, blinded study of adjusted-dose heparin in 20 patients with venous sinus thrombosis. At 3 months after therapy, 80% of the heparin-treated patients were normal, 60% had neurological deficits, and 30% were dead. The author went on to a retrospective study involving 102 patients with thrombosis, 43 of whom had intracranial hemorrhage. Twenty-seven of the 43 were treated without heparin, 9 of whom (56%) died and 3 had a normal recovery [31]. The authors concluded from this study that treatment with heparin was not only beneficial but also safe, even in the face of intracranial hemorrhage.

Other practitioners have advocated the use of fibrinolytic agents, with the goal of rapid clearance of thrombus from the venous system. In 1971, Vines and Davis [11] used urokinase and heparin in the treatment of 4 patients with sinus thrombosis, all of whom improved. In 1988, Scott et al. [33] catheterized the SSS via a frontal burr hole and infused urokinase over an 8-hour period. The patient, who was initially decerebrate, had only a mild dysphasia 4 weeks after therapy. In 1989, Higashida et al. [35] reported treatment of TS thrombotic occlusion in a newborn child with seizures by directed SSS puncture and instillation of urokinase 12,000 IU over a 12-hour period. The thrombus cleared, and the child remained neurologically normal 3 years later. Nevertheless, the safety and efficacy of urokinase therapy have not been established in pediatric patients. There are case reports of urokinase infusions to treat thrombus catheters or right atrial thrombi in infants. The dosage has ranged between 2,000 and 8,800 IU/kg/h [38–43]. Bolus doses of 5,000–10,000 IU have been used [42, 43], as well as low-dose infusions of 70–500 IU/kg/h [42]. There are also published reports of urokinase for treatment of arterial occlusions. Strife et al. [43] used it in neonates to treat four cases of central thrombosis via umbilical artery catheterization of the abdominal aorta. The urokinase dose used was a loading bolus of 4,400 IU/kg followed by 4,000–20,000 IU/kg/h maintenance dose. The duration of therapy for these neonates was 3–9 days.

In 1990, Persson and Lilja [25] performed an open thrombectomy and instilled urokinase into the SSS. Despite formation of a small cerebellar hematoma, the patient gradually improved, although never to baseline. In 1991, Barnwell et al. [32] reported the treatment of 3 patients with transjugular catheterization and instillation of urokinase, and Tsai et al. [34] reported five additional cases from the same institution in 1992. Seven of the 8 patients in these two studies had excellent neurological recoveries, and none had complications related to the therapy. Additionally, Smith et al. [36] described similar results in 7 patients in 1994, 2 of whom had previously been reported by

Barnwell et al. [32] (Dowd, pers. commun.). All patients in this last study did well. In total, we found 13 cases in the English literature of transjugular cerebral venous sinus catheterization and urokinase instillation.

Our series of 13 patients treated with transfemoral transvenous urokinase infusions directly into the cerebral dural sinuses demonstrates the efficacy that can be achieved using present catheter technology (table 2). Twelve of the 13 individuals reported had significant radiographic improvement (reestablished venous sinus drainage) or complete resolution of their thrombus along with rapid neurological improvements. One failure was in a patient with at least a 2-month history of sinus thrombosis and protein C deficiency. We can only speculate that the clot was organized to the extent that it was resistant to urkinase's thrombolytic properties. This concept is supported by a number of studies concerning thrombolysis for deep venous and pulmonary thrombosis and lower-extremity arterial occlusions. Genton and Wolf [44] noted that emboli estimated to be less than 72 h old responded well to fibinolysis, while lesions older than 2 weeks responded less well. Lesions at 6 weeks showed no appreciable change after therapy. Amery et al. [45] confirmed these findings in patients with lower-extremity arterial occlusions. The frequency of thrombus clearing was significantly higher in patients treated within 72 h than in those treated later (68 vs. 7%). The urokinase-pulmonary embolism trial also showed an advantage for acute treatment [4]. While venous and arterial thrombi are most susceptible to thrombolytic therapy early in their course, Duckert et al. [47] did achieve patency in 1 of 7 patients (14%) treated 22–56 days after the onset of deep venous thrombosis symptoms.

In addition to demonstrating the effectiveness of selective fibrinolytic therapy, this series also suggests that the techniques described here are safe even in individuals with hemorrhagic and nonhemorrhagic venous infarcts. No significant complications from therapy, especially those of intracerebral hemorrhage, pulmonary embolism, and vessel damage were seen in our 13 patients despite the apparent risks.

Patient Selection and Thrombolytic Technique

Thirteen patients (5 males, 8 females), ages 6 weeks to 65 years, presented with venous sinus thrombosis involving the SSS and at least one TS (see table 3). After adequate patient pronation, a 6-french sheath was placed into a femoral vein, and another was inserted into the contralateral femoral artery using a single wall puncture needle and the Seldinger technique. The artery and vein in a single leg were not catheterized because of the risk of creating an arteriovenous fistula when the sheaths were removed. Whenever possible,

Table 2. Patients treated with intrasinus urokinase

Urokinase Bolus dose (IU)	Infusion/hr	Clinical Outcome	Radiographic Outcome	Complications	Presumed Etiology	Pretreatment intraparenchymal Hemorrhage/infarct	Warfarin at discharge
250,000	80,000	Excellent	All sinuses patent, deep venous system patent	None	Dehydration	Bilateral occipital lobe 1 cm hemorrhages	Yes
250,000–500,000	100,000	Excellent (slight residual headache)	All sinuses patent, residual occlusion left JB	None	Oral contraceptives	No	Yes
400,000	60,000	Excellent	Sinus patent	None	Malignancy	Biparietal hemorrhages	Yes
?	?	Death secondary to pulmonary emboli	No change from pretreatment	Hematuria, groin hematomoas, death	Malignancy, protein C deficiency, antiphospholipid antibody syndrome	No	Yes
?	100,000	Excellent	Sinuses patent	Transient worsening of exam after initial improvement	Dehydration, mastoiditis	No	Yes
?	200,000	Excellent	Sinuses patent	Groin hematoma	Latrogenic-balloon migration in interventional therapy case	No	Yes

250,000	80,000	Excellent	Sinuses patent	Bilateral groin hematomoas	Unknown	No	Yes
250,000	80,000	Good; residual visual loss	Sinuses patent	None	Unknown (febrile illness?)	Right occipital lobe hemorrhage	Yes
50,000	10,000-20,000	? Follow-up period inadequate	Sinuses almost completely patent	None	Dehydration	Thalamic hemorrhage	Yes
500,000	60,000	Excellent; headache resolved	Good; anterograde drainage in sinuses reestablished	Retroperitoneal hematoma, blood transfusion	SLE	Right temporal lobe infarct	Yes
250,000	80,000	Good; cranial nerve VI paresis improved but not resolved	Good; SSS opened, TS remained occluded	? Bacteremia due to sheath	Ulcerative colitis, oral contraceptives, tooth abscess	No	Yes
250,000	80,000–100,000	Excellent; headache resolved	Good; anterograde from SSS to left TS reestablished, small residual clot SSS, torcula, right TS	Small groin hematoma	Sinusitis	No	Yes

Table 2. (continued)

Urokinase Bolus dose (IU)	Infusion/hr	Clinical Outcome	Radiographic Outcome	Complications	Presumed Etiology	Pretreatment intraparenchymal Hemorrhage/infarct	Warfarin at discharge
250,000	80,000	Excellent; headache resolved, returned to neurological baseline, papilledema minimally improved 1 wk posttherapy, visual fields restricted	Sinuses patent, right sigmoid sinus still with moderate thrombus	None	Medroxy-progesterone acetate injections	Right parietoccipital venous infarct	Yes

JB = jugular bulb.

Table 3. Certain predisposing factors and conditions in intracranial venous thrombosis

Case	Sex	Age	Symptom duration	Physical and neurological status	Heparin	Occlusion site	Treatment duration h	Total dose IU
1	M	26[a]	3 days	Diffuse headache, somnolent, left homonomous hemianopsia	Yes	SS, SSS, ICV, VG, BVR, bilateral TS	36	−3,380,000
2	F	27[a]	<2 days	Headache, nausea, vomiting, neck pain	Yes	SSS, bilateral TS, VG, SS, left JB	72	−4,500,000
3	F	65[a]	2 weeks	Decline in mentation, dysarthia, right hemiparesis	Yes	SSS	48	−3,280,000
4	F	36[a]	2 months	Right orbital swelling, blurred vision, right eye pain, pulmonary embolus, cardiac failure	Yes	SSS, bilateral TS, deep venous system	48	−4,000,000
5	M	38[a]	5 days	Headache, right hemiparesis, seizures	Yes	SSS, right TS	17	−2,600,000
6	M	35[a]	<1 h	Hemiparesis, altered mental status	Yes	TS	12	−2,400,400
7	M	35[a]	32 days	Seizure, change in mental status	Yes	TS, SSS	42	−3,600,000
8	M	32[a]	2 weeks (?)	Seizure, papilledema, bilateral cranial nerve VI palsies	Yes	SSS	48	−4,590,000

Table 3. (continued)

Case	Sex	Age	Symptom duration	Physical and neurological status	Heparin	Occlusion site	Treatment duration h	Total dose IU
9	F	6[b]	0–5 days (?)	Seizures	Yes	VG, ICV, SS, SSS, TS	84	−1,500,000
10	F	12[a]	3 months	Headache, papilledema, chorea	Yes	SSS, SS, ICV, VG, TS	72	−4,320.00
11	F	43[a]	2 days	Headache, left cranial nerve VI paresis, papilledema	Yes	SSS, right TS	~48	−2,750,000
12	F	27[a]	−1.5 months	Headache, bilateral papilledema	Yes	SSS, TS	~70	−7,000,000
13	F	22[a]	2 weeks	Headache, nausea, vomiting, blurred vision, atrophic papilledema, confusion	Yes	Posterior 2/3 SSS, torcula, right/left TS, right SgS, partial left SgS	~72	−5,800,000

BVR = Basal Vein of Rosenthal; JB = jugular bulb.
[a]Years.
[b]Weeks.

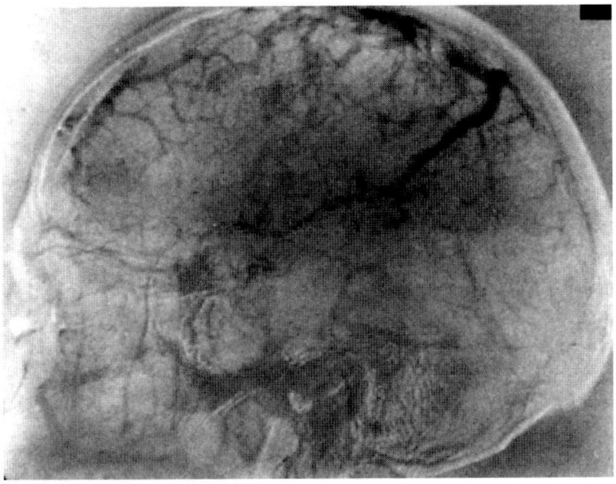

Fig. 1. Lateral arteriogram showing late venous phase with poor SSS opacification.

the right femoral vein was used because it would be closer to the interventionalist during microcatheter manipulations. A 5-french angiographic catheter and guidewire were then used to perform a complete cerebral angiogram, with imaging carried out into the late venous phase. Once the diagnosis of sinus thrombosis was made, the catheter was removed. A catheter and wire were then advanced via the femoral vein through the right atrium and into the superior vena cava. The decision of which internal jugular vein (IJV) to catheterize was made depending on the location of the sinus thrombosis. (Given a choice, the right IJV is generally the easier of the two to locate and negotiate.) Having entered the IJV, the catheter was placed at the C-1 level. A 0.018-inch microcatheter was advanced coaxially over a guidewire through the jugular bulb and into the appropriate sinus or sinuses. The catheter and wire sometimes made several loops and turns as it passed through and around the thrombus. Advancement sometimes required many back and forth rotary motions of the wire as the clot was macerated by the wire tip. During the advancement, we generally instilled urokinase in 50,000 IU aliquots approximately every 15 min to bathe the thrombus as we transversed its length. A total dose of 250,000–500,000 IU was given during a single sitting. The catheter was eventually positioned near the distal end of the thrombus, with careful attention not to leave it at a point where the urokinase would drain preferentially through venous collaterals. The system was then secured to the patient's thigh with an occlusion dressing, and the patient was returned to the intensive care unit (ICU) with a continuous urokinase infusion through the microcatheter at 60,000–100,000 IU/h.

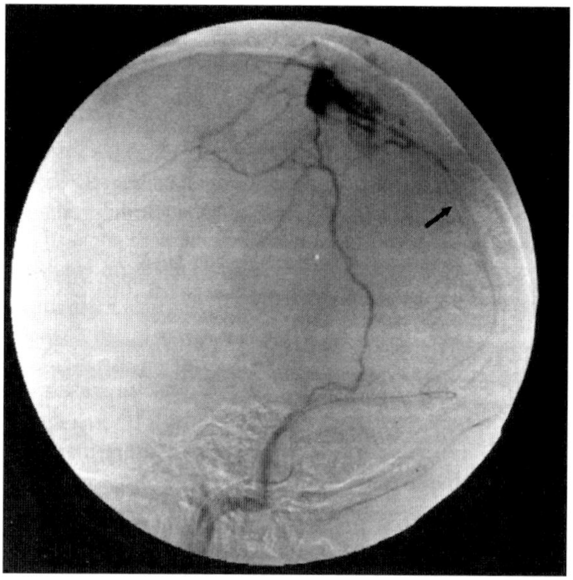

Fig. 2. Lateral venogram showing microcatheter positioned in SSS (arrow).

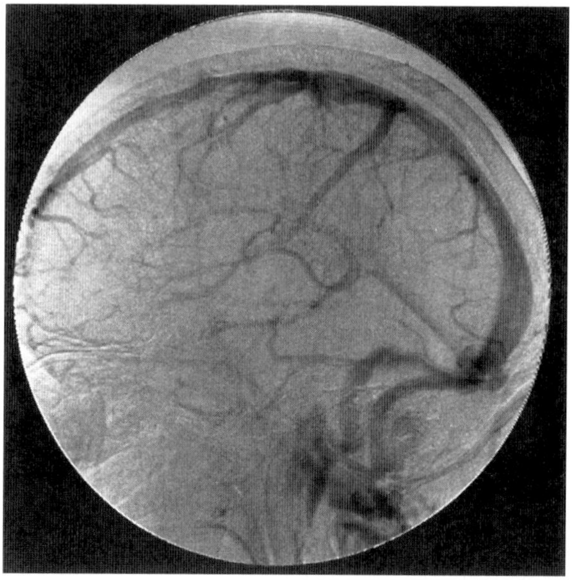

Fig. 3. Lateral arteriogram showing recanalization of SSS following intrasinus thrombolysis.

Approximately 18–24 h later, the patient was returned to the angiography suite where a repeat venogram was performed. If the sinuses appeared patent, a single common cartoid arteriogram was obtained to visualize the arterio-venous relationship and transit time. When thrombolysis was not adequate, additional boluses were administered, the catheter was repositioned, and the patient was continued on the urokinase infusion. Follow-up venograms and arteriograms were obtained at 24-hour intervals until the desired effect was achieved. Once the infusions were completed, the catheters were removed. The patient remained on heparin and was eventually converted to warfarin. Anticoagulant therapy was continued for 3–6 months.

Mechanical Clot Evacuation

An alternative to thrombolytic therapy is mechanical clot evacuation; while balloons and stents can be used to open a thrombosed sinus we have favored using a rheolytic thrombectomy catheter. In the angiography suite, a juglar vein is catheterized via the femoral vein approach using standard 5-french systems. Typically, the initial venogram images of the IJV will show occlusion beginning immediately caudal to the mastoid. A microcatheter (Tracker-18 turbo, Target Therapeutics, Freemont, Calif., USA) and wire are placed into the thrombus. Difficulty getting through the length of the thrombus is common and persistent manipulation of the microcatheter and wire is required to advance into the clot. The tip of the microcatheter is advanced as far as possible and then the microcatheter and base catheter are exchanged over an 0.014-inch exchange guidewire for a 7-french guide catheter and a rheolytic thrombectomy catheter (CF105 AngioJet, Possis Medical, Minneapolis, Minn., USA). Several similar alternative thrombectomy catheters are available if the initial choice proves unsatisfactory. Regardless, the rheolytic thrombectomy catheter is advanced over the 0.014-inch exchange guidewire. Usually, it will advance easily even if the clot had been resistant earlier. The rheolytic thrombectomy catheter is positioned in a distal location and then activated while it is being slowly withdrawn at 1–2 mm/s. A retrograde venogram can be obtained via the base catheter to show progress. Additional passes can be made with the thrombectomy catheter if the guidewire is first removed. However, unless the tip of the thrombectomy catheter is in a distal position, we would not recommend this for fear that we would be unable to reinsert the guidewire through residual clot.

Initially, the patient is administered and maintained on heparin systemically. The patient is later converted to Coumadin in order to reach a target INR of 2.0–3.0 for a minimum of 3 months of anticoagulant therapy.

Selected Case Reports

Case One

A 26-year-old right-handed man presented 72 h after the onset of diffuse headache and gradually increasing somnolence. He had a history of working outdoors in extreme heat over the previous days and may have become dehydrated. Neurological examination demonstrated the above findings plus a partial left homonomous hemianopsia. A head CT scan revealed density in the SS, SSS, torcular, TS, internal cerebral veins (ICV), and vein of Galen, as well as a cord sign in the left ambient cistern consistent with the location of the basal vein of Rosenthal. A 1-cm diameter hemorrhagic venous infarct was visible in the cortical and subcortical occipital lobes bilaterally. Cerebral MRI demonstrated subacute thrombus in the venous sinuses and an abnormal signal in the left centrum semiovale and occipital lobes. A diagnosis of venous sinus thrombosis was made. The patient was referred for cerebral angiography, which confirmed the above findings. After systemic heparinization, transfemoral catheterization of the right IJV was achieved, and a Fast Tracker-18 catheter was placed coaxially and advanced into the anterior SSS with minimal difficulty. Venograms obtained during the catheter positioning revealed diffuse thrombus within the right jugular bulb, right TS and SSS. The left TS was not opacified. Retrograde venous flow was seen from the anterior SSS into dilated cortical veins. A bolus dose of urokinase 250,000 IU in 50,000-IU aliquots administered every 5–10 min was infused into the anterior SSS with minimal effect on thrombus appearance. The patient was returned to the ICU with the microcatheter in the SSS just anterior to the coronal suture. Urokinase was infused over the next 18 h at a rate of 80,000 IU/h. The following day, repeat interval angiography demonstrated near-complete clearing of the SSS and right TS, although small filing defects representing a residual clot remained. We were unable to pass the catheter across the torcular to assess the left TS, SgS and left IJV. An additional 250,000 IU of urokinase were administered in boluses of 50,000 IU each, and the patient was infused over the next 18 h with 80,000 IU/h. Follow-up venography and angiography 18 h later revealed patency of the venous sinuses with decreased collateral drainage. Follow-up cerebral CT demonstrated resolution of the occipital hemorrhage and small infarcts in the deep left parietal white matter. Within 48 h of treatment, the patient's headaches had almost completely resolved, and visual fields were grossly normal to confrontational testing. He was discharged on warfarin. Coagulation studies investigating hypercoagulability were all within normal limits.

Case Two

A 27-year-old woman with a history of tobacco and oral contraceptive use presented with less than 24 h of headache, nausea, vomiting, and neck pain.

Cerebral CT and MRI studies revealed hyperdensity within the SSS, SS, and VG. No hemorrhages or infarcts were visible. Systemic heparinization was instituted. A cerebral angiogram and transvenous catheterization were performed (as described in case 1), revealing SSS and bilateral TS thrombosis. Over the next 72 h, three venograms were performed. Bolus urokinase injections of 250,000–500,000 IU were made during each procedure, and the patient remained on a continuous infusion of 100,000 IU/h in the ICU. After 3 days, near-complete resolution of the thrombosis was achieved, except for residual occlusion of the left jugular bulb, which was compensated for by significant posterior fossa venous collateralization. The patient's nausea and vomiting abated and her headaches improved, although they never completely resolved even at 3-month follow-up. Warfarin was discontinued after 3 months.

Case Three

A 65-year-old woman presented with a 2-week history of a gradually declining level of consciousness along with progressive dysarthia, right-sided weakness, and right facial paresis. Prior to therapy, the patient was stuporous with right lower-extremity plegia and severe right upper-extremity paresis. Cerebral CT revealed biparietal hemorrhages, parietal edema, and sulcal effacement. Hyperdensity was seen in the torcular and SSS. Angiography confirmed the above and in addition demonstrated slow arterial flow and dilated cortical veins. A Tracker catheter was placed into the SSS, and a 400,000-IU urokinase bolus was infused over 40 min. A 48-hour infusion at 60,000 IU/h was carried out. The patient improved markedly over the next 12 h such that she was alert and oriented with good right lower and upper extremity movement. Repeat angiography at 48 h demonstrated near-complete thrombus resolution with only small filling defects remaining. The patient was converted from heparin to warfarin and at the time of discharge was ambulating with the assistance of a walker, had minimal right-handed weakness, and was capable of independent living. The patient returned 6 months later with an angiographically documented pulmonary embolus. Routine workup for a hypercoagulable state was negative (antithrombin III, proteins C and S, urine homocystine, and anticardiolipin/antiphospholipid antibody). An occult colon malignancy was discovered shortly afterward.

Case Four

A 32-year-old black man with a history of a febrile illness 3 weeks before admission to our institution presented with a single tonic-clonic seizure, bilateral papilledema with flame hemorrhage, and mild bilateral sixth nerve palsies. A cerebral CT scan revealed a small right occipital lobe parenchymal hemorrhage, while MRI demonstrated increased signal within the SSS suggestive of venous sinus thrombosis. Cerebral angiography confirmed the diagnosis. Utilizing a transfemoral transvenous approach, a Tracker-18 catheter was advanced into the SSS, and urokinase 250,000 IU was infused over 60 min (50,000 IU every 12 min) with immediate lysis of clot surrounding the catheter tip. The catheter was left in position in the SSS, and 80,000 IU/h were infused over the next 48 h. The patient had interval angiography at 24 h, at which time an additional 500,000 IU was infused into the SSS and TS. At 48 h after initiation of therapy, all venous sinuses were widely patent. A follow-up CT scan at 48 h showed resolution of the hemorrhage. A coagulopathy study revealed normal protein C and S levels. Antiphospholipid antibodies were also within normal limits. The patient was discharged on warfarin 7.5 mg/day.

Case Five

A 6-week-old girl was admitted, suffering from dehydration and malnutrition. On the 5th hospital day, she experienced two focal seizures localized to the left hemisphere. Cerebral CT revealed a right thalamic hemorrhage, and thrombus within the VG, ICV, SS, SSS, and TS. The anterior fontanelle was tense. MRI confirmed the above findings and transfemoral transvenous selective catheterization and thrombolysis were initiated. A 3-french left common femoral sheath was placed, with the tip of the sheath in the inferior vena cava. This was exchanged for a 5-french sheath. A Tracker-18 catheter was advanced coaxially into the mid-SSS. A venogram confirmed the presence of complete thrombosis with venous collaterals via both cortical and scalp veins. An infusion of urokinase 50,000 IU was delivered within 1 h. Follow-up venography demonstrated minimal improvement, and the patient was transferred to the ICU with the Tracker catheter in place infusing urokinase 10,000 IU/h. The following day a venogram demonstrated minimal improvement. The infusion was increased to 20,000 IU/h. This rate was maintained for the next 72 h, and subsequent venograms revealed gradual thrombolysis of the SSS, TS, and SgS. Normal venous drainage was restored, and abnormal venous collateral flow disappeared. A follow-up MRI obtained 3 days after the termination of therapy showed patency of the SSS, left TS, left SgS, and SS, along with residual clot in the ICV and VG. Multiple CT scans were obtained during the thrombolysis procedure, and there was no enlargement of the right thalamic hemorrhage.

Conclusion

The management of cerebral venous sinus thrombosis is controversial. This series does not establish which patients warrant intervention and which can be followed conservatively with expectant care or systematic heparinization.

As a result of our favorable experience with dural sinus urokinase infusions, we tend to favor aggressive interventional management because it is impossible to predict which patients will succumb to the ravages of venous infarction. Unlike heparin therapy, which inhibits thrombus progression while the body lyses the clot in a natural fashion, thrombolytic therapy hastens clot dissolution, thus opening venous channels in a more timely fashion. Though outcome improvement with urokinase has not been definitively shown, we believe rapid restoration of venous outflow by clot dissolution should be to the patient's benefit.

Acknowledgments

This series was initially accepted in March 1995 for publication in the *Annals of Neurology* and entitled 'Treatment of Cerebral Dural Sinus Thrombosis Using Selective Catheterization and Urokinase Infusion'. Many thanks to Robert A. Fishman, MD, Editor, *Annals of Neurology*, for permitting its publication in textbook format.

Thanks to Leslie Mihal for her help in preparing this manuscript; to Bill Perkins, MD, Mike Graber, MD, and Preston Harrison, MD, for patent referral; to Carol Zimmerman, MD, for ophthalmologic management, and to George Carstens, MD, Hal Unwin, MD, Joe Hise, MD, Tom Kopitnik, MD, Hunt Batjer, MD, Nancy Rollins, MD, and Duke Samson, MD, for assistance in patient management.

References

1 Carrol JD, Leak D, Lee HA: Cerebral thrombophlebitis in pregnancy and the puerperium. Q J Med 1966;35:347–368.
2 Gowers WR: Manual of Diseases of the Nervous System, ed 2. London, Churchill, 1888, p 416.
3 Holmes G, Sargent P: Injuries of the superior longitudinal sinus. BMJ 1915;ii:493–498.
4 Lhermitte J, Lereboullet J, Kaplan B: Ramollissement hémorragipare d'origine nerveuse chez un enfant, attaint de malformations cardiaques. Rev Neurol (Paris) 1936;65:305.
5 Martin JP, Sheehan HL: Primary thrombosis of cerebral veins (following childbirth). BMJ 1941;i:349.
6 Diaz JM, Schiffman JS, Urban ES, Maccario M: Superior sagittal sinus thrombosis and pulmonary embolism: A syndrome rediscovered. Acta Neurol Scand 1992;86:390–396.
7 Ehlers H, Courville CB: Thrombosis of internal cerebral veins in infancy and childhood. Review of the literature and report of five cases. J Pediatr 1936;8:600–623.
8 Kalbag RM, Woolf AL: Cerebral Venous Thrombosis. London, University Press, 1967.
9 Ameri A, Bousser MG: Cerebral venous thrombosis; in Barnett HJM, Hachinski VC (eds): Cerebral Ischemia: Treatment and Prevention. Neurol Clin 1992:10:87–111.
10 Osborne A: Diagnostic Neuroradiology. St Louis, Mosby, 1994.
11 Vines FS, Davis DO: Clinical-radiological correlation in cerebral venous occlusive disease. Radiology 1971;98:9–22.
12 Barnett HJM, Hyland HH: Non-infective intracranial venous thrombosis. Brain 1953;76:36–49.
13 Atkinson EA, Fairburn B, Heathfield KWG: Intracranial venous thrombosis as a complication of oral contraception. Lancet 1970;i:914–918.
14 Shende MC, Lourie H: Sagittal sinus thrombosis related to oral contraceptives. J Neurosurg 1970;33:714–717.
15 Estanol B, Rodriguez A: Intracranial venous thrombosis in young women. Stroke 1979;10:680.

16 Strauss HS, Diamond LK: Elevation of factor VIII during pregnancy in normal persons and in a patient with von Willebrand's disease. N Engl J Med 1963;269:1251.
17 Marlar RA, Kleiss AJ, Griffin JH: Protein C: Inactivation of factors V and VIII in plasma. Ann NY Acad Med 1981;370:303.
18 Roos AI, Pascuzzi RM, Kuharik M: Prior intracranial venous thrombosis associated with dysfunctional protein C and deficiency of protein S. Obstet Gynecol 1990;76:492.
19 Cros D, Loup PC, Beltran G, Gum G: Superior sagittal sinus thrombosis in a patient with protein S deficiency. Stroke 1990;21:633–635.
20 Levin SR: Cerebral venous thrombosis with lupus anticoagulants. Report of 2 cases. Stroke 1987;18:801–804.
21 Hacker H: Normal supratentorial veins and dural sinuses; in Newton TH, Potts DG (eds): Radiology of the Skull and Brain. St Louis, Mosby, 1974.
22 Fincher RME, Swift TR: Case report: Improvement in sagittal sinus thrombosis by MRI. Am J Med Sci 1991;301:262–264.
23 Taha JM, Crone KR, Berger TS, Becket WW, Prenger EC: Sigmoid sinus thrombosis after closed head injury in children. Neurosurgery 1993;32:541–546.
24 Estanol B, Rodriguez A, Conte G, Aleman JM, Loyo M, Pizzuto J: Intracranial venous thrombosis in young women. Stroke 1979;10:680–684.
25 Persson L, Lilja A: Extensive dural sinus thrombosis treated by surgical removal and local streptokinase infusion. Neurosurgery 1990;26:117–121.
26 Stansfield FR: Puerperal cerebral thrombophlebitis treated by heparin. BMJ 1942;i:436–438.
27 Brown JIM, Coyne TJ, Hurlbert RJ, Fehlings MG, Ter Brugge KG: Deep cerebral venous system thrombosis: Case report. Neurosurgery 1993;33:911–913.
28 Bousser MG, Chiras J, Borias J, Castaigne P: Cerebral venous thrombosis. A review of 38 cases. Stroke 1985;16:199–213.
29 Gettelfinger DM, Kokmen E: Superior sagittal sinus thrombosis. Arch Neurol 1977;34:2–6.
30 Fairburn B: Intracranial venous thrombosis complicating oral contraception: Treatment by anticoagulant drugs. BMJ 1973;2:647.
31 Einhaupl KM, Villringer A, Meister W, et al: Heparin treatment in sinus venous thrombosis. Lancet 1991;28:135–142.
32 Barnwell SL, Higashida RT, Halbach VV, Dowd CF, Hieshema GB: Direct endovascular thrombolytic therapy for dural sinus thrombosis. Neurosurgery 1991;28:135–142.
33 Scott JA, Pascuzzi RM, Hall PV, Becker GJ: Treatment of dural sinus thrombosis with local urokinase infusion. J Neurosurg 1988;68:284–287.
34 Tsai FY, Higashida RT, Matovich V, Alferi K: Acute thrombosis of the intracranial dural sinus: Direct thrombolytic therapy. Am J Neuroradial 1992;13:1137–1141.
35 Higashida RT, Helmer E, Halbach VV, Hieshema GB: Direct thrombolytic therapy for superior sagittal sinus thrombosis. Am J Neuroradiol 1989;10:S4–S6.
36 Smith TP, Higashida FT, Barnwell SL, et al: Treatment of dural sinus thrombosis by urokinase infusion. Am J Neuroradiol 1994;15:801–807.
37 Alexander LF, Yammamoto Y, Ayoubi S, Al-Mefty O, Smith R: Efficacy of tissue plasminogen activator in the lysis of thrombosis of the cerebral venous sinus. Neurosurgery 1990;26:559–564.
38 Pongiglione G, Marasini M, Ribaldone D, Silvestri G, Tuo P, Cantoni-Garello L: Right atrial thrombosis in two premature infants: Successful treatment with urokinase and heparin. Eur Heart J 1986;7:1086–1089.
39 Zureikat GY, Martin GR, Silverman NH, Newth CJL: Urokinase therapy for a catheter-related right atrial thrombus and pulmonary embolism in a 2-month-old infant. Pediatr Pulmonol 1986;2:303–306.
40 Delaplane D, Scott JP, Riggs TW, Silverman BL, Hunt CE: Urokinase therapy for a catheter-related right atrial thrombus. J Pediatr 1982;100:149–152.
41 Winthrop AL, Wesson DE: Urokinase in the treatment of occluded central venous catheters in children. J Pediatr Surg 1984;19:536–538.
42 Ragnall HA, Gomperts E, Atkinson JB: Continuous infusion of low dose urokinase in the treatment of central venous catheter thrombosis in infants and children. Pediatrics 1989;83:963–966.
43 Strife JL, Ball WS, Towbin R, Keller MS, Dillion T: Arterial occlusions in neonates: Use of fibrinolytic therapy. Radiology 1988;166:395–400.

44 Genton E, Wolf PS: Urokinase therapy in pulmonary thromboembolism. Am Heart J 1968;76:628.
45 Amery A, Deloof W, Vermylen J, Verstraete M: Outcome of recent thromboembolic occlusion of limb arteries treated with streptokinase. BMJ 1970;4:639–644.
46 Urokinase-Pulmonary Embolism Trail. A National Cooperative Study. Circulation 1973; 47/4(suppl 2):1–108.
47 Duckert F, Muller G, Nyman D: Treatment of deep venous thrombosis with streptokinase. BMJ 1975;1:479–481.
48 Scarrow AM, Williams RL, Jungreis CA, Yonas H, Scarrow MR: Removal of a thrombus from the sigmoid and transverse sinuses with a rheolytic thrombectomy catheter. AJNR Am J Neuroradiol 1999;20:1467–1469.

Michael B. Horowitz
Department of Neurosurgery
Director, Neuroendovascular Surgery
UPMC Presbyterian
Suite B-400, 200 Lothrop Street, Pittsburgh, 15213-2582, USA
Tel. +1 412 647 3685, Fax +1 412 647 7000, E-Mail horowitzmb@upmc.edu

Horowitz MB, Levy EI (eds): Neuroendovascular Surgery.
Prog Neurol Surg. Basel, Karger, 2005, vol 17, pp 216–231

Vein of Galen Aneurysms: A Review and Current Perspective

Michael B. Horowitz, Charles A. Jungreis,
Ronald G. Quisling, Ian Pollack

Center for Cranial Nerve Disorders, UPMC Presbyterian, Pittsburgh, Pa., USA

The term vein of Galen aneurysm encompasses a diverse group of vascular anomalies sharing a common feature, dilatation of the vein of Galen. The name, therefore, is a misnomer. Although some investigators speculate that vein of Galen aneurysms comprise up to 33% of giant arteriovenous malformations (AVMs) in infancy and childhood [1], the true incidence of this anomaly remains uncertain. A review of the literature reveals fewer than 300 reported cases since the clinical description of Jaeger et al. [2] in 1937. As we will outline below, our understanding of the embryology, anatomy, clinical presentation, and management of these difficult vascular malformations has progressed significantly over the past 50 years.

Embryology and Vascular Anatomy of the Vein of Galen

The development of the human cerebral vascular system is complex: a thorough analysis has been conducted by Padget [3]. Cerebral vascularization begins during gestational week 4, at the time of neural tube closure. By the end of week 5, the choroidal and quadrigeminal arteries, the main afferents to the vein of Galen, are well developed [4]. During week 6 the circle of Willis is completed. The anterior cerebral artery supplies the choroid plexus of the lateral ventricles, and the middle cerebral artery supplies the striatum [4]. Meanwhile, at the roof of the diencephalons, the median prosencephalic vein, or primitive internal cerebral vein, develops as the main draining structure for the telencephalic choroid plexus. By week 10 the median prosencephalic vein is largely replaced by the paired internal cerebral veins, which then become the predominant means of choroidal drainage [4]. Although the median prosencephalic regresses, its most caudal portion joins the internal cerebral vein to form the vein of Galen [4].

Differentiation of the venous sinuses occurs concurrently with the development of the arterial and venous drainage system. By week 4, a primitive capillary network is drained by anterior, middle, and posterior meningeal plexi [3, 4]. Each plexus has a stem that drains into one of the paired longitudinal head sinuses, which in turn drain into the jugular veins [3, 4]. Atresia of the longitudinal sinuses leads to the development of the transverse and sigmoid sinuses by week 7 [3, 4]. At birth only the superior and inferior sagittal, straight, transverse, occipital, and sigmoid sinuses remain, along with a still plexiform torcula [3, 4]. On occasion, a transient falcine sinus presents persistent intradural channels located within the falx cerebri.

Under normal circumstances, the mature vein of Galen persists as a bridge between the deep parenchymal venous system and the venous sinuses. As such, it serves as a conduit between the internal cerebral veins, basal veins of Rosenthal, precentral cerebellar vein, vermian veins, and straight sinus [5].

Lying within the subarachnoid space in an area known as the great transverse cleft, the vein of Galen is bordered superiorly by the free margin of the falx, posteriorly by the tentorium cerebelli, anteriorly and inferiorly by the roof of the third ventricle, and laterally by the choroidal fissures of the lateral ventricles [4].

Arterial Supply

In a series of 23 patients with vein of Galen aneurysms, Raybaud et al. [4] found posterior choroidal arteries to be the primary feeders. The anterior cerebral arteries were the second most commonly involved vessels, generally providing bilateral blood supply. The anterior thalamoperforators were common secondary tributaries, joining primary afferents at the level of the choroidal fissure. Perimesencephalic vessels were constantly involved in neonates and frequently involved in older children. Distal branches of the posterior cerebral arteries and posterior thalamoperforators supplied the malformations in a moderate number of neonates. In approximately 50% of patients, the meningeal arteries were significant.

Venous Drainage

In healthy persons the vein of Galen drains the internal cerebral veins, basal vein of Rosenthal, posterior mesencephalic vein, superior vermian vein, precentral cerebellar vein, and superior cerebellar veins [5]. Sixty-eight percent of the patients of Raybaud et al. [4] had major venous anomalies including absent or interrupted straight sinuses, straight sinuses divided into two segments, and straight sinuses judged too small in relationship to the sacs. A small number of patients demonstrated both falcine and patent straight sinuses. An equally small number presented with falcine sinus draining the sac into the superior sagittal sinus. From the superior sagittal sinus, blood flowed posteriorly into the torcula and then into one transverse sinus. Some blood, however, flowed anteriorly within the superior sagittal sinus, entered a second falcine sinus, which angiographically seemed to cross the first (in a separate dural sheet), and finally discharged into the torcular or another transverse sinus. In these situations blood may drain via petrosal and tentorial venous channels into the cavernous sinus. Falcine sinuses were generally associated with high-flow shunts. Five of the cases of Raybaud et al. revealed an angiographic absence of straight, falcine, transverse, and sigmoid sinuses with stasis of contrast within the sacs and lack of jugular vein opacification. In terms of nonsinus venous drainage, the authors at no time demonstrated dilation of the internal cerebral veins, although they did see retrograde flow in these structures. Large choroidal veins and an engorged subependymal system drained into the basal veins, uncal veins, and cavernous sinuses. Lateral mesencephalic venous drainage entered the transverse sinus.

Categorization

Yasargil [6] divided vein of Galen aneurysms into four categories. Type 1 contains pure fistulas between arteries and the vein of Galen with the nidus of the lesion being the ampulla of the vein. This entire lesion is extrinsic to the brain parenchyma. Type 2 is composed of thalamoperforators that travel through normal parenchyma and supply both brain tissue and give branches to the vein of Galen. These lesions are both intrinsic and extrinsic to the central nervous system. Type 3 malformations are mixed lesions with characteristics of both type 1 and type 2 lesions. Type 4 lesions have malformations proximal to the vein of Galen aneurysms that drain into veins that then empty into the veins of Galen.

A further modification of these classifications has been provided by Quisling and Mickle [7], who categorized galenic vascular malformations on the basis of several factors: nidus complexity, afferent supply, and efferent drainage patterns. Type 1 consists of 'true' galenic fistulas with direct arteriovenous communication via a unilateral, choroidal arterial trunk. As it approaches the vein of Galen aneurysm this trunk can be divided into as many as five smaller distal branches. When an angiomatous matrix is present it is usually less than 1 cm in greatest diameter and is typically in direct continuity with the galenic aneurysm. Type 2 galenic fistulas are actually 'ordinary' deep AVMs located within the thalamus and/or hypothalamus. They are supplied by the thalamoperforating arteries and drain via the superior thalamic veins and galenic system. AVM matrix size in such cases ranges from 1 to 2 cm in greatest diameter. Type 3 galenic vascular malformations are similar to type 1 fistulas but have significantly more afferent vascular complexity. Instead of single feeding arteries, type 3 malformations are supplied by both anterior and posterior chorodial arteries and the persistent embryonic remnants of the distal anterior cerebral arteries. The authors observed that their angiographic distinctions correlated with the clinical presentation of the lesion. For example, no patients in categories 1 or 2 had overt cardiac decompensation [7], whereas the type 3 galenic fistulas, which as a group exhibited the most shunting, were more likely to present with high-output cardiac failure in the newborn period.

In addition to categorizing the arterial supply to the vein of Galen aneurysm, these authors also favored using a grading system for the venous aspect of the malformation. In grade 1, the degree of ectasia of the straight sinus is proportional to that of the vein of Galen, with both being only minimally enlarged. Grade 2 occurs when the vein of Galen is more dilated than the straight sinus, with both structures moderately increased in size. Grade 3 lesions demonstrate marked dilation of both structures, and grade 4 lesions have a significant enlargement of the veins of Galen with normal, stenotic, or absent straight sinuses [7]. These angiographic findings correlated well with measurements of venous pressure within the malformation. Whereas the mean venous pressure within galenic aneurysms in individuals with venous restrictions was 40 cm of water, the pressure in patients without venous restrictions averaged 25 cm of water [3]. These angiographic findings and pressure measurements were related in a logical way to a number of clinical features. For example, no patient with obstructed drainage was in cardiac failure at the time of presentation, thus confirming that some measure of cardiac protection is provided by the restriction of venous outflow from the malformation. Conversely, no case in which the efferent venous pressure was less than 20 cm of water had brain calcifications, implicating elevated venous pressure in the development of the finding. Finally, grade 4 patients with severe outflow restriction were more likely to undergo spontaneous thrombosis of their malformations, which suggests that a lower flow rate is present in those fistulas that have high-grade efferent stenosis. Taken together, these observations provided the rationale for initial attempts to treat galenic malformations via the venous route particularly in patients with high-output cardiac failure.

Developmental Theory

Raybaud et al. [4] propose that vein of Galen aneurysms are not a result of dilation of the vein of Galen, but rather a consequence of the dilation of persistent median prosencephalic veins. The evidence they cite supporting this statement includes the following: (1) the vein of Galen develops late and lacks connections to the choroidal branch of the anterior cerebral artery, which is a primary feeder in most vein of Galen aneurysms, and (2) the typical vein of Galen aneurysm directly drains both prosencephalic and mesencephalic arteries in a pattern typical of the median prosencephalic vein, but the normal mature vein of Galen does not. Anomalous venous drainage as described in previous sections probably represents persistent fetal drainage that remains intact because it effectively deals with the high-flow system [4]. Such persistent fetal drainage may prevent the development of the normal sinus system [4]. Alternatively, persistent falcine sinuses may be a consequence of straight sinus occlusion early in the developmental period [4].

Lasjaunias et al. [8] have proposed additional theories concerning the development of vein of Galen aneurysms. They agree that these aneurysms may develop secondary to proximal angiomatous malformations. However, they also point out the frequency of sinus obstruction (especially the straight sinus) associated with vein of Galen malformations, thus speculating that increased resistance to outflow at an early stage may lead to proximal venous ectasia. These authors felt that venous agenesis was a more likely mechanism of outflow obstruction than was sinus thrombosis, because acquired thrombosis usually fails to produce subsequent vein of Galen aneurysms. Mayberg and Zimmerman [9], however, have reported a case of a 64-year-old man with a dural AVM, vein of Galen aneurysm. They felt straight sinus thrombosis was the primary event leading to the development of both vascular abnormalities.

Clinical Presentation

The association in neonates of intractable congestive heart failure and a cranial bruit provides the most striking manifestation of vein of Galen aneurysm; however, less fulminant modes of presentation are the norm in older infants, children, and adults. Although attempts have been made to subdivide clinical presentation on a strictly age-related basis, it is readily apparent that, between age groups, signs and symptoms overlap [10, 11]. For example, in the classification schema of Amacher and Shillito [10], group 1 consists of neonates with cranial bruits and severe congestive heart failure, and group 2 consists of neonates and infants with mild heart failure who develop craniomegaly and cranial bruits within 1–6 months. Group 3 comprises children 1–12 months old with craniomegaly and cranial bruits, but no heart failure, and group 4 consists of persons 3.5–27 years of age who present with headaches, exercise syncope, and subarachnoid hemorrhage. In addition, certain presenting signs such as visual deterioration, proptosis, seizures, hemiparesis, developmental retardation, facial vein enlargement, epistaxis, and vertigo do not necessarily coincide with age-related groupings. Nonetheless, the above classification schema provides a useful basis for categorizing patients with vein of Galen aneurysms.

Congestive Heart Failure

Congestive heart failure is the major cause of mortality and morbidity in neonates and infants harboring vein of Galen aneurysms. In severe cases, as much as 80% of left ventricular output may be delivered to the head as a consequence of the low vascular resistance within the malformation [12]. Because this output returns directly to the right ventricle, right heart failure from volume and work overload may ensue. Myocardial ischemia is further promoted by decreased afterload induced by the AVM. Consequent reduction in diastolic pressures jeopardizes myocardial perfusion [8]. Other cardiac anomalies reported in association with vein of Galen aneurysms include transposition of the great vessels and aortic stenosis [13, 14].

Heart failure generally presents not before, but shortly after birth. The explanation for this may reside in the fact that in utero, the placenta's low vascular resistance reduces the amount of blood, which is 'stolen' by the abnormal, low-resistance cerebral shunt [12]. On examination, the neonate or infant with cardiac decompensation from a vein of Galen aneurysm may manifest cyanosis, decreased peripheral pulses, and in some cases audible cranial bruits [12]. In the absence of an obvious bruit, the correct diagnosis initially may be missed unless a high index of suspicion is maintained.

Hydrocephalus

The etiology of hydrocephalus is multifactorial and includes sylvian aqueduct obstruction, resorptive blocks, hydrocephalus ex vacuo (a consequence of encephalomalacia and cerebral atrophy [15]), and abnormal transependymal cerebrospinal fluid resorption. Resorptive blocks may be attributable to increased pressure within the sagittal sinus [7, 8].

Developmental Retardation

Developmental retardation is common with vein of Galen aneurysms and is often used as an argument against offering treatment to severely affected infants. Mechanics implicated for such damage are arterial steal, ischemia caused by compression from engorged draining veins and an enlarged vein of Galen, and increased venous pressure with subsequent venous infarction after spontaneous, partial, or complete aneurysm thrombosis [7, 8, 16]. Grossman et al. [17] recognized the role of arterial steal after noting resolution of optic disc pallor in 2 patients undergoing vein of Galen aneurysm excision. They concluded that early surgery might abort ischemic brain damage in those fortunate enough to be born with normal parenchyma.

Failure to Thrive

Many neonates and infants with vein of Galen aneurysms fail to thrive. Cardiac decompensation undoubtedly plays a tremendous role in such failure. However, hypothalamic and hypophyseal dysfunction secondary to venous congestion within these structures also must be considered a potential mechanism [8].

Vein of Galen Aneurysm Thrombosis

Spontaneous thrombosis of vein of Galen aneurysms may be heralded by the development of obstructive hydrocephalus or by the onset of intraventricular hemorrhage [18–24]. Heinz et al. [20], the first to describe thrombosis of a vein of Galen aneurysm, felt it occurred in utero or during birth. However, later reports clearly indicated that thrombosis could take place throughout infancy and, in some cases, in adulthood [18, 25]. There is no typical presentation of a thrombosed vein of Galen aneurysm except the nearly ubiquitous presence of hydrocephalus and its attendant signs and symptoms.

Associated Illnesses

Both Turner syndrome and blue rubber bleb nevus syndrome have been reported to occur in conjunction with vein of Galen aneurysms [26, 27]. The former involves the absence of a single X chromosome in female patients and has been associated with other vascular anomalies including coarctation of the aorta and pulmonic stenosis. The latter presents with blue, nipple-like, compressible skin lesions composed of blood-filled venous and cavernous angiomas. Whether the association of these diseases with vein of Galen aneurysms is a chance occurrence is not known at this time. Other malformations reported in association with vein of Galen aneurysms include supernumerary digits, hypospadias, transposition of the great vessels, and aortic stenosis [13, 14, 28].

Evaluation and Diagnostic Studies

Ultrasound

Ultrasound is an excellent method of screening for and evaluating vein of Galen aneurysms, both in utero and during the neonatal period [29–31]. Ultrasonic demonstration of vascular pulsations helps differentiate vein of Galen aneurysms from other possible midline structures [30]. Color Doppler ultrasound permits the characterization of blood flow within the malformation and, although useful in delineating feeding and draining vessels, is especially valuable in evaluating the effectiveness of therapy [32, 33].

Chest Radiographs

Chest radiographs may reveal cardiomegaly with right-sided chamber enlargement, widening of the superior mediastinum, retrosternal fullness, posterior displacement of the upper trachea, and retropharyngeal soft tissue prominence caused by encroachment on this space by dilated carotid arteries and jugular veins [34].

Skull Radiographs

Radiographs of the skull are of minimal utility in the diagnosis and evaluation of suspected vein of Galen aneurysms. Occasionally they demonstrate rims of calcium corresponding to a calcified aneurysm sac [35].

Computed Tomography

Computed tomography images of vein of Galen aneurysms generally reveal round masses lying in the quadrigeminal cistern behind the posterior border of an anteriorly displaced third ventricle. High density within the lesion may suggest vein of Galen aneurysm thrombosis [5, 22, 36]. After administration of contrast, dense, homogeneous opacification of both the vein of Galen aneurysm and the adjacent tentorial vessels and draining sinuses is seen [5, 36]. When the malformation is thrombosed contrast tends to enhance the aneurysm wall and opacify small zones within the aneurismal pouch [5, 36]. A ‘target sign' has been described in this circumstance. Calcification of the malformation wall, seen in approximately 14% of patients, is rarely seen in patients younger than 15 years of age [18]. Cerebral parenchymal calcifications are generally attributed to ischemia especially when located in watershed regions and, as such, may be an index of cerebral damage.

Magnetic Resonance and Magnetic Resonance Angiography

The ability of magnetic resonance (MR) to image noninvasively in sagittal, coronal, and axial planes makes it an invaluable tool in the characterization of arterial afferents, venous drainage, malformation position and size, and appearance of surrounding brain. MR allows the early identification of sinus abnormalities and venous drainage patterns, which not only facilitates therapeutic planning of transvenous or transtorcular endovascular approaches, but also helps guide the angiographer toward the most important vessels for study [37]. This is particularly critical in neonates in whom venous access is difficult, and total acceptable contrast loads are low. However, MR has not obviated the need for catheter angiography, especially when intervention is planned [38, 39]. MR angiography, on the other hand, has begun to provide substantial insight into the anatomy of many vascular diseases and with improvement may become the primary tool for the evaluation of vein of Galen aneurysms.

Angiography

Angiography remains the standard of reference for the evaluation of vein of Galen aneurysms.

Treatment

The primary indication for treating neonates with vein of Galen aneurysms is congestive heart failure refractory to medical treatment. Surgery or endovascular treatment can in many cases be postponed by medical care until the child is older, at which point intervention is safer and easier. In those patients requiring invasive treatment, the goal of therapy is not necessarily the complete obliteration or extirpation of the aneurysms, but rather the arrest of congestive heart failure. Relative contraindications to treatment include medically controlled systemic failure. Finally, imaging evidence of brain damage has been considered a contraindication by some [40].

Surgery

Jaeger et al. [2] performed carotid ligation in an attempt to control the degree of blood flow through a galenic malformation. This procedure provided no clear protection against further cardiovascular compromise and eventual death. Subsequent to that initial case report, numerous other reports have described surgical approaches to galenic malformations [6, 11, 15, 41, 42]. Certain issues must be considered before undertaking any planned ablative procedure. The delicacy of the poorly myelinated neonatal brain makes the retraction necessary to visualize and treat the vein of Galen aneurysm and its arterial supply potentially more dangerous than in older children. Moreover, the risk of life-threatening blood loss is accentuated in such patients because of their limited blood volumes. Accordingly, where feasible, every attempt should be made to treat such lesions nonsurgically in this age group with the thought that if surgery is required, it can be undertaken more safely in an older patient.

Theoretical risks of normal perfusion pressure breakthrough must be considered when planning any treatment of vascular malformation. After obliteration of some vascular malformations, previously hypoperfused peripheral brain tissue has increased blood flow. Sudden increases in blood flow to these regions has been reported to result in brain swelling, hemorrhage, and seizures [43, 44]. Normal perfusion pressure breakthrough has been associated with malformations greater than 4 cm in largest dimension, angiograms showing steal, and individuals with possible steal-related neurological deficits. [45]. Many surgeons and interventionalists, therefore, feel that staged treatment of complicated galenic malformations should be considered, especially when the above-mentioned risk factors are present.

The need for and timing of ventricular drainage in conjunction with primary treatment of vein of Galen aneurysms remains controversial. Schneider et al. [46] have described a number of complications associated with ventriculoperitoneal shunts in children with hydrocephalus and vein of Galen aneurysms. These included status epilepticus, intraventricular hemorrhage, subdural collections, and new neurological deficits. In the series of Yasargil et al. [42] two postoperative deaths were heralded by intraventricular hematomoas in hydrocephalic patients who had shunts placed at surgery. The authors felt that all patients requiring shunts should have catheters placed before malformation ablation, because after ablation the subependymal veins may become distended and thus possibly prone to rupture if a catheter is passed through the ventricular wall. Distended ependymal veins, however, may be present before malformation ablation, and the risks of shunt placement may be high at this time as well.

In many patients, particularly those with obstructive hydrocephalus secondary to thrombosed vein of Galen aneurysms, cerebrospinal fluid shunting is the only therapy required [21]. In such patients, attempts to resect the thrombosed aneurysm sacs have been associated with unacceptable morbidity [20–23, 25, 42].

Endovascular Approaches

Advances in catheter design and embolization materials have brought neuroradiologic endovascular approaches to the forefront of therapeutic options in the treatment of vein of Galen aneurysms. The indications of Berenstein and Epstein [47] for embolization include: (1) preoperative obliteration of less surgically accessible feeding vessels in the hope of reducing surgical morbidity, (2) postoperative obliteration of smaller feeding vessels after surgical ligation of major arterial suppliers, and (3) definite therapy of vein of Galen aneurysms using a staged technique. Lasjaunias et al. [40] have made an important distinction in their discussions of the endovascular treatment of vein of Galen aneurysms. In those patients with vein of Galen aneurysms secondary to a parenchymal or choroidal AVM, they feel venous embolization should be limited. Approaches to such malformations should be from the arterial side to avoid venous hypertension and congestion and their associated morbidity and mortality.

Various techniques have been described for obliteration of vein of Galen aneurysms, including transarterial, transvenous, and transtorcular embolization [8, 40, 47–52]. The specific endovascular approach has depended on the specific anatomy of the given case. Arteriovenous fistulas can be occluded on the arterial side from either a transarterial or transvenous approach using embolic agents such as coils, acrylics (cyanoacrylates), and endovascular balloons. Fistulas pose the technical challenge of depositing emboli at the site of the shunt in such a way as to maintain their positions. High-flow fistulas are notorious for transmitting even large emboli to the venous side and to the pulmonary circulation with fatal results. As a consequence of such pass-through phenomena, venous occlusion therapy has gained popularity. In cases of multiple fistulas converging on the vein of Galen, the transvenous and transtorcular approaches have even more appeal. The goal in these approaches is to occlude the outflow in the vein of Galen, thus inducing retrograde thrombosis and obliteration of the fistulas. Many embolic agents have been used, although coils are currently the primary agents used in this approach. Complete cure is not usually required, and partial occlusion of the dilated vein frequently reverses the cardiovascular compromise.

When approaching these lesions from a transarterial route with primary arterial embolizations, the interventionalist must be aware of the risks of normal perfusion pressure breakthrough. Mickle and Quisling [51] tried to avoid normal perfusion pressure breakthrough by reducing blood flow by 50% in stage 1 and then returning 3–21 days later, if necessary, to completely eliminate all residual flow. If total obliteration could not be achieved, embolization was aimed at stabilizing the patient's cardiovascular status in the hope of converting a neonate or infant into an older-age-group member in whom surgery or embolization has a better outcome [47].

An unusual but potentially fatal complication of endovascular therapy is a consumptive coagulopathy manifested by a precipitous postembolization thrombocytopenia that is followed by intracranial hemorrhage. The cause of such coagulation abnormalities may rest in the rapid deposition of large amounts of thrombus within the recently treated vascular anomaly. As in the related Kasabach-Merritt syndrome [53], treatment consists of clotting factors and platelet replacement.

Outcome

Johnston et al. [41] reviewed 232 cases of vein of Galen aneurysms reported in the literature before 1987 and recorded cases involving 80 neonates, 82 infants (1–12 months of age), 39 children (1–5 years), 22 children and young adults (6–20 years), and 22 adults (older than 20 years). Of these patients, 110 presented with congestive heart failure, 94 with increased intracranial pressure, 57 with cranial bruits, 37 with focal neurological deficits, 26 with seizures, and 25 with hemorrhage. Ninety-one patients underwent direct surgical treatment; 29 received shunts and remote vessel ligation; 46 had medical treatment alone, and 79 had no therapy or no details of therapy in their reports. Overall mortality was 55.6% with 37.4% mortality for surgical cases and a 46.3% incidence of significant morbidity in postoperative survivors. Neonates had 91.4% surgical mortality, which approximated the nonsurgical outcome. The 1- to 12-month age group suffered 31.7% surgical mortality, and the older-than-1-year age group had 25.6% surgical mortality and 42.3% major morbidity. The series of Yasargil [6] consisting of 70 patients showed 67% neonatal (younger than 1 month old) postoperative mortality and 27% child and adult postoperative mortality. Total survival in this series of patients was 10% for neonates, 47% for infants, and 56% for children and adults. An inescapable conclusion from these studies, which include cases spanning many eras of neurosurgical, medical, and radiologic advances, is that neonates have profoundly worse outcomes than other age groups, most likely as a consequence of cardiac decompensation with resultant multisystem failure.

Fortunately, in the current era of endovascular therapy, morbidity and mortality rates have improved. Lasjaunias et al. [40] have reported 36 cases treated by endovascular approaches (78% pediatric, 22% adult) with a mortality of 13%. Casasco et al. [54] reported 100% survival in seven infants treated via transvenous embolization. Dowd et al. [52] reported transvenous approaches to the venous and/or arterial sides of vein of Galen aneurysms in 3 neonates who survived and were stable at 9- to 12-month follow-up. The experience of Mickle [55] with transtorcular embolization in 15 infants and older children and

9 neonates was favorable. Fourty-four percent of the latter and 93% of the former survived. Lylyk et al. [56] used endovascular therapy in 28 children. Forty-five percent of those younger than 1 year of age had good outcomes, 61.5% of those aged 1–2 years had good outcomes, and 100% of those older than 2 years had good outcomes.

Summary and Conclusions

The approach to treating a patient with a vein of Galen aneurysm should be influenced greatly by the age of the patient, the clinical symptoms, and the angiographic architecture of the malformation. Therapeutic options are primarily based on whether a true AVM is present or the malformation represents an arteriovenous fistula involving the vein of Galen. Arterial endovascular approaches, microneurosurgery, and/or radiosurgery are preferred for management of the former; the transvenous endovascular approach has become the cornerstone of treatment in the latter. The most critical group, however, is the neonate in medically refractory cardiovascular distress. In this case therapeutic intervention is initially endovascular from the venous side, either transfemoral or transtorcular. The immediate goal is to increase resistance to right ventricular output. Advantages of this approach over a transarterial approach include a shorter anesthesia time, minimal fluid and/or contrast administration, and creation of a wire 'basket' or 'bird's nest' on the venous side that helps prevent emboli that may be deposited on the arterial side in subsequent embolizations from passing through the malformation. The transvenous approach can be easily repeated multiple times and may be supplemented by transarterial embolizations. Fibered endovascular coils have been the mainstay for such venous embolizations. The end point of treatment is not necessarily complete occlusion of the fistula but improvement in cardiac function. Often, more than one stage is required to reach this goal.

The results in recent years have been encouraging and are to a large degree attributable to advance in endovascular approaches. With future improved tools for diagnosis and treatment, perhaps the prognosis for this difficult malady also will continue to improve.

References

1 Long DM, Seljeskoge EL, Chous SN, French LA: Giant arteriovenous malformations and childhood. J Neurosurg 1974;40:304.

2 Jaegar JR, Forbes RP, Dandy WE: Bilateral congenital cerebral arteriovenous communication aneurysm. Trans Am Neurol Assoc 1937;63:173–176.

3 Padget DH: Cranial venous system in man in reference to development, adult configuration and relation to arteries. Am J Anat 1956;98:307–355.
4 Raybaud CA, Strother CM, Hald JK: Aneurysms of the vein of Galen: Embryonic consideration and anatomical features relating to the pathogenesis of the malformation. Neuroradiology 1989;31:109–128.
5 Skirkhoda A, Whaley RA, Boone SC, Scatliff JH, Schnapf D: Varied CT appearance of aneurysms of the vein of Galen in infancy. Neuroradiology 1981;21:265–270.
6 Yasargil MG: Microsurgery IIIB. New York, Thieme, 1988, pp 323–357.
7 Quisling RG, Mickle JP: Venous pressure measurements in vein of Galen aneurysms. AJNR Am J Neuroradiol 1989;10:411–417.
8 Lasjaunias P, Ter Brugge K, Lopez Ibor L, et al: The role of dural anomalies in vein of Galen aneurysms: Report of six cases and review of literature. AJNR Am J Neuroradiol 1987;8:185–192.
9 Mayberg MR, Zimmerman C: Vein of Galen aneurysm associated with dural AVM and straight sinus thrombosis: Case report. J Neurosurg 1988;68:288–291.
10 Amacher AL, Shillito J Jr: The syndromes and surgical treatment of aneurysms of the great vein of Galen. J Neurosurg 1973;39:89–98.
11 Hoffman HJ, Chaung S, Hendrick EB, Humphreys RP: Aneurysms of the vein of Galen: Experience at the hospital for sick children, Toronto. J Neurosurg 1982;57:316–322.
12 Pellegrino PA, Milanesi O, Saia OS, Carollo C: Congestive heart failure secondary to cerebral arterio-venous fistula. Childs Nerv Syst 1987;3:141–144.
13 Gomez JR, Whitten CF, Nolke A, Bernstein J, Meyer JS: Aneurysmal malformations of the great vein of Galen causing heart failure in early infancy. Pediatrics 1983;31:400.
14 Hirano A, Solomon S: Arteriovenous aneurysm of the vein of Galen. Arch Neurol 1960;3:589.
15 Rosenfeld JV, Fabinyi GC: Acute hydrocephalus in an elderly woman with an aneurysm of the vein of Galen. Neurosurgery 1984;15:852–854.
16 Norman MG, Becker LE: Cerebral damage in neonates resulting from arteriovenous malformation of the vein of Galen. J Neurol Neurosurg Psychiatry 1974;37:252–258.
17 Grossman RI, Bruce DA, Zimmerman RA, Glodberg HI, Bilaniuk LT: Vascular steal associated with vein of Galen aneurysm. Neuroradiology 1984;26:381–386.
18 Chapman S, Hockley AD: Calcification of an aneurysm of the vein of Galen. Pediatr Radiol 1989;19:541–542.
19 Dean DF: Management of clotted aneurysm of the vein of Galen. Neurosurgery 1981;8:589–592.
20 Heinz RE, Schwartz FJ, Sears RA: Thrombus in the vein of Galen malformation. Br J Radiol 1968;41:424–428.
21 Mancuso P, Chiaramonte I, Pero G, Tropea R, Guamera F: A case of thrombosed aneurysm on the vein of Galen associated with superior sagittal sinus thrombosis. J Nuerosurg Sci 1989;33: 305–309.
22 Six EG, Cowley AR, Kelly DL Jr, Laster DW: Thrombosed aneurysm of the vein of Galen. Neurosurgery 1980;7:274–278.
23 Weir BK, Allen PB, Miller JD: Excision of thrombosed vein of Galen aneurysm in an infant. Case report. J Neurosurg 1968;29:619–622.
24 Whitaker JB, Latack JT, Venes JL: Spontaneous thrombosis of a vein of Galen aneurysm. AJNR Am J Neuroradiol 1987;8:1134–1136.
25 Lazar ML: Vein of Galen aneurysm: Successful excision of a completely thrombosed aneurysm in an infant. Surg Neurol 1974;2:22–24.
26 Jarrell HR, Schochet SS Jr, Krous H, Barnes P: Turner's syndrome and vein of Galen aneurysm: A previously unreported association. Acta Neuropathol 1981;55:189–191.
27 Rosenblum WI, Nakoneczna I, Konderding HS, Nochlin D, Ghatak NR: Multiple vascular malformation in the 'blue rubber bleb naevus' syndrome: A case with aneurysm of vein of Galen and vascular lesions suggesting a link to the Weber-Osler-Rendu syndrome. Histopathology 1978;2:301–311.
28 Eide J, Folling M: Malformation of the great vein of Galen with neonatal heart failure: Report of two cases. Acta Paediatr Scand 1978;67:529–532.
29 Jeanty P, Kepple D, Roussis P, Shah D: In utero detection of cardiac failure from an aneurysm of the vein of Galen. Am J Obstet Gynecol 1990;163:50–51.

30 Mendelsohn DB, Hertzanu Y, Butterworth A: In utero diagnosis of a vein of Galen aneurysm by ultrasound. Neuroradiology 1984;26:417–418.

31 Rodemyer CR, Smith WL: Diagnosis of a vein of Galen aneurysm by ultrasound. J Clin Ultrasound 1982;10:297–298.

32 Deeg KH, Scarf J: Colour Doppler imaging of arteriovenuos malformation of the vein of Galen in a newborn. Neuroradiology 1990;32:60–63.

33 Tessler FN, Dion J, Vinuela F, et al: Cranial arteriovenous malformations in neonates: Color Doppler imaging with angiographic correlation. AJR Am J Roentgenol 1989;153:1027–1039.

34 Swischuk LE, Crowe JE, Mewborns EJ Jr: Large vein of Galen aneurysms in the neonate: A constellation of diagnostic chest and neck radiologic findings. Pediatr Radiol 1977;6:4–9.

35 Agee OF, Musella R, Tweed CG: Aneurysm of the great vein of Galen. Report of two cases. J Neurosurg 1969;31:346–351.

36 Martelli A, Scotti G, Harwood-Nash DC, Fitz CR, Chaung SH: Aneurysms of the vein of Galen in children: CT and angiographic correlations. Neuroradiology 1980;20:123–133.

37 Seidenwurm D, Berenstein A, Hyman A, Howalski H: Vein of Galen formation: Correlation of clinical presentation, arteriography and MR imaging. AJNR Am J Neuroradiol 1991;12: 347–354.

38 Leff SL, Kronefeld G, Leondias JC: Aneurysm of the vein of Galen: Ultrasound, MRI and angiographic correlations. Pediatr Radiol 1989;20:98–100.

39 Roosen N, Schirmer M, Lins E, Bock WJ, Stork W, Gahlen D: MRI of an aneurysm of the vein of Galen. AJNR Am J Neuroradiol 1986;7:733–735.

40 Lasjaunias P, Rodesch G, Terbrugge K, et al: Vein of Galen aneurysmal malformations: Report of 36 cases managed between 1982 and 1988. Acta Neurochir 1989;99:26–37.

41 Johnston IH, Whittle IR, Besser M, Morgan MK: Vein of Galen malformations: Diagnosis and management. Neurosurgery 1987;20:747–758.

42 Yasargil MG, Antil J, Laciera R, Jain KK, Boone SC: Arteriovenous malformations of vein of Galen: Microsurgical treatment. Surg Neurol 1970;6:195–200.

43 Barrow DL: Intracranial vascular malformations; in Barrow DL (ed): Neurosurgical Topics. AANS, 1990, p 91.

44 Spezler RF, Wilson CB, Weinstein P, Mehdorn J, Townsend J, Telles D: Normal perfusion pressure breakthrough theory. Clin Neurosurg 1978;25:651–672.

45 Barrow DL: Intracranial vascular malformations; in Barrow DL (ed): Neurosurgical Topics. AANS, 1990, p 160.

46 Schneider SJ, Wisoff JS, Epstein FJ: Complications of ventriculopertioneal shunt procedures of hydrocephalus associated with vein of Galen malformations in childhood. Neurosurgery 1992;30: 706–708.

47 Berenstein A, Epstein F: Vein of Galen malformations: Combined neurosurgical and neuroradiologic intervention; in American Association of Neurological Surgeons (eds): Pediatric Neurosurgery, Surgery of the Developing Nervous System. New York, Grune & Stratton, 1982, pp 638–647.

48 Hawkins J, Quisling RG, Mickle JP, Hawkins IF: Retrievable Gianturco-coil introducer. Radiology 1986;158:262–264.

49 King WA, Wackym PA, Jinuela F, Peacock WJ: Management of vein of Galen aneurysms: Combined surgical and endovascular approach. Childs Nerv Syst 1989;5:208–211.

50 McCord FB, Shields MD, McNeil A, Halliday HL, McClure G, Reid MM: Cerebral arteriovenous malformation in a neonate: Treatment by embolization. Arch Dis Child 1987;62:1273–1275.

51 Mickle JP, Quisling RG: The transtorcular embolization of vein of Galen aneurysms. J Neurosurg 1986;64:731–735.

52 Dowd CF, Halbach W, Barnwell SL, Higashida RT, Edwards MSB, Hieshema EM: Transfemoral venous embolization of vein of Galen malformations. AJNR Am J Neuroradiol 1990;11: 643–648.

53 Kasabach HH, Merritt KK: Capillary hemangioma with extensive purpura: Report of a case. Am J Dis Child 1940;59:1063–1080.

54 Casasco A, Lylyk P, Hodes JE, Kohan G, Aymard A, Merland JJ: Percutaneous transvenous catheterization and embolization of vein of Galen aneurysms. Neurosurgery 1991;28:260–265.

55 Mickle AP: The transtorcular embolization of vein of Galen aneurysms and update on the use of this technique in twenty-four patients; in Marlin AE (ed): Concepts in Pediatric Neurosurgery. Basel, Karger, 1991, vol 11, pp 69–78.
56 Lylyk P, Vinuela F, Dion JE, et al: Therapeutic alternatives for vein of Galen vascular malformations. J Neurosurg 1993;78:438–445.

Dr. Michael B. Horowitz
Department of Neurosurgery
Director, Neuroendovascular Surgery
UPMC Presbyterian
Suite B-400, 200 Lothrop Street, Pittsburgh, 15213-2582, USA
Tel. +1 412 647 3685, Fax +1 412 647 7000, E-Mail horowitzmb@upmc.edu

Horowitz MB, Levy EI (eds): Neuroendovascular Surgery.
Prog Neurol Surg. Basel, Karger, 2005, vol 17, pp 232–238

Petrosal Sinus Sampling for Cushing's Disease

Michael B. Horowitz[a], *Elad I. Levy*[b], *Julie Genevro*[a], *Amin Kassam*[a], *Bartolome Burguera*[a]

[a] Center for Cranial Nerve Disorders, UPMC Presbyterian, Pittsburgh, Pa., USA
[b] Millard Filmore Hospital, Dept. of Neurosurgery, Buffalo, N.Y., USA

Definitions

The etiology of Cushing's syndrome (CS) can broadly be divided into two categories: adrenocorticotropic hormone (ACTH)-dependent and ACTH-independent. Of the ACTH-dependent forms, pituitary-dependent CS, Cushing's disease (CD), is the most common, accounting for 60–80% of all cases. CD involves a constellation of abnormalities secondary to elevated levels of serum cortisol as a consequence of a pituitary adenoma which produces excess ACTH. CS is also a result of hypercortisolism. Ectopic sources of ACTH derive from multiple tumor types such as pulmonary small-cell carcinoma, thymomas, pancreatic islet cell tumors, carcinoid tumors, medullary carcinoma of the thyroid, and pheochromocytoma. In such cases ACTH is usually more highly elevated than with pituitary adenomas. In addition, excessive autonomous cortisol secretion can occur from an adrenal adenoma or carcinoma. A pseudo-Cushing state can also exist and is secondary to hypothalamic release of corticotropin-releasing hormone (CRH). This condition is a heterogenous group of disorders, including alcoholism and depression, that share many of the clinical and biochemical features of CS.

Clinical Findings

Clinical findings in CD include: hypertension, ecchymoses and purple striae on flanks, breasts, and lower abdomen, hyperglycemia, amenorrhea, impotence, reduced libido, hypokalemia, hyperpigmentation of skin and mucous membranes, weight gain, atrophic tissue, depression, emotional lability, osteoporosis, muscle wasting, easy fatigability, and elevation of other adrenal hormones (androgens may cause hirsutism and acne).

Inferior Petrosal Sinus Sampling

Inferior petrosal sinus sampling (IPSS) has been the most important advance in the past two decades for the subtype evaluation of CS. IPSS was first described by Corrigan et al. [2] in its unilateral form as a means of identifying the pituitary as the central cause of hypercortisolism. In 1984, Doppman et al. [4] described synchronous bilateral measurements to establish an interpetrosal sinus gradient in order to lateralize the lesion within the gland. Further refinement has lead to the use of CRH to enhance and amplify the resulting gradients. Numerous techniques exist for performing IPSS. Our technique for catheterization and sampling is described below simply as a guide for those who have not performed this procedure before.

(1) Using the Seldinger technique two 5-french sheaths and one 4-french sheath are placed into the common femoral vein. We prefer using one femoral vein for all three sheaths to minimize postprocedural discomfort, although both the right and left veins may be used if so desired.

(2) Through each 5-french sheath a straight 5-french catheter is advanced over a wire (0.038-inch hydrophilic wire) using fluoroscopic guidance. One catheter is placed into the right internal jugular vein (IJV) while the other is placed into the left IJV. When traversing the right atrium from the inferior vena cava to the superior vena cava transient cardiac ectopy will be encountered; however, this usually ceases once the catheter and wire are in the superior vena cava. The left IJV is accessed via the left subclavian vein which arises from the superior vena cava at approximately the second or third intercostal space. Entering the left IJV may be difficult due to a valve located at the junction between the left IJV and left subclavian vein; however, with gently probing and wire manipulation this valve can be crossed.

(3) The catheters and wires are then sequentially advanced up the left and right IJV towards the skull base. At the C1-C2 level the wire is gently directed medially and anteriorly. Eventually the wire can be placed in the inferior petrosal sinus (IPS). A venographic run will generally opacify the IPS, cavernous sinus and contralateral IPS. If the contralateral IPS opacifies well a roadmap can be produced to help guide the placement of the contralateral wire and catheter.

Of note, we prefer using a 5-french straight catheter for sampling because the inner diameter allows for a rapid sampling of 5–10 ml of blood at the prescribed intervals. We also prefer using a straight catheter because we have found that

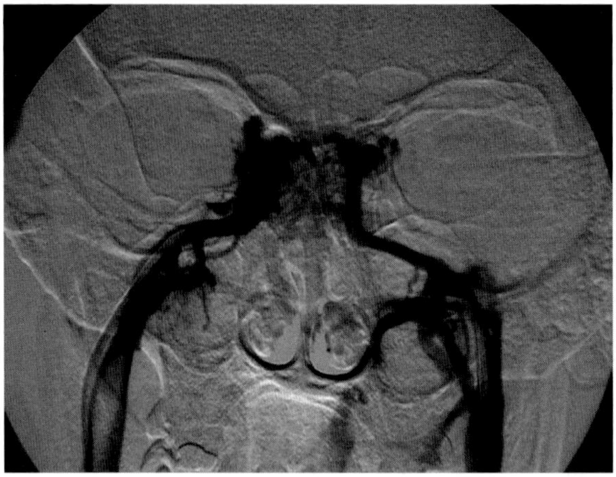

Fig. 1. AP renogram of right and left IPS and cavernous sinuses.

angle-tipped catheters often become transiently occluded as the tip comes in contact with the wall of the vein during syringe suction. We have tried using straight 0.018-inch microcatheters but have been disappointed with the volume of blood and the rate at which blood can be aspirated when sampling takes place.

(4) Once the catheters are in position sampling is carried out using a protocol designed by our endocrinologists. This sampling protocol is described on the record sheet below (see Appendix) with the goal being simultaneous removal of blood from the appropriate locations. The 4-french sheath is used for the peripheral blood draws.

(5) All catheters and sheaths are placed on continuous heparinized saline drips (6 units heparin/ml) so as to avoid catheter thrombosis between blood draws. The catheters are aspirated and saline-diluted blood is discarded prior to each sample being drawn. In addition, because the procedure takes approximately 90 min a Foley catheter is recommended in case the patient needs to void.

IPS Anatomy

IPS anatomy can vary with large or small anastomoses with the IJV. In some cases there will be no connection to the IJV but simply connections to a skull base venous plexus. In instances of small anastomoses or absent IJV connections the 5-french catheters may need to be placed at the C1–C2 level with sampling done from this location. Results of such testing may lead to spurious results due to transverse/sigmoid sinus contamination. While it may be difficult at first to catheterize the IPSS with experience and gentle persistence the

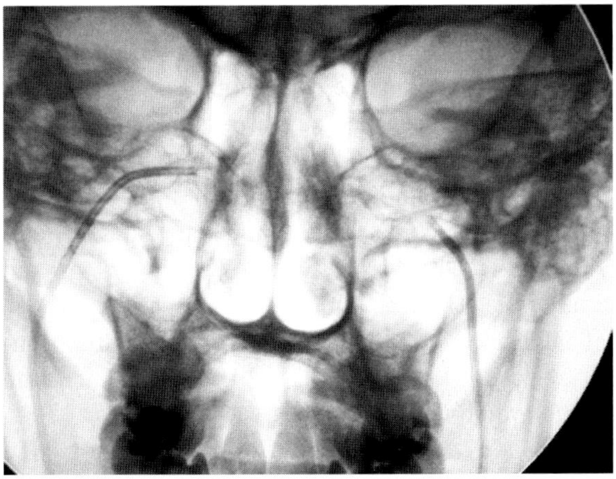

Fig. 2. AP skull view showing catheters positioned in right and left IPS.

interventionalist will find greater frequency of success. Even with experience, however, failure to cannulate the IPS occurs in 15–20% of cases.

Complications

IPSS is not a completely benign procedure. While complication rates are poorly reported they can include brainstem hemorrhage and brainstem stroke (presumably from venous thrombosis), venous subarachnoid hemorrhage, peripheral venous perforation (sublcavian vein, IJV), uncontrolled cardiac ectopy, and pulmonary embolism (from blood clot or inadvertent air injection).

Outcomes and Alternative Testing

Investigators have reported 55–99% success rates when performing IPSS in terms of carrying out the procedure and obtaining useful data. Most studies suggest a sensitivity in the order of 80% with accurate lateralization in 64–80% of cases and 88–90% accurate lateralization when CRH stimulation is utilized. If the IPSS results are negative, the MR is negative and an ectopic source of ACTH production is not identified it is recommended that the patient at the minimum be followed with MR since the IPSS might be falsely negative. Such false-negative studies have been reported to be due to poor technique or a hypoplastic or plexiform IPSS that makes accurate sampling difficult. False-negative studies have also been encountered in patients who exhibit periodic hormonogenesis. Therefore, it is important that the patient be hypercortisolemic at the time the IPSS is performed.

Alternatives to IPSS include superselective cavernous sinus sampling without CRF stimulation. This procedure is said to be as sensitive as IPSS with CRF stimulation and to provide near 100% correct lateralization. False lateralization with this technique can occur with midline tumors.

Noninvasive alternatives primarily involve MRI. While some studies point to a superior ability for IPSS to correctly diagnose a pituitary adenoma and lateralize it within the gland others feel MRI is equivalent or superior to IPSS. Reports supporting the use of MRI suggest that this modality may identify pituitary adenomas in 34–100% of cases. These reports also state that accurate lateralization with MRI is on the order of 90%.

Plasma Ratios

IPS must be sampled simultaneously because of the pulsatile secretion of ACTH. While we suggest leaving the interpretation of the IPSS results up to a trained endocrinologist it is felt that simultaneous bilateral IPSS that shows a central to peripheral gradient of >2:1 at baseline and >3:1 after administration of ovine CRF is consistent with pituitary-dependent disease. Ratios of gradients between each IPS >1.4 at 5 min after CRF stimulation correctly lateralize a lesion in approximately 80% of cases.

Conclusion

The need for IPSS and interpretation of the results should be determined by the endocrinologist, neurosurgeon, and neuroradiologist so as to maximize results and minimize the performance of unnecessary tests. Nevertheless, by understanding the rationale behind these decisions, the INR can better determine why testing is performed in a particular manner.

References

1 Boolell M, Mcneill P, Gilford E, Cummins J, Arnott R, Alford F: An overview of bilateral synchronous inferior petrosal sinus sampling (BSIPSS) in the pre-operative assessment of Cushing's disease. Aust NZ J Med 1990;20:765–770.

2 Corrigan DF, Schaaf M, Whaley RA, Czerwinski CL, Earll M: Selective venous sampling to differentiate ectopic ACTH secretion from pituitary Cushing's syndrome. N Engl J Med 1977;296:861–862.

3 de Herder WW, Uitterlinden P, Pieterman H, Tanghe HLJ, Kwekkeboom DJ, Pois JAP, Singh R, van de Berge H, Lamberts SWJ: Pituitary tumor localization in patients with Cushing's disease by magnetic resonance imaging. Is there a place for petrosal sinus sampling? Clin Endocrinol 1994;40:728–735.
4 Doppman JL, Oldfiled EH, Krudy AG, et al: Petrosal sinus sampling of Cushing syndrome: Anatomical and technical considerations. Radiology 1984;150:99–103.
5 Doppman JL, Frank JA, Dwyer AJ, et al: Gadolinium DTPA enhanced MR imaging of ACTH-secreting microadenomas of the pituitary gland. J Comput Assist Tomogr 1988;12:728–735.
6 Findling JW, Aron DC, Tyrerell JB, et al: Selective venous sampling for ACTH in Cushing's syndrome: Differentiation between Cushing's disease and the ectopic ACTH syndrome. Ann Intern Med 1981;94:647–652.
7 Kaye TB, Crapo L: The Cushing syndrome: An update on diagnostic tests. Ann Intern Med 1990; 112:434–444.
8 Kley HK, Stolz L, Kruskemper HL: Juglar vein sampling of ACTH (letter). N Engl J Med 1977; 300:679.
9 Kucharcyzk W, Davis DO, Kelly WM, Sze G, Norman D, Newton TH: Pituitary adenomas: High-resolution MR imaging at 1.5-T. Radiology 1986;161:761–765.
10 Kulkarni MV, Lee KF, McArdle CB, Yeakeley JW, Haar FL: 1.5-T MR imaging of pituitary microadenomas: Technical considerations and CT correlations. AJNR Am J Neuroradiol 1988; 9:5–11.
11 McCance DR, Mcilrath E, McNeill A, et al: Bilateral inferior petrosal sinus sampling as a routine procedure in ACTH-dependent Cushing's syndrome. Clin Endocrinol 1989;30:157–166.
12 Miller DL, Doppman JL, Nieman LK, Cutler GB, Chrouse G, Loriaux DL, Oldfield EH: Petrosal sinus sampling: Discordant lateralization of ACTH-secreting pituitary microadenomas before and after stimulation with corticotrophin-releasing hormone. Radiology 1990;176:429–431.
13 Nichols DA, Laws ER, Houser OW, Abbound CF: Comparison of magnetic resonance imaging and computed tomography in the preoperative evaluation of pituitary adenomas. Neurosurgery 1988;22:380–385.
14 Peck WW, Dillon WP, Norman D, Newton TH, Wilson CB: High-resolution MR imaging of pituitary microadenomas at 1.5-T: Experience with Cushing's disease. AJR Am J Roentgenol 1989;152:145–151.
15 Pojounas KW, Daniels DL, Williams AL, Haughton VM: MR imaging of prolactin secreting microadenomas. AJNR Am J Neuroradiol 1986;7:209–213.
16 Greenberg MS: Handbook of Neurosurgery, ed 4. Lakeland, Greenberg Graphics, 1997.

Dr. Michael B. Horowitz
Department of Neurosurgery
Director, Neuroendovascular Surgery
UPMC Presbyterian
Suite B-400, 200 Lothrop Street, Pittsburgh, 15213-2582, USA
Tel. +1 412 647 3685, Fax +1 412 647 7000, E-Mail horowitzmb@upmc.edu

Appendix

Record Sheet Sent to the Lab with All Tubes

Date:					Petrosal Venous Sampling With CRH Stimulation					
Sample	Time Drawn	Right IPS **ACTH**	Left IPS **ACTH**	Peripheral **ACTH**	Peripheral **CORTISOL**	Right Jugular **ACTH**	Left Jugular **ACTH**	SVC **ACTH**	IVC Hepatic **ACTH**	IVC Renal **ACTH**
−15 minutes		1	2	3	4					
−5 minutes		5	6	7						
0 (1.0 mcg/kg of CRH given)		8	9	10	11					
+2 minutes		12	13	14						
+5 minutes		15	16	17						
+10 minutes		18	19	20	21	22	23	24	25	26
+20 minutes				27	28					
+30 minutes				29	30					
+60 minutes				31	32					
+90 minutes				33	34					

All ACTH samples (Tubes 1–3, 5–7, 8–10, 12–14, 15–20, 22–26, 27, 29, 31, 33) are to be placed in purple top tubes and all Cortisol samples (Tubes 4, 11, 21, 28, 30, 32, 34) are placed in red top tubes. All tubes must be kept on ice until delivered to the lab. Tubes must also be numbered and labeled accordingly so that the lab cannot mix up the samples. This table is sent to the lab with all tubes at the end of the case for reference as to what time each sample is drawn.

Author Index

Subject Index